MEDICINE HANDS

MASSAGE THERAPY FOR PEOPLE WITH CANCER

Gayle MacDonald, MS, LMT

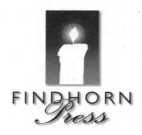

FINDHORN
Press

IMPORTANT, PLEASE READ:

Prior to initiating the use of massage or any other touch modalities, consult with the patient's doctor. *Medicine Hands* is designed to be a resource; it is not a substitute for medical advice. Different state or municipal licensing boards have jurisdiction over the practice of massage. These regulating bodies may have a policy or recommendation with regard to massaging people with cancer. Practitioners should become knowledgeable about these regulations by contacting the licensing board.

© Gayle MacDonald 1999, 2007

First published 1999.
This new, revised and expanded edition (60% new material) published 2007.

ISBN 978-1-84409-090-6

A CIP catalogue record for this title is available
from the British Library

Edited by Jean Semrau
Layout by Pam Bochel
Cover design by Damian Keenan

Printed and bound in the USA

1 2 3 4 5 6 7 8 9 10 11 12 13 14 13 12 11 10 09 08 07

Published by

Findhorn Press

305a The Park, Findhorn,
Forres IV36 3TE
Scotland
Tel +44 (0)1309 690582
Fax +44 (0)1309 690036
eMail: info@findhornpress.com
findhornpress.com

Dedicated to Marcella MacDonald,
mother, teacher, guide, sounding board,
and the one I can tell my stories to.

ACKNOWLEDGMENTS

Findhorn Press originally published *Medicine Hands* in 1999 on the spur of the moment. To Thierry Bogliolo and Karen Bogliolo, who hold their responsibilities as publishers to be sacred, thank you! Your willingness to print *Medicine Hands* changed the lives of thousands of cancer patients, their families, touch practitioners, and the massage profession.

The first edition of *Medicine Hands* was a reflection of what my students and I had learned in five years of working on the oncology unit at OHSU. At that time I didn't know Tracy Walton, Lonnie Howard, Cheryl Chapman, Tina Ferner, Liz Davidson, Sandy Canzone, Toni Creazzo, Charlotte Versagi, Cynthia Myers, Lyse Lussier, Shay Beider, Isabel Adkins, Wendy Miner, and many, many more. Eight years later, there is a vast network that brings us together. This edition, while built upon the foundation of the first book, is a reflection of what many of us have learned over the past decade.

Many people have contributed in seen and unseen ways to this edition. Huge THANK YOU's to Jamie Elswick for her contribution on "Scars," Isabel Adkins for material on the use of acupressure and reflexology for symptom management, and Shay Beider for her insight into working with pediatric patients. Thanks, too, to Tracy Walton for sharing so many aspects of her work in *Medicine Hands*. It is an example of the generous spirit and comraderie that exist between the people in this field.

Kitty Leonard, nurse massage therapist, spent many hours proofreading Chapters 2, 4, and 5, making them as accurate as possible. Chris Montgomery made the review of research easy by helping gather articles. Thanks to Joan Pinkert for organizing the Research Tables; Joseph Carter, of the Acupressure Institute, for revision of the acupressure points; and Nicki Hansen-Dix for being graphic designer, sounding board, and typesetter for Chapter 6. Thanks also to Amanda Scheerer and Alexandra Jackson for support work on Chapter 6. Thanks to David J. Lawton, Providence St. Vincent medical photographer, Portland, Oregon, and Andy Aryapour, Aryapour Design, Inc., Santa Monica, California. And a very special thanks to Pam Bochel from Findhorn Press for the care she gave to the layout.

Mary Malinski and Tony Borcich from Providence St. Vincent, Portland, Oregon, took part of a day from their work to participate in a photo shoot, as did Allison Krizner and Alexandra Haines, the two massage therapists who appear in Chapter 7. Gratitude also to Lisa Brubaker, Good Samaritan Medical Center in Phoenix, Arizona, and Joe Bubalo, pharmacist at Oregon Health and Science University, Portland, Oregon, for checking facts. Bruce Hopkins, thanks for sharing your research on the Cytoxan and gloving question.

Two final acknowledgments. Gratitude to all of the therapists and patients who contributed anecdotes and quotes. They show the human face behind the clinical facade. And another thanks to all of the therapists who have been in the oncology massage trainings. You are part of advancing the knowledge that has been gained.

G.M.

Table of Contents

Preface

The first edition of *Medicine Hands* was written in complete isolation at my dining room table. Seven years later I am writing in front of a window that looks out onto orange and pecan trees. Every hour or two I stop to check e-mail, my other window to the world. There is no more isolation. I am in contact with more people than I could have imagined – hundreds of massage therapists and students, oncology nurses, patients and their friends and family.

So much has changed since *Medicine Hands* was first published. Fewer massage schools teach that cancer is a contraindication to massage. Only rarely do I receive long-distance phone calls or e-mails from terrified therapists worried that they may have done harm to someone with a history of cancer. Hundreds of touch therapy programs exist in hospitals, clinics, and cancer resource centers; the NIH now funds massage research projects; and there are beginning to be conferences devoted to oncology massage. In a few short years, oncology massage has become a specialty. Students start massage school now already knowing that they want to specialize in massage for people with cancer.

In preparing the new manuscript, I read back through old journals in which I recorded the stories of patients, therapists, family and health care providers. There were funny stories, sad, glad, and maddening ones. One patient felt as if she were being touched by the hands of God, another was glad to find out that there are oncology massage specialists. This helped her to relax into the session. One woman told of being turned away a number of times while looking for a massage therapist who would work with her following treatment for breast cancer. This so infuriated her that she went to massage school to become a therapist so that cancer patients in her community would have a place to turn.

I recorded stories of therapists who cried while telling me that in this work they found the place where they belong. I have also heard how they have sent patients away when told about their cancer, of broken hearts, and of learning kindness toward the body. And consistently, practitioners have shared their experience of answering "The Call" that drew them to this field and how of their hearts ache to be able to give their gift.

Malidoma Some, an African medicine man, writes about the responsibility to our gift and the responsibility of the village to help one another discover and express those gifts. *Medicine Hands* is hopefully one way to help therapists in our community express their true purpose. The world needs their gift because there are literally millions of people who need the support of touch therapists as they endure the rigors of cancer treatment.

The book's title came from the comment of a hospital nursing assistant to whom I was giving a seated massage. "You have medicine hands," she said. In Native American cosmology, medicine exists in everything – the wind, animals, the sea, and even rocks. Something is medicinal if it creates a connection with the energy of the universe. Personal power comes from connecting with energies that bring to us that which is needed for healing. These medicinal energies are unique to each individual. They may be in the breath, the flute, the bear, or the hands. We all have medicine to offer through our hands. Touch is a way of connecting with the healing energies of the universe, of creating a conduit that helps patients re-connect with themselves.

ROOTS

This book is the result of working with cancer patients and supervising massage students since 1994 on the oncology unit at Oregon Health and Science University (OHSU). OHSU is a large teaching and research hospital, which means many of the patients are referred there because of a severe or unusual form of cancer. The students and I, therefore, have been blessed to assist a number of very sick people and to witness the undeniable benefits of massage in a wide variety of situations – for patients just out of surgery, those undergoing stem cell transplants, people admitted for bowel problems due to the side effects of pain medication, or patients who have lost part of a colon, a kidney, breast, lung, arm, or part of their face. We have found ways to touch those healing from radiation burns, struggling for breath, or enduring a bone marrow biopsy. The oncology social workers have sought us out to comfort the mother of a 21-year-old man who was being intubated in the ICU, to calm a family who just learned of the mother's breast cancer diagnosis, and to ease the way for a man told by the doctors that they could do nothing more for him.

Additionally, *Medicine Hands* is the accumulated knowledge and experience of therapists I have met since 1999 in my continuing education classes. As part of those classes, we work with cancer patients on Sunday afternoons. Thus I have heard the stories of more than a thousand therapists, many of whom have been personally affected by cancer, and more than a thousand patients who have been treated for cancer.

DEFINING MASSAGE

Before we continue, it is important to clearly define what is meant by the term "massage." In this book, massage is defined as "any form of systematic touch." This opens the possibilities greatly. Within this definition, nearly all clients, despite their infirmity, qualify for touch therapies of some sort.

When "massage" is part of a specific modality, such as Swedish Massage, it will be capitalized to set it apart from the generic meaning of the word. For the sake of variety, the words "touch" and "bodywork" are used synonymously with "massage." Such terms as gentle massage, low impact massage (borrowed from Tracy Walton), and skilled touch all refer to the type of massage that is at the center of *Medicine Hands* – comfort-oriented massage. "Therapist," "practitioner," and "body-worker" are used interchangeably, as are "client" and "patient." Two words that are never used instead of "patient" are "victim" and "sufferer," labels which evoke a sense of pity toward people who are ill. The sick don't want pity; they seek companions who can take the journey with them.

OVERVIEW

Medicine Hands is for the private practitioner who wants to know how to approach a client with a colostomy or to understand how steroids relate to bodywork. It is for the massage therapist seeking data to substantiate the benefits of massage for proposals to hospital boards. It is for the lay practitioner whose friend has lost hair, energy, and appetite from chemotherapy. It is for the massage therapist who has been trained to believe that all massage will contribute to metastasis. It is for the social worker or pastoral counselor who never before considered massage as an intervention for loneliness or for the burnout of a caregiver. And it is a resource for the nurse and physician in determining what kind of touch is possible and appropriate for their patients.

One of the main focuses of the original edition was First Do No Harm. This is the cornerstone of all bodywork. Safety, along with the incredible good that happens through massage, are still the primary messages of the second edition. In this version, however, I take the vision forward and include not just safety considerations and the benefits of massage, but also the ways in which touch therapies can support the person who is in treatment or post-treatment. We expand our notion of massage as a comfort measure to include massage as an intervention that strengthens the body and mind. To be sure, it is not a treatment for cancer, but a support for the person whose organs are affected by chemotherapy, whose tissue is bound down from the adhesions caused by radiation, or who has limited function due to the scars from surgery.

Readers of the first edition will recognize vestiges of the original manuscript, but much is new. The first edition, which was written for my hospital students, contained many pages of hospital-related information. Some of that material has not been included in this edition. An entire book, *Massage for the Hospital Patient and Medically Frail Client* (Lippincott, Williams, and Wilkins, 2005) has been devoted to hospital massage, leaving no need to repeat the information in *Medicine Hands*.

Several chapters may appear to be the same when comparing the initial Table of Contents to the new one. But major remodeling has been done on many sections of the book. The introductory chapter has been reconstructed from the foundation up. The premises from which we now work are so different from those of 1999 that an entirely new foundation was required. Gone is the atmosphere of fear and uncertainty, replaced by increased confidence and maturity.

Chapter 2, Understanding Metastasis, contains much of the original material with new information woven in. The basic message of the chapter remains the same – metastasis is a complex set of biochemical interactions that is driven by genetic mutations or hormonal influences; it is not a mechanical event. The material in Chapter 8 (formerly Chapter 7), too, remains the same. Its subject, massage for those at the end of life, will change little over the years. No matter how cancer treatments improve and change, death is immutable.

The number of research studies to report in Chapter 3 has expanded greatly, requiring the chapter to be torn down to its foundation and rebuilt completely. Massage research in general has exploded and many of these new studies have looked at the effect of various bodywork modalities on people undergoing cancer treatment. In the 1999 edition, ten studies were reported. Seven years later, there are at least 60 completed research projects with more in the works.

Chapter 4 focuses on the need to be less demanding. This more gentle approach centers around the philosophy of beginning slowly and inching forward as the client and practitioner discover a state of "new normal." For some, a less demanding approach is needed both during and immediately after treatment. Others require special care for the remainder of their lives, no matter how short or long that may be.

Chapter 5 is the core of *Medicine Hands*. In it, the common side effects from cancer treatment are listed alphabetically and described relative to massage. For each side effect, instruction is given that will allow the safe administration of bodywork. The guidelines revolve around three categories of adjustment – pressure adjustments, site restrictions, and positioning. Thanks to Jamie Elswick, a section on work with scars and adhesions was added to this chapter.

New chapters have been added, thanks in part to the expertise of two colleagues, Isabel Adkins and Shay Beider. Chapter 6 presents information from Isabel Adkins on the use of acupressure and reflexology to support and strengthen people with cancer through both the treatment and recovery periods. Chapter 7, written by Shay Beider, focuses on massaging children with cancer. A third new chapter, Chapter 10, gives readers guidance in the gathering of a patient's medical history. The need to be skillful at performing a client intake cannot be overemphasized. It is the therapist's responsibility to elicit information from the client, not the client's job to know what the practitioner needs.

Naturally, the focus of this book is on patients, but one way to indirectly care for patients is to attend to the family caregivers. Chapter 9 does just this. The role of caregivers is physically and emotionally arduous. Bodyworkers who are serving a cancer patient, especially one in the hospital or in hospice, should consider family members as an equal part of the "unit of care." The stress of watching a loved one endure cancer and its treatment can be even higher than for those actually experiencing the disease itself. Massage can serve as a momentary respite from the anxiety and soften a body that has become exhausted and armored.

The final subject of *Medicine Hands* is the importance of being a companion on the journey. Although few in pages, Chapter 11 speaks to an aspect of this work that is fundamental and often under-developed: our presence. This intangible factor is as important as our clinical knowledge and hands-on massage skills.

The original book contained appendices of vocabulary, abbreviations, types of cancer, styles of bodywork, and other lists. This edition has included some of this information in the various chapters in Info Boxes. The reason for eliminating the appendices is purely practical – page count. The more pages devoted to appendices meant the fewer pages available for actual massage information. Although many medical terms are defined the first time the word is used, readers are encouraged to have a medical dictionary nearby when they read. I know this suggestion is a bit old-fashioned, but by giving you, the reader, more responsibility for searching out such things as types of cancer, I was able to devote more pages to material that actually counts.

There are a number of topics not covered in *Medicine Hands* – for example, breathing and relaxation techniques, exploring and coping with grief, communication skills, and the use of intuition. Each of these subjects is important to our work, but because they are already superbly presented in other sources, no attempt is made to replicate or improve upon them in this book. Business information, such as writing proposals, billing, or fund raising, is also not presented. *Medicine Hands* confines itself mainly to the clinical information needed for both professional and non-professional bodyworkers wishing to massage clients, friends, or family members with a history of cancer.

No attempt is made to teach any style of bodywork or touch techniques. It is assumed that the reader is already skilled in a chosen modality, whether it is Reiki, Swedish Massage, Shiatsu, Polarity Therapy, Therapeutic Touch, reflexology, or any of the multitude of other techniques.

PERSONAL NOTE

When I began giving massage to people with cancer, it was in the hospital, and I knew next to nothing. I was not trained as a nurse, physical therapist, or social worker. I was a teacher and a bodyworker who had no formal preparation for hospital work, but had a desire to be with the seriously ill and a fearlessness about asking questions. I learned from scratch, making more than a few mistakes in the process. That experience helped greatly when it was time to assist massage students in learning to apply their bodywork skills in the hospital setting. It was beneficial in teaching massage students and in writing this book to have no formal training in health care. This allowed me to experience the hospital and the patients much as students would, and to know exactly what instruction the average bodyworker needed.

I wasn't completely without advantages when embarking on this path. My mother is a nurse, and I was conceived at about the time she started her first nursing job, which was in a hospital. During those nine months I was being acclimatized unconsciously, *in utero*, to the hospital milieu. Strange as it may sound, being around sick people seemed natural to me.

For all of my professional life, my mother has filled the gaps in my education. She has been a mentor and teacher whom I could call upon day and night to answer the little questions that arise in the course of a day's work. This has been a huge blessing. Even after nearly 35 years of various health-related teaching assignments, I still phone my mother at least once a week with a question. Not everyone is so lucky. In case your mother isn't a nurse, and you have no one to help fill the gaps in your education, I have tried to write this book in sufficient detail so that you can call upon it to answer your "nuts and bolts" questions.

Often before bodyworkers start their training, they massage family, friends, and sweethearts with a joyful innocence. Massage school can take that away, replacing it with fears about causing harm, lawsuits, or how to correctly relate to clients. Being mindful of these concerns is important, but a balance must be struck so that the pure delight of giving touch to another human being does not get lost. It is easy when presenting material about disease to create fear instead of confidence. I have tried to present this information in a way that will give you the assurance to proceed, mixed with an appropriate amount of caution.

It has been an honor and a labor of love to be with both the patients and the students on their intersecting journeys. They have been inspiring teachers and companions as I explored my own healing. The reciprocal giving and receiving has been its own reward. I hope *Medicine Hands* assists you on your journey. It is a privilege to be with you.

Chapter 1

Introduction

A New Era in Oncology Massage

In 1971, Richard Nixon signed the National Cancer Act which committed the United States to what has been known as the "war on cancer." Since then, dramatic technologies have been created in cancer detection and care. "Smart" drugs that target only the cancer cells are being developed, radiation machines are becoming more and more refined, causing less damage to surrounding tissue, and each year since 1993 the survival rates have improved. In 1975, the five-year survival rate for Americans was 50%. In 2001, the last year figures were available, the rate has improved to 65%.[1] This trend is similar for most developed nations.[2-7]

And yet, despite the advances made in the last few decades, the rate of cancer incidence remains sobering. At some point in their lives, usually later in life, a staggering number of people will be diagnosed with cancer. For instance more than a third of American women and nearly half of men are stricken.[1] One in four Australian women and one in three men develop cancer by the age of 75.[3,4] And in the U.K., more than one in three will be diagnosed at some point in their lives.[5] These numbers will only rise as the baby boomer generation ages because cancer, by and large, is a disease of aging. As the population grows older through the early 21st century, the number of people with cancer will also increase.

Many thought that cancer would be solved by now. But, when readers stop to realize that cancer is not one disease but instead is a myriad of different diseases, it is little wonder that a cure still evades scientists. (The common cold is still a riddle, so it is not surprising

The cancer experience is a time of renewal, not a battle.

— WENDY KANTOR,
MASSAGE THERAPIST AND CANCER
SURVIVOR, CINCINNATI, OHIO

INFO BOX	Worldwide 5-year survival rates for breast cancer:[7]	
U.S.		81%
Japan		75%
Western Europe		74%
Eastern Europe		58%
South America		67%
India		46%
Sub-saharan Africa		32%

that cancer is a dilemma.) The discovery of the proverbial "big one" sometimes seems to be just around the corner, the one haywire gene, evasive enzyme, or biochemical cascade. But the end is not in sight. The search will require more plodding, one step after another. There will be tiny victories on good days, dead ends on other days. "And yet," as Stephen Sener, MD, points out, "...there is no question that cancer can be controlled. Declining incidence and mortality rates in the developed nations prove it."[6]

USE OF COMPLEMENTARY AND ALTERNATIVE MEDICINE

When the National Cancer Act was signed, the only concern was to cure the disease. Scant attention was paid to the physical, emotional, and social issues created by the toxic treatments. The aim was to keep people alive. Now, more than three decades later, the vision of cancer care has changed. The focus has broadened to include not only eradication of the disease, but also to improve quality of life, particularly since many varieties of cancer are being managed as a chronic condition, as with diabetes and heart disease. Cancer survivors, numbering nearly 10 million in the U.S., not only want to be cured from their cancer; they also want to live well.

As part of enhancing quality of life, cancer patients have turned toward complementary and alternative medicine (CAM), also referred to as integrative medicine. These therapies include such interventions as exercise, prayer, aromatherapy, acupuncture, guided imagery, massage, diet, and nutritional supplementation. When used as an alternative therapy, these modalities are used in place of allopathic care or in conjunction with it to promote a cure. When used in a complementary fashion, these therapies are used alongside mainstream medicine, usually to ameliorate the side effects of the curative treatments and to improve quality of life.

Studies from countries all over the developed world paint a common picture: cancer patients are flocking toward the use of complementary and alternative medicine.[8-18] An internet search of studies on CAM usage will yield studies not only from the U.K., Europe, Australia, New Zealand, and the U.S., but from China, Japan, Israel, and Turkey. David Eisenberg, MD, the most well-known American researcher on the use of CAM, states that "CAM use is widespread and here to stay."[19]

Consistently, massage is reported as one of the most popular complementary modalities. Multiple studies show that approximately 20% of cancer patients use massage.[9,13,15,21] In one study of a group of breast cancer patients, the percentage was as high as 53%.[12] Patients say that they use complementary modalities to enhance their quality of life, to feel more in control, to strengthen the immune system, to reduce stress, and to manage the side effects of treatment.[8,12,16,17] According to Morris, et al., "Our cancer patients are using complementary therapies with specific goals in mind as opposed to using them merely to obtain refuge from the 'uncaring world of allopathic medicine,' as many people in the lay press believe."[12] Massage helps people heal, it moves them toward wholeness. For a day or an hour, they forget about cancer.

Some patients surveyed also believe that CAM therapies could prevent a recurrence of the cancer.[17] But, to be sure, massage is not a cure for cancer, it is a complement to the treatments being used to cure the disease. These curative treatments are notorious for their side effects, such as nausea, fatigue, weight changes, or immuno-suppression. Touch therapies lessen the severity of chemotherapy, radiation, and surgery, making the treatment process easier to tolerate.

Genevieve

When called to meet with a new client, you never know what lessons await behind the curtain. Genevieve was an amazing teacher. She didn't have all the answers. No, she had endless questions. She taught me that the heart of the lesson lies in the question. She asked why our massage sessions left her feeling so alive – as alive as she could feel in the moment. I worked with her in bottling those moments so she could carry them into her countless radiation and chemo treatments.

You see, Genevieve discovered empowerment in those moments of healing. She healed into life while still facing potential death. She also maintained a wicked sense of humor. She'd wear black clothes to the radiation treatments in mourning for the death of her cancer cells. She donned fancy, dangling earrings to the chemo clinic for the so called "cocktail parties."

During one particular in-home session, I placed my hands beneath her low back and sacrum, offering support so she could let go of the pain and tension she often felt in this area. I encouraged her to breathe deeply through her belly. While focusing on her breath, she slowly started to lift her hips and move them around in circles. She bridged her pelvis upward with amazement. She opened like a flower blooming for the first time.

I witnessed Genevieve relax and then tap into the healing process by way of her inner power. Each session was a new gift that she'd open with child-like eyes of wonderment. Cancer offered Genevieve an opportunity to unpeel the layers of her authentic self and feel peace with the result. She summed it up after the ground breaking hip-circling session: "I haven't felt so good since I was diagnosed with cancer."

Genevieve's lesson taught me that each moment has potential for healing. Once the layers are unpeeled, discovery unfolds. She showed me that there's joy in the discovery, regardless of the outcome.

— EILEEN HICKEY, LMT, PORTLAND, OREGON

Patients are leading the way in the use of CAM therapies. Health care providers are in the process of catching up to this consumer-driven trend so that they can advise their patients about the safety and efficacy of therapies such as massage. Many nursing and medical school curriculums now include basic training in the area of integrative medicine. Journals aimed at nurses, nurse practitioners, and doctors regularly feature articles on patient use of CAM practices. On-line education is even available.

A 2005 survey of physicians showed that nearly two-thirds of them have recommended CAM therapies to their patients. In this survey, massage therapy ranked higher than other CAM therapies with the doctors: 57% felt massage can be effective. [22]

 INFO BOX The research has also given us a profile of the CAM user. More often they are female, younger in age with a higher level of education, income, and private insurance, and they attend a support group. [13,18,20]

SLOW, STEADY PROGRESS

Over the past 20 years, massage has been making slow, steady progress as a complementary therapy in hospitals, hospices, cancer wellness centers, medical spas, and chemotherapy and radiation oncology clinics. Large well-established institutions such as Dartmouth Hitchcock Medical Center, Memorial Sloan Kettering, Massachusetts General Hospital, and Stanford Hospital and Clinics provide a variety of bodywork services for their oncology patients; so, too, do small, lesser-known hospitals in Toledo, Ohio, The Dalles, Oregon, Anchorage, Alaska, Mesa, Arizona, and Boulder, Colorado.

Massage is provided at special events, such as The Race for the Cure sponsored by the Komen Foundation, World Survivor's Day, and Relay for Life, an American Cancer Society event. Cancer resource centers around the world (such as the Charlotte Maxwell Center in Oakland, California, Clan House, Aberdeen, Scotland, and the Leucan Association, a group in Quebec, Canada, that provides oncology massage to children) make massage available to those receiving cancer treatment. Therapists in Australia work at the Run for Your Life event and massage the Pink Ladies, a group of breast cancer survivors who race dragon boats. St. Vincent Medical Center in Toledo, Ohio, sponsors a special "survivor's day" celebration, inviting those who have had or are in treatment for cancer for a special day of yoga, neck massages, Tai Chi, and music therapy. In fact, a handful of massage businesses have "spa nights" for their cancer clients.

The American Cancer Society and the National Cancer Institute advocate massage and manual pressure as ways to relieve pain without medicine.[23] The National Comprehensive Cancer Network recommends massage in its treatment guidelines as a treatment for refractory cancer pain.[24] In addition, an article in the prestigious *Annals of Internal Medicine* rated massage as an "acceptable" CAM therapy for people with cancer as long as certain precautions were followed.[25]

Pioneers in the massage field have worked with oncology patients for more than two decades and have given the profession a large body of experience and wisdom to draw upon. Therapists are no longer required to guess or just intuit how to safely administer massage in the oncology setting because the needs of people with cancer histories are clearly known. Rather than using primarily their intuition for guidance and hoping for the best, bodyworkers can be given clinical training in how best to adjust their touch techniques for cancer patients.

In addition to the years of anecdotal evidence, scientific research is now well underway and will begin to shape the practice of massage for people with cancer. Two of the side effects of cancer and its treatment, pain and anxiety, are clearly improved by massage. Data on the effect of massage on fatigue is hopeful but not yet conclusive. Nausea has shown mixed results, while many other conditions, such as sleep and medication use, have not yet been studied enough to make firm conclusions. However, what is clear, is that by making the right adjustments, the benefits of massage can be enjoyed by nearly all persons affected by cancer.

A New Training Paradigm

In order to massage cancer patients, advanced training is often thought to be needed. Just the opposite is true: the ability to work with this population should be part of a basic curriculum and should be taught to all therapists who use manual interventions. Because the rate of cancer is so high, a lifetime risk of approximately 40% in the U.S. and over 30% in Canada, Britain and Australia, all bodyworkers will eventually come into contact with people who are in treatment for cancer or who have a history of it. Therefore, all touch therapists need to have a fundamental understanding of how to administer bodywork to cancer patients.

Students of massage should be taught from the start that bodywork for people with a history of cancer is extremely beneficial. When properly given, it is an incalculable blessing. But, working with those affected by cancer is complex and students should not perform massage on this group until they have received training. Preferably, this training includes supervised experience.

Advising students at the start of their training that cancer is a contraindication for massage plants seeds of fear. Once students are indoctrinated toward this view, it takes longer to unseat the anxiety. A number of therapists have worked with a cancer client who later died. Because they didn't understand the process of the disease and because of the fear that had been instilled in them during their schooling, some of them carry around a conscious or semi-conscious level of guilt that perhaps something they did in the massages contributed to their client's death. This is an unnecessary burden.

Sometimes, therapists who have been instilled with apprehension during their formal training, turn cancer patients away. One massage therapist recounted a story about a spa client who was assigned to her. The woman had been given a gift certificate from friends for a day at the spa. A day away from "cancer" was what the client was looking forward to. A massage session was scheduled first, to be followed by a facial and a pedicure. When she arrived, the massage therapist, who had been so thoroughly indoctrinated in school to never massage a cancer patient, told the client she couldn't massage her because massage might spread the cancer, but that she could give her a session of cranialsacral therapy or Reiki. The client burst into tears when told this. Her upset was so deep that she left the spa without even the facial or pedicure. All she had wanted was a day to feel normal.

An attitude of trepidation is injurious to patients and practitioners. It is harmful to patients because it denies them access to a service which is beneficial and further stigmatizes an already branded group. Practitioners are damaged because of an atmosphere of apprehension,

CHAPTER 1
INTRODUCTION: A NEW
ERA IN ONCOLOGY MASSAGE

5

INFO BOX

By the time the age of 64 is reached, citizens of the following areas have the following percentage chance of being diagnosed with cancer. (Between 64 and 85, the rate becomes even higher.)[7]

	Men	Women
Australia/ New Zealand	15.0%	15.6%
Northern Europe	11.7%	14.0%
Southern Europe	14.2%	12.0%
North America	18.2%	16.7%
South America	9.9%	10.8%
Eastern Asia (China/Japan)	11.2%	8.0%

Learning to massage people with cancer put the heart back into my learning. I learned as much about life as I did about technique.

— D. F., MASSAGE STUDENT, PORTLAND, OREGON

I'm contemplating a career change into massage therapy. My mother and sister were both diagnosed with cancer about 3 years ago. Massage therapy played a vital role in my sister's care. She had an outstanding therapist. Whenever she came home from a session, my sister was filled with hope and comfort. I want to be able to help people this way.

— FROM A LETTER TO THE AUTHOR

so even when bodyworkers do embark on working with cancer patients, they often do so with a lack of confidence that carries through their being and into their hands.

Bodywork training institutions must also evaluate their policies regarding the massage of people with a history of cancer. Some clinics turn away anyone in treatment for cancer, a very hurtful practice to those patients. Other schools allow the massage of cancer clients without providing training to the student practitioners. Both of these policies are unsound. Ideally, all therapists would be educated in the adjustments necessary for massaging clients with a cancer history.

Curriculums must be reexamined to determine if the needed coursework is being included in students' training that will allow them to safely work with cancer patients. For instance, all touch practitioners should understand such cautions as the risk for lymphedema, low platelets, compromised immune systems, the toxicity to vital organ systems from chemotherapy and radiation, and neuropathy. Practitioners should graduate with the ability to administer gentle, soothing bodywork. Not only do cancer patients need this; so do the elderly or pregnant client, the person on anti-inflammatory medications, the one who bruises easily. These clients present themselves to bodyworkers every day in every setting. All of this should be part of the core curriculum. The focus given to deep tissue techniques by many massage schools must be expanded to teach students how to work with all types of clients using a variety of rhythms and pressures appropriate to the physical and emotional condition of each client.

There will be touch therapists who specialize in massage for people with cancer. Specialists like this are needed. But EVERY therapist needs to be trained to confidently and carefully minister to people with a history of cancer.

FINAL THOUGHTS

People with cancer or a history of it receive massage in the same places as others – at health fairs, in chiropractic offices, with private practitioners, at spas, and through employee seated massage programs. Practitioners cannot avoid working with clients affected by cancer; the numbers are too great. In light of this, all massage therapists must be knowledgeable about working with this population, even those practitioners who "just do relaxation massage."

Bodywork is unique in its ability to simultaneously provide healing in many areas of the patient's life. Skilled touch can increase quality of life, lend emotional support, and decrease pain and other physical discomforts. Receiving comforting, attentive bodywork reminds the patient that the body can still be a source of pleasure. As they relax, pain, fatigue, and nausea diminish. Touch reminds them they are still lovable and worthwhile. For a moment, this person who may be disfigured, lonely, or without hope feels whole again.

People who are seriously ill look for hope wherever they can find it. This is one reason that people with cancer are coming in huge numbers to CAM providers. Cancer patients have become the bridge between complementary care practitioners and conventional, allopathic health care providers. Each side must now walk onto the span created by the patients and learn what the other has to offer, so that complementary and conventional medicine may work together to better the lives of those who have survived.

REFERENCES

1. Jemal A, Siegel R, Ward E, et al. Cancer Statistics 2006. *CA: A Journal for Clinicians*. 2006;56(2):106-130.

2. Latest cancer statistics released by Canadian Cancer Society – cancer incidence and death rates dropping. Available at: http://www.cancer.ca/ccs/internet/mediareleaselist/0,3208,3172_21050 4884_39119674_langId-en,00.html. Accessed February 22, 2005.

3. Cancer death rates falling, survival up. Available at: http://www.aihw.gov.au/mediacentre/2001/mr20011122.cfm. Accessed January 6, 2006.

4. Cancer death rates low in Australia compared to overseas, but incidence high. Available at: http://www.aihw.gov.au/mediacentre/2004/mr20041215a.cfm. Accessed January 6, 2006.

5. Statistics: Cancer facts and figures. Available at Cancer Research UK. Available at: http://www.cancerresearchuk.org/aboutcancer/statistics/. Accessed Dec. 21, 2005.

6. Sener SF. Disease without Borders: The Growing Global Burden of Cancer. *CA: A Cancer Journal for Clinicians*. 2005;55(1):7-9.

7. Parkin DM, Bray F, Ferlay J, et al. Global Cancer Statistics, 2002. *CA: A Cancer Journal for Clinicians*. 2005;55(1):74-108.

8. Sparber A, Bauer L, Curt G, et al. Use of Complementary Medicine by Adult Patients Participating in Cancer Clinical Trials. *Oncology Nursing Forum*. 2000;27(4):623-630.

9. Berstein BJ, Grasso T. Prevalence of complementary and alternative medicine use in cancer patients. *Oncology*. 2001 Oct;15(10):1267-72.

10. Yates JS, Mustian KM, Morrow GR, et al. Prevalance of Complementary and Alternative Medicine Use in Cancer Patients During Treatment. *Supportive Care in Cancer*. 2005;13(10):806-11

11. Lengacher CA, Bennett MP, Kipp KE, et al. Frequency of use of complementary and alternative medicine in women with breast cancer. *Oncology Nursing Forum*. 2002 Nov–Dec; 29(10):1445-52.

12. Morris KT, Johnson N, Homer L, et al. A comparison of complementary therapy use between breast cancer patients and patients with other primary tumor sites. *American Journal of Surgery* 2000 May;179(5):407-11.

13. Lee MM, Lin SS, Wrensch MR, et al. Alternative therapies used by women with breast cancer in four ethnic populations. *Journal of the National Cancer Institute*. 2000 Jan 5;92(1):42-7.

14. Kao GD, Devine P. Use of complementary health practices by prostate carcinoma patients undergoing radiation therapy. *Cancer*. 2000 Feb 1;88(3):615-9.

15. Crocetti E, Crotti N, Feltrin A, et al. The Use of Complementary Therapies by Breast Cancer Patients Attending Conventional Treatment. *European Journal of Cancer*. 1998;34(3):324-28.

16. Lewith GT, Broomfield J, Prescott P. Complementary cancer in Southampton: a survey of staff and patients. *Complementary Therapy Medicine*. 2002 June;10(2):100-6.

17. Henderson JW, Donatelle RJ. Complementary and alternative medicine use by women after completion of allopathic treatment for breast cancer. *Alternative Therapy Health Medicine*. 2004 Jan–Feb;10(1):52-7.

18. Cope D. News Briefs: Complementary and Alternative Medicine: Two-thirds of Breast Cancer Survivors Seek Nontraditional Therapy. *Clinical Journal of Oncology Nursing*. 2001 July/August;5(4):134.

19. Eisenberg DM. The Institute of Medicine Report on Complementary and Alternative Medicine in the United States-Personal Reflections on Its Content and Implications. *Alternative Therapies*. 2005 May/June;11(3):10-15.

20. Ashikaga T, Bosompra K, O'Brien P, et al. Use of complementary and alternative medicine by breast cancer patients: prevalence, patterns and communicating with physicians. *Support Care Cancer*. 2002 Oct;10(7);542-8.

21. Oncology Nursing Society Position Paper. The Use of Complementary and Alternative Therapies in Cancer Care. October 2004.

22. Allopathic doctors divided on benefits and advantages of complementary and alternative medicine. Available at: http://www.newstarget.com/011778.html. Accessed December 1, 2005.

23. Questions and Answers about Pain Control. National Institutes of Health. 1995.

24. Grossman SA, Benedetti C, Payne R, et al. NCCN practice guidelines for cancer pain. *Oncology* 1999;13(A11):33-44.

25. Weiger WA, Smith M, Pharms MR, et al. Advising Patients who Seek Complementary and Alternative Medical Therapies for Cancer. *Annals of Intenal Medicine*. 2002;137:889-903.

26. Parkin DM, Bray F, Ferlay J, et al. Global Cancer Statistics, 2002. CA: *A Cancer Journal for Clinicians*. 2005;55(2);74-108.

Acknowledgment: Parts of the chapter were adapted from "Bodywork for Cancer Patients: The Need for a Less-Demanding Approach." *Massage and Bodywork*, June/July 2005.

Chapter 2

Understanding Metastasis

Putting "Old Wives' Tales" to Rest

At one time it was thought that the pressure from massage strokes would cause cancer cells to release from the primary tumor and recolonize (metastasize) at distant sites. Some therapists accepted this guideline as gospel; others wondered where the notion came from. During this prohibition, many people with cancer who wanted massage were either turned away or given sessions on the sly. Neither of these approaches was healthy.

The caution against massage for people with cancer can perhaps be traced back to an image planted in Western psyches more than two thousand years ago by Hippocrates, the well-known Greek physician. He described cancer as a disease that spread out like the arms of a crab and grabbed on to other body parts.[1] This view of cancer might have led health care providers of the day to predict that mechanical force could break off the crab-like appendages of the tumor, setting them loose to travel to new places in the body and eventually implant there. If mechanical pressure were thought to be a causal factor in the spread of cancer, it would make sense to avoid forceful activities such as massage.

Fortunately, those days have passed. Researchers have shown that genetic alterations are the driving forces behind metastasis. Pressure alone is not sufficient to cause a tumor to become invasive (i.e., invade other areas of the body).[2] If this were the case, how could some tumors grow to a significant size, exert considerable pressure, but never invade or metastasize? Obviously, there is more to the picture than mechanical pressure.

Today, science is discovering more and more about how cancer starts and spreads. Even though there are still many pieces missing in the puzzle, it is apparent that previous fears about massaging people with cancer are unfounded. Metastasis, the spread of cancer to distant sites, is a complex, biochemical process that is orchestrated by genetic alterations. Generally, the changes are the result of mutations in the cells' DNA. It is not a mechanical process spurred on by exercise, walking the dog, or massage. If this were the case, oncologists would instruct their patients to stay in bed to minimize circulation and muscle contraction. If metastatic tumors were caused by mechanical motion of the body, hospitals would not allow oncology patients to exercise or have physical therapy.

Cancer is a common term for many different diseases that have the same underlying mechanism. Just as "bacterial infection" is an umbrella for many different illnesses such as pneumonia, meningitis, and staph infections, "cancer" is an all-encompassing term for more than 200 separate diseases. Breast cancer is a different disease from lung or colon cancer. Indeed, the term "breast cancer" describes more than 20 different diseases, each of which depends on the type of cell within the breast which developed cancer. Kidney cancer is unique and completely different from liver cancer. And yet, like bacterial infections, cancers have many processes in common.

It is the purpose of this chapter to explain in a simplified way some of the commonalities of these diseases that reside under the heading of "cancer." It is important to put practitioners' minds at rest about this old wives' tale that has plagued the massage profession, so that nothing will stand in the way of fully touching people with cancer.

THE ROLE OF GENES

In 1953, four English researchers, Watson, Crick, Wilkins and Franklin, cracked the "double helix" structure of DNA. The first three were given the Nobel Prize in 1962 for this discovery; Rosalind Franklin died of cancer in 1958 and could not receive the honor.[3] Their discovery, that DNA molecules consisted of double strands which spiraled, allowed scientists to understand the molecular basis for genetics and this decoding allowed scientists to discover the underlying mechanisms of many diseases, including cancer. Their discoveries also led to the field of molecular genetics, which is now fueling a new biological view of humanity, albeit a somewhat one-dimensional view that has genetics at the hub. The human being is more than just its genes.[4] But genes are central to the story of cancer, so this Chapter will focus on that component.

The genetic material of the body is contained within each cell's nucleus. This specialized area is the control center for each cell. The nucleus tells the cell when to grow and when to rest; when to make

Massage therapy is not contraindicated in cancer patients, massaging a tumor is, but there is a great deal more to a person than their tumor.

— BERNIE SIEGEL, MD

certain proteins or other material; how to communicate with other cells near and far; along with all other functions it needs to survive and thrive. When the cell can no longer function properly, the genetic material directs the mechanisms of its own destruction, known as apoptosis.

The genetic material that provides the body's blueprint is contained on chromosomes, of which there are 23 pair in each human cell (46 total chromosomes, except in the sperm and the egg cells which contain only 23 chromosomes – one copy of each). Chromosomes are composed of deoxyribonucleic acid (DNA). Four fundamental constituents compose DNA – adenine, thymine, cytosine, and guanine (A, T, C, and G). Each is attached to a backbone of a sugar-based compound called ribose and phosphate, a type of salt. The backbone of each A, T, C or G joins with other backbones to form an elaborate "spine" along which each of these molecules is fixed.[5] These four components are arranged in pairs along a double helix formation and can be aligned in a nearly infinite number of arrangements. The millions of minute processes necessary for life are contained in this code.

MECHANISMS OF GENETIC DAMAGE

Epithelial cells are some of the highly active cells referred to in the text immediately above. It is here that the majority of cancers, approximately 80–90%, have their origin.[8,9] These cancers are referred to as carcinomas. Epithelial cells are found throughout the body. They line the tract of the gastrointestinal system, the lungs, heart, blood and lymphatic vessels and the cavities of the body. Epithelium covers surfaces of glandular organs as well as the entire human body. These cells are especially vulnerable to mutation because they replicate over and over in a period of days.[10] It is this constant replication that puts them at risk for genetic mutation and explains why the majority of tumors appear in the epithelium.[4,10] Fast-growing blood and lymph cells are also at risk for developing cancer.

Two classes of genes play a major role in the development of cancer:

- **Proto-oncogenes,** which control growth and tissue repair. The defective versions of these genes are known as oncogenes. Their expression results in excessive cell proliferation. Mutations within the control genes also cause failure of the cell's regulatory system that induces apoptosis (programmed cell death) when the cell senses it cannot repair damage to its own DNA.

- **Tumor suppressor genes** normally regulate cell growth in an orderly, measured fashion; they stifle tumor growth by acting as a braking system that halts inappropriate growth. When they are inactivated by mutations, uncontrolled cell proliferation is allowed to go unchecked.[11]

INFO BOX

Through the cell's ability to read the code, the DNA directs all the activities of growth, development and maintenance. To do this, the DNA must "unzip" itself along the middle of the rungs of the DNA ladder, allow various other molecules to "read" the code of in the genes, then re-zip themselves together again when the gene is "decoded." They must do this as many times as needed for various functions. At any given time within cells, different portions of chromosomes are unwinding from their spirals, unzipping, allowing decoding, and re-forming. Highly active cells such as those which line the digestive tract, lungs, or form the surface of organs such as the liver are required not only to maintain their functions, but also to replenish themselves frequently. Nerve and muscle cells, on the other hand, have a much lower demand to replenish themselves, and so they rarely if ever make new cells.[6,7]

Genetic material can be damaged in many ways. Parts of the DNA can be deleted during copying or extra copies can be made; chromosomes can break or be incorrectly repaired; or a carcinogen such as a pesticide or virus can bind to the DNA causing damage to it. These injuries or copying mistakes reshuffle the genetic pack, so to speak.[4]

Approximately 10% of defective genes are inherited, while the remainder are acquired over the course of a lifetime.[11] Inherited genes are passed through sperm or ova and are found in every cell of the body. Acquired mutations are located in selected cells of the body and often happen as a result of environmental factors. Through the years, the strands of DNA can be damaged by chronic inflammation, carcinogens such as smoke, pesticides, UV rays, chemicals produced by the body, or microbes such as bacteria, parasites, and viruses. A surprising variety of viruses has been implicated in certain cancers – human papilloma virus (HPV) in cervical cancer, hepatitis B in liver cancer, and Epstein-Barr virus with lymphomas.

Genetic damage is also acquired because cells naturally make mistakes in the copying of DNA even without the influence of environmental agents.[4] No matter what the origins of genetic injury, if the mutations occur in the growth-controlling genes, the cell is given misinformation about how it should reproduce, which eventually can result in a tumor. Some tumors will remain encapsulated, or benign, while others will become invasive, also known as cancerous.

More recently, scientists have theorized that some cancers may have their origins in stem cell mutation. Research has shown potential stem cell implication in leukemia, breast cancer, and brain cancer. According to this idea, stem cells within tissues serve as a repository for each tissue's ability to regenerate itself. If stem cells are involved in the rise of cancer, it would explain why some treatments, especially chemotherapy, ultimately fail (the target of chemotherapy is large quantities of fast-growing cells). While the cancer may be tamed momentarily, the real culprit remains alive to re-trigger the cancer at a later time. If the theory about stem cell mutations is correct, even for only some cancers, it could lead scientists to create new treatments that target the mutated stem cells.[13]

The cancer burden differs regionally, in large part because of lifestyle factors and exposure to infectious agents. Throughout most of the developed world, the four deadliest cancers – lung, breast, colorectal, and prostate – are strongly influenced by tobacco use, diet, reproductive patterns, and sedentary lifestyle. In much of the developing world, cancers related to infection – stomach, liver, and cervix – remain leading killers but lung cancer is now the major cause of cancer death in developing countries.[14]

— STEPHEN F. SENER, MD

PRECANCEROUS GROWTH PATTERNS

Cancerous growths don't happen overnight. In most cases, neoplasms have their beginnings decades before patients present to their physician with a palpable tumor or with symptoms associated with an established cancer, such as severe fatigue or blood in the stool. By the time of the initial diagnosis, approximately 60% of patients with solid tumors already have metastatic lesions, also known as metastases. It is these secondary lesions that most often cause death, not the original tumor.[9,15]

A single mutation rarely causes cancer in an adult. It is necessary to have a number of injuries to the DNA. Hahn, et al. have identified three as the minimum number of injuries required to turn a normal cell into a cancer cell.[16] In *Cancer: The Evolutionary Legacy*, Mel Greaves posits that five to ten mutations are necessary.[4] Weinberg states half a dozen or so are needed.[2]

Before a cancer develops, it passes through a number of stages on its way to becoming invasive. Initially, cells may become enlarged; this is known as hypertrophy. Commonly, this condition results from an increased workload, hormonal over-production, or compensation for other tissue that is functioning poorly. Cigarette smoke is an example of an agent that can trigger hypertrophy due to increased workload. The inflammatory response is triggered in the mucosal lining of the lungs which leads to fibrosis and thickening in the membranes and bronchioles.[9]

A mass will begin when a normal cell mutates, increasing its propensity to over-produce when normally it would rest.[2] These transformed cells look normal, but they reproduce at a higher than usual rate. This stage is referred to as hyperplasia. It is important to note that the cells in a tumor all originate from a single cell whose DNA has mutated. The proliferating cells are clones of the original.

At times, one cell type substitutes for another, a condition known as metaplasia. The uterine cervix is a common place for this to occur. The process is reversible if the stimulant is removed. Inflammation, irritation, chemicals, or dietary insufficiencies are common triggers.

If the cause of the metaplasia is not removed, years later, one in a million of these cells may be affected by another genetic mutation, causing further malfunctions in cell growth. At this stage, cells not only continue the excess growth, but the descendants take on an abnormal shape and orientation referred to as dysplasia. One of the ways of determining how advanced a tumor might be is by the degree to which it has lost its resemblance to the cells in the original tissue.

After a time, if another mutation damages the cell's DNA, the growth and appearance of the tumor cells becomes even more abnormal. At this point, the neoplasm makes the transition from benign to cancerous. Although it is still contained within the boundaries of the original tissue, it is considered to be an *in situ* cancer. These encapsulated cancers can become problematic because of their sheer size. They may remain in this state indefinitely, or may eventually accumulate the mutations required to become metastatic.[9]

QUALITIES OF TUMOR CELLS

Although cancer cells appear to be inconscionable rogues or rebels that violate the body's regulatory system of growth and proliferation, in reality they are part of a well-orchestrated process in which a single normal cell undergoes changes that give it special

Vocabulary Basics

Angiogenesis – The creation of new blood vessels

Benign – Non-invasive tumor

Cancerous – A tumor that has the capacity to be invasive; malignant

Carcinoma – A cancer that has its start in epithelium

Emboli – A detached mass in the blood stream that may consist of bits of tissue, tumor cells, fat globules, air bubbles, clumps of bacteria, and foreign bodies

Endothelim – A type of epithelium that lines the heart, blood vessels, lymphatic vessels, and serous cavities

Epithelium – The layer of cells that lines the GI tract, hollow organs, blood vessels, and forms the skin and part of glandular organs. It has the ability to regenerate frequently

Growth Factors – Proteins that regulate a variety of cellular processes. They typically act as signaling molecules

In situ – A cancer that is localized

Malignancy – A cancerous tumor

Metastasis – The process by which cancer spreads from the original site to a distant one

Metastases – The new tumors formed at a distant site

CANCER
deep, angry red
yearning
burning
twisting
turning
eating bones and flesh
screaming to heard
without uttering a word

— Dana Doolin, LMT,
Portland, Oregon

abilities.[4,9] Normal cells conduct themselves in an orderly manner, adhering to one another, stopping growth when contact is made with another cell, dividing only when attached to an anchor point. Cancer cells are rowdy renegades in which the inhibition mechanisms have failed. They grow and divide, crowding the space they occupy, until the cells are piled on each other in an unorganized mass.

Another quality of malignant cells that is responsible for their ability to spread is a lack of adhesiveness. Normally, cells adhere to one another and to a mesh of proteins known as the extracellular matrix. Metastatic cells are able to drift away from their original site and reattach to unlike cells because of changes in certain cell surface receptors. E-cadherin is an example. When it is compromised or missing from the surface of the cell, researchers have found that many cancers, such as breast, prostate, esophageal, gastric, colon, skin, kidney, lung, and liver progress. Cancer cells not only lack adhesiveness, these aberrant cells are "anchorage independent" and can divide while suspended in a liquid medium. When normal cells are denied anchorage, they stop reproducing and commit "cellular suicide," thereby safeguarding the integrity of tissues.[8,9,10,15]

Tumor cells are able to accomplish their feats on only a fraction of the growth factors normal cells would require. Some cancer cells even grow in the absence of these factors, which would seem to indicate that they make their own growth factors. In addition, they sometimes induce surrounding tissue cells to produce more growth factors.[4]

The lining of body cavities, blood and lymphatic vessels, the outer part of the skin, interiors of the respiratory and digestive tracts, and glandular tissue are made of epithelial cells. These cells are designed to protect the body's underlying tissues, or in the case of glandular epithelium, they constitute the secreting portion of glands. This layer of cells forms a barrier that most normal cells cannot breach. However, invading tumor cells have the ability to secrete enzymes (collagenases) that degrade the basement membrane and other extracellular matrices. The cells are then able to digest their way through surrounding tissue. This ability to penetrate the epithelial basement membrane and enter the underlying interstitial stroma, allowing them to gain access to lymphatics and blood vessels, is a major difference between invasive and non-invasive tumors.[17]

Breakdown of the basement membrane was thought to be required for tumor cell invasiveness. However, researchers have found that some cells are able to adapt their shape into an amoeba-like form and squeeze through gaps in the extracellular matrix.[18] This ability to so drastically change their morphology puts tumor cells at an incredible metastatic advantage. It also explains how some cancer cells are able to pass through capillary beds that are smaller than themselves and migrate to outer reaches of the body.

Tumor cells that possess the ability to induce new capillary growth, or neovascularization, are much more apt to become metastatic. Usually, by the time a tumor is large enough to detect, neovascularization, also known as angiogenesis, is well underway.

Without a blood supply to provide the needed nutrients, neoplasms cannot grow more than a few millimeters. Tumors that lack this ability remain *in situ*, a steady state in which the number of new cells equals the number of dying cells.[8,19] But, for unknown reasons, an *in situ* tumor can suddenly induce new capillary growth, allowing the mass to continue growing and invade adjacent tissue. Evidence shows that some cancers progress due to decreased oxygen availability, or hypoxia. The lack of oxygen triggers a chemical response that in turn creates neovascularization and other processes that allow tumor cells to survive or escape their oxygen-deficient environment.[20]

Once angiogenesis occurs, scores of new capillaries converge on the tiny tumor. According to Hawkins, "…each vessel soon has a thick coat of rapidly dividing tumor cells."[15] Within months the tumor may grow to a cubic centimeter, containing about one billion tumor cells. To make matters worse, the endothelial cells of the new capillaries release different proteins that can stimulate excess cell proliferation or the cell's ability to move, increasing the likelihood that cancer cells will leave the primary tumor and migrate into the bloodstream.[15]

It is these qualities of uncontrolled proliferation, lack of adhesiveness, anchorage independence, diminished need for growth factors, the ability to secrete degradative enzymes and induce new capillary growth that are associated with cancer cells' ability to spread. The spreading occurs irrespective of patients' activities. It happens while watching TV, cooking dinner, playing with the children, or even sleeping. Avoiding massage will not stop these rogue cells from slipping away from the original tumor. This is not to say that bodyworkers are free to work without inhibition. As shall be seen in later chapters, there are reasons for adjusting the sessions a cancer patient receives, but the adjustments do not center around the potential for metastatic spread. They are, by and large, a result of the patient's treatment history.

THE SPREAD OF CANCER

Cancer does not spread in a random, willy-nilly way. It is a logical, orchestrated event. Malignant cells spread from the primary tumor by two major processes: 1) direct spreading to adjoining areas, or 2) metastatic spread to distant sites. The dissemination may be by one or both processes, since spread via one route may create access to the other.

DIRECT SPREAD

It is not yet understood why certain malignant masses remain *in situ*, some are locally invasive but limit their growth to the surrounding tissue without metastasizing, and others become aggressively malignant and metastasize to often distant tissues. Researchers believe

Chronic Inflammation and Cancer

Many inflammatory diseases are considered to be precursors to cancer – inflammatory bowel disease, gastritis, pancreatitis, rheumatoid arthritis, and reflux, to name just a few. Some of these conditions are triggered by diet, others by infectious agents such as *H pylori* or the inflammatory disease itself. For instance, a high intake of traditionally-preserved salted foods such as meats and pickles increases the risk for gastritis. Therefore, people in countries such as Russia and Japan, where consumption of pickled foods is high, have greater rates of gastric cancer than do North Americans. (North Americans are plagued by different cancers, such as breast and prostate.) *H pylori* infection is another cause of gastritis and can also lead to cancer of the stomach. In fact, the evidence linking it to gastric cancer was considered sufficient to classify *H pylori* as carcinogenic. Evidence has shown that rheumatoid arthritis sufferers are more susceptible to a type of skin cancer known as malignant melanoma.[12,21]

The inflammatory response releases a variety of substances – macrophages, white blood cells, prostaglandins, and growth factors, to name some. It is a high-energy process that produces potentially damaging by-products. Temporarily the body can cope with this metabolic overdrive, but the by-products of persistent inflammation can damage DNA and/or create an environment that is rich with growth factors that fuel tumor cells.[4]

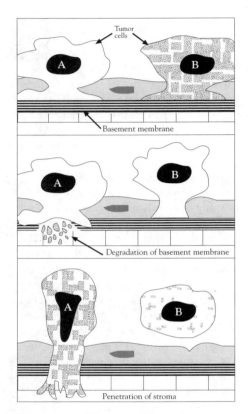

Figure 2.1 The use of degradative enzymes.

After a metastatic tumor cell adheres to the endothelium and penetrates to the subendothelial basement membrane, it releases enzymes that degrade elements of the basement membrane. (Cell A) Cells that cannot degrade the extra-cellular matrix cannot invade the organ and eventually move on to another site or die in the bloodstream. (Cell B)[22]

that tumors are propelled toward invasiveness by another accumulation of genetic transformations.

Direct spread, the penetration and destruction of adjacent tissue, is the result of many factors. Local invasion is enhanced by the ability of malignant cells to stimulate new capillary formation. This greatly increases the tumor's growth rate. Rapid proliferation produces densely packed, expanding masses of cells that exert pressure on adjacent tissues, forcing fingerlike projections into neighboring areas. Tumors then spread into spaces that separate in response to pressure, such as interstitial or cerebrospinal spaces or the abdominal cavity.[2,9,11]

Malignant cells may also invade by secreting enzymes that break down the basement membrane of tissues, resulting in the penetration of body cavities (see Figure 2.1). After spreading into neighboring areas and penetrating body cavities, such as the pleura or peritoneum, cancer cells can attach to the surfaces within the cavity.[9]

METASTATIC SPREAD

Fortunately, even if a malignant cell is released due to increased pressure or has slipped away from the primary site, the formation of a secondary tumor is not an automatic outcome. Once a tumor cell has left the parental mass, it must successfully complete a series of steps to establish a metastatic lesion. (A lesion is tissue that is pathologically changed.) The inability to complete any of the following steps will stop the metastatic cascade:

1. Detach from the original tumor
2. Invade the blood system or lymph vessels
3. Survive in the circulatory system and travel to a distant site
4. Arrest in a congenial site
5. Adhere to the endothelial lining of the blood vessels in the new organ
6. Re-invade the distant organ or tissue
7. Establish a blood supply[15]

Despite their many capabilities, it is so difficult for the migrating cells to complete all of these requirements that very few manage to colonize a distant site. The spread to distant sites occurs via two entryways, lymphatic channels or blood vessels. Often, because the vascular and lymphatic systems are interconnected, both are involved.[2,9,11]

LYMPHATIC DISSEMINATION

For many types of cancer the first evidence of spreading is a mass in the lymph nodes that drain the area where the primary tumor is located. The spread of malignant cells into the lymph nodes is a significant occurrence, as lymph nodes are involved in about half of all fatal cancers. Lymphatic metastases indicate the tumor is able to leave the primary site and are predictors that distant metastases are likely to be found.[10] Extension into the lymph nodes can be fast or slow, depending on the tumor. Once malignant cells lodge in lymph nodes they have several possible fates: 1) die of a local inflammatory reaction; 2) wither and die because of a lack of the proper environment; 3) grow into a mass; 4) remain dormant.[9]

At one time, the filtering action of the lymph nodes was believed to be the cause of nodal metastasis. Research, however, has shown filtration to be only a minor influence. Most likely the interaction between physiochemical changes on the cancer cell's surface and the lymph node determines whether and where the cancer cells will lodge in the lymphatic system. Logically, it might follow that the nearby lymph nodes that drain the primary tumors would test positive before more distant nodes. While this sometimes is the case, other metastatic cells bypass local lymph nodes and settle in distant ones, indicating that other influences are at work. Just as blood-borne metastases are not random or completely the result of anatomical flow routes, neither are nodal metastases. Most likely, site specific recognition plays a part in the location of these cancers.[9]

Until recently, researchers were unaware that tumors are able to form new lymph vessels. A protein known as vasoendothelial growth factor-C has been found to stimulate the formation of lymph vessels, a process known as lymphangiogenesis.[23] The formation of new vessels facilitates the spread of cancer to nearby lymph nodes. These new vessels do not, however, appear to spread the cancer to distant sites. Other factors are responsible for that.[10]

BLOOD-BORNE SPREAD

The local spread of cancer occurs predominantly through the lymphatic vessels, but spreading to remote organs and tissues is almost always via the bloodstream. Lymphatic metastases are rarely in and of themselves the cause of death in people with cancer. When the spread is to critical distant organs, such as the liver, lung. bone, or brain, cancers are most dangerous.[10]

Tumor cells that enter the blood stream circulate until one of three things happens: 1) they are killed, 2) they are trapped in the capillary bed of another organ, or 3) they invade the blood vessel wall into the tissue of a distant organ. Only the latter group can ever form metastatic colonies. Cells that remain in the blood stream or are trapped inside the tiny vessels of a capillary bed die fairly quickly, often within hours.[10]

It is so difficult for the migrating cells to complete all of the requirements that very few ever manage to colonize at a distant site. It is estimated that fewer than one in 10,000 cancer cells that enter the bloodstream live to reach another organ. Even fewer successfully implant themselves.[9-11] At every step they must escape the many controls that keep normal cells in place. But, because the process

---

Metastatic Potential

A woman with lymphoma came to a massage practitioner with a doctor's order for massage. The practitioner, however, told the woman she would not work with her because massage increased lymphatic flow, which would speed up the flow of cancer cells in the lymph. The massage therapist explained to the client that she didn't want to be responsible for contributing to her cancer. The woman pleaded with the practitioner, saying that she was certain massage would help. When the bodyworker called the client's doctor, he urged her to proceed with the massage. He supported the idea that beliefs are powerful and can bring about positive outcomes. The physician went on to explain that the spread of cancer is not brought about by speeding up lymphatic flow, but is dependent on the metastatic potential of the tumor cells.

— AUTHOR

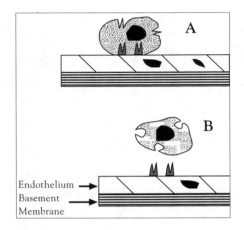

Figure 2.2 Site specific cell adhesion.

Tumor cells that adhere to certain sites do so in part because they possess receptors for those organs. (Panel A) Tumor cells that lack receptors for a specific organ will fail to bind and thus pass through the organ vasculature into the collecting veins (Panel B).[22]

occurs over and over for many days, some metastatic growths eventually form.[10]

While in the circulatory system cancer cells face many threats, such as the mechanical forces of blood turbulence. Hemodynamics has been suggested as a possible factor in that vascular pressure and flow rate may be too high in certain areas, such as skin and skeletal muscles, to allow cancer cells to come to rest there.[15] On the other hand, tumor cells often adhere to other tumor cells and blood cells, especially platelets. Platelets produce their own growth factors which may help the cancer cells survive in the blood.[17] Adhering to other cells also helps protect the tumor cells from circulating immune cells and produces enlarged emboli, increasing the likelihood they will arrest in the target organ.[4,9]

It is hypothesized that the location of over half of metastatic deposits can be predicted from the blood flow route. In this model of prediction, the first organ encountered would be the site of the greatest tumor cell arrest. This might account for the higher number of lung tumors, as the lung is the first organ the shed cells encounter after entering the venous circulation. How, though, do tumors travel past the initial organ and implant farther afield? There is evidence that cells can pass through capillaries smaller in size than themselves,[18] so it is not enough to passively trap tumor emboli that are too big to pass. Other factors dictate where metastatic colonies will develop.

The ability of cancer cells to flourish at a specific site is dependent on the interactions between the cancer cell and the organ. One characteristic that might make an organ congenial to tumor growth is the presence of specific growth factors found at those sites. Other evidence points toward an idea of adhesive-specificity, where particular cancers bind to certain types of tissue. In part, this happens because they home in to certain sites that contain the molecular address system that matches to the surface of certain tissues or organ. Figure 2.2 illustrates this "lock and key" configuration known as site specific recognition. Migration to these sites appears to be under the influence of chemical messengers that guide the tumor cells to travel in the direction of certain growth factors rather than moving about in hit-or-miss fashion. Some researchers have put forward the idea that the preference for certain metastatic sites may be genetically determined.[17]

After the tumor cell embolus has arrested, a number of things must happen in order for the sequence to continue. It must adhere to the endothelial lining, and then invade that wall to pass through to the basement membrane surrounding the tissue or organ. Then the metastatic cells must invade that protective wall. This happens either directly through thin-walled capillaries, or by producing enzymes that degrade the basement membrane. Degradation of the basement membrane damages the tissue, which in turn stimulates an inflammatory response. Prostaglandins, one of the substances released during the inflammatory process, causes vasodilation, which increases the permeability of the affected vessels. Cancer cells use these leaky vessels and the subsequent creation of an inflammatory reaction at the site to further escape from the vascular system.[9,17]

A number of things can happen once cancer cells invade remote tissue. They may die, or lie dormant for years and then grow to a large size long after the primary tumor has been removed, or they may begin growing to a large size immediately. It is not known what causes cancer cells to remain in a dormant stage, or what causes them to eventually become active. Possibly small populations of tumor cells remain in an avascular phase for prolonged periods, until a new biochemical message stimulates them into action. Breast cancer, for example, has been known to metastasize to the vertebrae 30 years later.[9]

The final ability needed to create a new growth is the capacity of the tumor to establish its own blood supply. This is done when the metastatic cell sends a chemical message to the host tissue, such as the lungs, that stimulates capillary growth. Without the ability to perform angiogenesis, the tumor would wilt and die after a short period of time.[19]

HOST FACTORS

Exposure to a cancer-causing agent doesn't mean a person will get cancer. The development of cancer is a complex interaction that is influenced by how often, how long, and how much exposure the person had, and his or her genetic predisposition to developing cancer. The way in which tumors of the same type metastasize varies from one person to the next. This has led some researchers to conclude that factors related to the host contribute to metastatic potential. Besides genetics, diet and other lifestyle choices, the immune system, age, and hormones can determine the way in which the cancer process unfolds.[9]

The capacity of a person's immune system influences whether and how cancer will develop. Some researchers believe that cancer cells are continually being created in our bodies, and then destroyed, and that it is when the "surveillance system" breaks down that malignancies occur. Stress, age, or certain medications can be the cause of the immune system's becoming suppressed. In experiments with animals, cancer cells that normally wouldn't metastasize will do so in animals whose immune systems are suppressed. Human evidence bears this out, too. Immunocompromised individuals are many times more likely to develop cancer than those in the general population.[9]

Surprisingly, certain processes of the immune system, such as inflammation, assist in the establishment of metastatic disease. Some tumors can induce an immune response when their growth causes injury to surrounding tissue. This sets the inflammatory cells of the immune system into motion. Along with the tumor, these inflammatory cells also produce enzymes that degrade the basement membrane of surrounding tissue as well as blood vessels. Tumor cells

Cortisol, commonly known as the stress hormone, has been connected to increased tumor growth. In her doctoral thesis, "The Effect of Therapeutic Massage on Post Surgical Outcomes," Martha Brown Menard posits that "massage may actually have a protective effect against tumor growth."[25] She hypothesizes that interventions known to lower elevated cortisol levels may have an inhibitory effect on tumor growth. Cortisol levels, a yardstick commonly used in research to measure physical and psychological stress, have consistently been shown to decrease as a result of massage in the Touch Research Institute studies. Wouldn't it be ironic if, after years of being contraindicated for fear of spreading cancer, massage was actually found to be a deterrent to the disease?

also form emboli in collaboration with elements of the immune system, such as leukocytes and macrophages, as well as elements of the blood, like platelets. This embolization is facilitated by products of the activated inflammatory cells, such as procoagulants, which trigger the blood to coagulate, and prostaglandins,[9] which cause vasodilation and increased permeability of blood vessels.[22]

Another determinant in the development of cancer is the age of the host. The longer a person's lifespan, the more opportunity for DNA mistakes to occur and go unrepaired or misrepaired.[4] A look at the rates of incidence provides proof of this. The chance of an American male between the ages of 40 and 59 developing cancer is one in 12. Between ages 60 and 69, the chance rises steeply to one in six.[23]

Certain types of tumors appear to increase, regress, or arrest because of hormones. For example, women who breast fed their children have a decreased incidence of breast cancer, possibly due to less estrogen exposure. On the other hand, those who have children late in life or not all have increased rates of gynecological cancers. This can be explained by the change in women's reproductive lives. European and North American women start menstruating earlier, delay having children, and have fewer of them. The result is more ovulatory cycles, which translates into increased estrogen exposure. Men, too, can stress the prostate by having sex past the normal reproductive age. This increases testosterone levels, which impacts the prostate. It is important to note, though, that while chronic hormonal stress may promote the expansion of a cancerous growth, many scientists believe that an external, carcinogenic event is still needed to trigger the initial process.[4]

IMPLICATIONS FOR BODYWORK

The examination of metastasis in this chapter has remained relatively simple. The focus has centered on the role genetic alterations play in the rise and spread of cancer. In no way can massage contribute to the mutation of genes. There are, however, some obvious implications with regard to the metastatic process and bodywork:

- It is not possible to know at a any given time whether a client is cancer free. There are always aberrant cells present in the body. Cancer cells can lie dormant and then years later become active. Despite following intake protocols to the letter, many bodyworkers have unknowingly massaged someone with cancer. Patients often times do not present to their physician until a tumor is well established, and by the time of the initial diagnosis, a high percentage already have metastases. However, massage practitioners have acted in a judicious manner if they performed an adequate intake, obtained physician approval for clients whose medical condition warranted it, and observed appropriate safety precautions.

- Denying gentle massage to a patient will not prevent metastasis. Cancer spreads even while patients are involved in completely sedate activities such as sitting or sleeping.

- Massaging the site of a tumor is contraindicated, as the mechanical force on the tumor may contribute to the pressure build-up already taking place with the uncontrolled growth of the neoplasm. It can also be uncomfortable to have the tumor site massaged if for no other reason than the tissue is prone to inflammation and highly sensitive or is mechanically exerting pressure on underlying structures.

- Deep massage, which is known to create an inflammatory response, is contraindicated. Inflammatory cells produce enzymes that degrade surrounding tissue as well as facilitate embolization by some of the substances they produce. Both of these processes factor heavily into metastatic potential. It is also imperative not to injure tissue, thereby causing bruising, which then leads to blood clotting. Cancer cells combine with blood constituents present in the clotting process, such as platelets and fibrin, to form emboli which more easily come to rest in a distant capillary bed.

- Teachers of lymph drainage modalities advise that their techniques are contraindicated for patients with cancers of the lymphatic system. Many oncologists fail to see how this style of bodywork would contribute to the spread of cancer. Lymphatic circulation occurs naturally as a result of skeletal muscles contracting, which compresses lymph vessels and forces the movement of lymph. Another major factor that contributes to lymph flow is the simple act of breathing. Comfort-oriented massage does not increase lymphatic circulation any more than do activities of daily life such as exercising, shopping, or caring for children, activities which doctors urge their patients to engage in.

I have treated many, many cancer patients using CranioSacral Therapy and SomatoEmotional Release over about a 25-year period. I have yet to see anything that arouses the slightest suspicion in me that any of this work contributes to metastases. I have seen it do a lot of good however, even complete remission in some cases. Further, I do not believe that massage contributes to metastasis unless it is very deep, traumatic massage.

— DR. JOHN UPLEDGER,
ORIGINATOR OF CRANIOSACRAL
THERAPY

FINAL THOUGHTS

After reading this chapter, some readers may be shaking their head and muttering, "This is too complicated for me to understand!" This is a reasonable reaction; the development of cancer and its metastasis is a complex process involving enzymes, growth factors, genetics, adhesion-specificity, and a myriad of other biochemical processes. If all that the reader takes away from this chapter is that metastasis is a complex process which will not be accelerated by gentle, nurturing massage, that is enough. When the complexity of the process is seen, it becomes clear that simple mechanical pressure is not the source of metastasis. And massage is not responsible for genetic alterations that trigger excess proliferation, invasiveness, or the metastatic sequence.

There has been no evidence that massage therapy can spread cancer, although direct pressure over a tumor is usually discouraged.[26]

— *Lisa Corbin, MD*

There is no evidence to suggest that touch or gentle, caring massage causes metastasis, but there is proof that it greatly benefits many cancer patients, both physically and emotionally. Research and anecdotal evidence has shown low-impact massage to positively affect symptoms related to cancer or side effects from treatment regimens, such as nausea, fatigue, insomnia, and pain. Patients report an increased sense of well-being, with reduction in anxiety and the sense of isolation, as well as increased relaxation and decreased muscle tension. As *Medicine Hands* proceeds, it will become apparent that care, caution, and a soft touch are the watch words when massaging people with cancer. This is not to say that metastasis is a trivial matter. It is a very serious one. However, it is not the main issue where massage is concerned.

This does not mean there are no cautions to be observed when working with those in or recovering from cancer treatments. Therapists must be alert to the many side effects of chemotherapy, radiation, and surgery, such as low blood counts, the risk for lymphedema, and body image changes. And the cancer itself will cause cautions. These are the real issues that must be attended to rather than the imagined issue of metastasis. The following chapters go into depth in discussing these issues and how to adjust sessions to ensure client safety and comfort.

REFERENCES

1. Leaf C. Why We're Not Winning the War on Cancer and How to Win It. *Fortune*. March 22, 2004. P.77-98.

2. Weinberg, RA. How Cancer Arises. *Scientific American*. 1996; 275(3):62-70.

3. Chemical Achievers, The Human Face of the Chemical Sciences: James Watson, Francis Crick, Maurice Wilkins, and Rosalind Franklin. Available at: http://www.chemheritage.org/classroom/chemach/pharmaceuticals/watson-crick.html. Accessed July 3, 2006.

4. Greaves M. *Cancer: The Evolutionary Legacy*. Oxford, England: Oxford University Press, 2000.

5. Introduction to DNA Structure. Available at: http://www.blc.arizona.edu/Molecular_Graphics/DNA_Structure/DNA_Tutorial.HTML#Backbone. Accessed July 3, 2006.

6. Structure of DNA. Available at: http://chemistry.hull.ac.uk/lectures/kjw/Structure%20of%20DNA.pdf. Accessed October 8, 2006.

7. DNA Molecular Animation. Available at: http://www.wehi.edu.au/education/wehi-tv/dna/dna.html. Accessed October 8, 2006.

8. Cell Adhesion and Metastasis. Mayo Clinic College of Medicine. Available at: http://mayoresearch.mayo.edu/mayo/research/mcj/AnastasiadisLab.cfm. Accessed June 5, 2006.

9. Pfeifer KA. *Pathophysiology in Oncology Nursing,* 4th Ed. St. Louis, MO: Mosby, 2001.

10. Tumor Metastasis. Zetter Research Lab. Available at: http://www.zetterlab.org/research/tumor_metastasis.html. Accessed June 5, 2006.

11. Oncogenes and Tumor Suppressor Genes. Available at: http://www.cancer.org/docroot/ETO/content/ETO_1_4x_oncogenes _and_tumor_suppressor_genes.asp. Accessed July 3, 2006.

12. Schottenfeld D, Beebe-Dimmer J. Chronic Inflammation: A Common and Important Factor in the Pathogenesis of Neoplasia. CA: *A Journal for Clinicians.* 2006;56(2):69-83.

13. Travis J. The Bad Seed: Rare stem cells appear to drive cancer. *Science News Online.* 2004;165(12).

14. Sener SF. Disease Without Borders: The Growing Global Burden of Cancer. CA: *A Cancer Journal for Clinicians.* 2005 Jan/Feb;55(1):7-9.

15. Hawkins R. Mastering the Intricate Maze of Metastasis. *Oncology Nursing Forum.* 2001;28(6): 959-965.

16. Hahn WC, Counter CM, Lundberg AS, et al. Creation of human tumor cells with defined genetic elements. *Nature.* 1999; July Volume 400:464-468.

17. Ruoslahti E. How Cancer Spreads. *Scientific American.* 1996;275(3):72-77.

18. Wolf K, Mazo I, Leung H, et. al. Compensation mechanism in tumor cell migration: mesenchymal-amoeboid transition after blocking of pericellular proteolysis. *Journal of Cell Biology.* 2003;160(2):267-277.

19. Folkman J. Fighting Cancer by Attacking its Blood Supply. *Scientific American.* 1996;275(3):150-154.

20. Vaupel P. *The Role of Hypoxia-Induced Factors in Tumor Progression.* Available at: http://theoncologist.alphamedpress.org/cgi/reprint/9/suppl_5/10. Accessed July 3, 2006.

21. Ekstrom K, Hjalgrim H, Brandt L, et al. Risk of Malignant Lymphomas in Patients with Rheumatoid Arthritis and in Their First-Degree Relatives. *Arthritis and Rheumatism.* 2003;48(4):963-970.

22. Zetter BR. The Cellular Basis of Site-Specific Tumor Metastasis. *Seminars in Medicine of the Beth Israel Hospital.* 1990:41(5):301-305.

23. Achen MG, Mannz GB, Stackeri SA. Targeting Lymphangiogenesis to Prevent Tumour Metastasis. *British Journal of Cancer.* 2006;94;1355-60.

24. Jemal A, Siegel R, Ward E, et al. Cancer Statistics 2006. CA: *A Cancer Journal for Clinicians.* 2006;56(2):106-130.

25. Menard M. The Effect of Therapeutic Massage on Post Surgical Outcomes. Doctoral dissertation, University of Virginia, 1995.

26. Corbin L. Safety and Efficacy of Massage Therapy for Patients with Cancer. *Cancer Control.* 2005;12(3):158-164.

Chapter 3

Touch — Rx for Body, Mind, and Heart

A Review of the Research

Massage changes people's lives. The accounts of how it has affected those with cancer are dramatic, unexpected, and sometimes inspiring. Anxiety is curbed, pain dulled, and nausea made manageable. Patients describe feeling whole again, hope is restored, or connection to self is reestablished. For one woman it was like being "held in the hands of God." Another patient, who received massage following chemotherapy, was able to plod through her treatments without having to be in bed the first few days following chemo. This was important, as she is the mother of a four-year-old.

There is a plethora of rich anecdotal evidence from patients and therapists that illustrates the effectiveness of touch therapy. This type of proof is told via written case histories or by word of mouth from therapist to therapist, patient to doctor, and teacher to student.

The loving touch, like music, often utters the things that cannot be spoken.

— ASHLEY MONTAGU

Anecdotal evidence is the story of individuals – of Laura, whose fever dropped from 103.6 to 98.6 after 30 minutes of light effleurage; or Mary Ellen, who said that touch therapy provided a safe space for healing.

Another form of evidence is gleaned through scientific research. This type of inquiry tells the story of groups rather than individuals. For instance, Hernandez-Reif and her colleagues at the Touch Research Institute systematically examined the effect of Swedish Massage on a group of 34 women who were treated for stage 1 or 2 breast cancer three months previous. The women received a 30-minute Swedish Massage three times a week for five weeks. The results showed a decrease in depression and anger and an increase in vigor.[1] This information can help predict how women in the earlier stages of breast cancer might respond to this specific application of touch therapy, but it can't tell us how any one individual may be affected.

Both types of evidence, anecdotal and scientific, help therapists, clients, family, and health care providers to understand the effects of massage on people with cancer. However, the scientific research paradigm is given greater credence by mainstream medicine. Therefore, it is important for touch practitioners to be knowledgeable of this research so that they can accurately represent· what is scientifically known about the benefits of massage for people with a history of cancer. This is not meant to undervalue anecdotal evidence. Readers will find examples of it liberally placed through the entire book.

The studies presented here are a snapshot of the state of research at the moment this manuscript was being prepared. Oncology massage research is accumulating so quickly that by the time this book is published, there will be another batch of studies to consider. Readers will need to search further for the new studies that will be released in future years. A list of additional resources can be found on pages 35 and 39.

"... The debate in this area has shifted from 'convention versus alternative,' 'modern versus ancient,' and 'dominant versus marginal' to one in which we collectively embrace the complex challenges of redefining healthcare nationally and internationally in the 21st century, all the while being guided by science. Clearly, more research in complementary and integrative medicine is warranted and necessary to meet these objectives.[2]

— DAVID EISENBERG, MD

RESEARCH LITERACY

Research literacy has just begun within the massage community. Becoming conversant in this area is especially important for massage practitioners who are working within mainstream medicine; it is part of learning to interact with members of the allopathic health care team. Mainstream health care providers have a vastly different orientation than do many complementary care practitioners. Each group values different aspects of care. Massage therapists, for instance, understand the importance to patients of having a place to share their story. A massage session provides a natural place for this. For the medical provider, blood counts and MRI results are of primary importance. The latter place stock in randomized, controlled trials, whereas massage therapists are often at the other end of the spectrum, tending to overglorify anecdotal evidence. Touch practitioners often use anecdotal evidence to support claims that massage causes such benefits as shorter hospital stays, lower medication use, improved sleep, or quicker wound healing. Scientific evidence, however, does not exist for these assertions. Touch therapists, therefore, need to be discriminating between anecdotal and scientific evidence, especially when talking to the allopathic community.

Massage literature is often lax in the way it reports the effects of massage. The benefits of massage are commonly listed without credible citations or are based on anecdotal evidence which is then generalized to the entire population. It is important to paint a precise picture of what is known about the benefits of massage. Rather than making sweeping generalizations, such as, "Massage improves immune function," a more accurate statement would be, "A few studies have looked at the effect of massage on immunity. The findings were promising, but firm conclusions cannot yet be drawn." Or, perhaps a statement such as, "Little research has been done on that variable, but the experience of some massage therapists and clients shows that massage helps patients' blood counts return to normal more quickly."

Oncology massage research is still at the apples and oranges stage. (Actually, bananas and watermelon are a better comparison!) With the exception of studies from the Touch Research Institute (TRI), comparing various studies is impossible because the massage protocols are all different. The pressure used in massage strokes is not consistent, nor are the length of sessions; the modalities vary from study to study as do the personality traits and training level of the therapists; and there is no consistency in the design of the studies or the statistical analysis. Only the TRI studies use a standard massage protocol, with consistency in design and analysis.

Massage does not easily lend itself to the randomized, controlled format. Because of this, CAM researchers are trying to create tools and research models that truly measure the bodywork experience. This is important with cancer patients as the outcomes may not always be numerical.

Until new ways are devised to measure massage, there is existing scientific evidence that shows some of the effect of massage. Most often studied are pain and anxiety, which consistently improve immediately following a skilled touch session. Fatigue has not yet been examined enough, but there is every reason from the present studies to be hopeful. The jury is still out out on nausea. And all of the other measures usually assumed to improve because of massage, such as medication use, immune function, and sleep, have had minimal study. Solid claims cannot yet be made.

Research Vocabulary

Control group: The group that did not receive the experimental treatment, used to compare to the treatment group.

Crossover design: Two groups are used. Each receives the experimental intervention and serves as the control, but in opposite order from the other. Halfway through, the groups switch.

Experimental group: The participants who received the intervention being tested.

Meta-analysis: A way to statistically analyze a group of studies that meet certain criteria.

Outcome: A variable to be measured, such as insomnia.

Randomized controlled trial: A method that randomly places participants into the control or the experimental group.

Retrospective study: A study that looks at previously-collected data. The data could have been collected expressly for research or to evaluate patient care.

Statistical significance: Analysis that proves the results are not due to chance or error.

Trend: Results that are leaning toward a positive outcome but haven't reached statistical significance.

Touch was never meant to be a luxury. It is a basic human need. It is an action that validates life and gives hope to both the receiver and the giver. The healing of touch is reciprocal.

— IRENE SMITH,
FOUNDER OF EVERFLOWING

INCLUSION CRITERIA

CAM researchers are grappling with how best to evaluate the effects of massage. The right tools, methods of design, and analysis still must be worked out. For now, practitioners must familiarize themselves with the studies that have been performed to this point. Despite the lack of standardization among the trials, the scientific research gives some understanding of the effects of skilled touch.

How to examine the 60 or so research projects is a sticky question. Should only those studies with a certain sample size be included? or those that were randomized? or those that utilize certain techniques? Often the people who analyze the research are very exclusive in what they examine or report. For example, an article in the *Annals of Internal Medicine* reviewed the CAM research for physicians for the purpose of teaching them how to advise their patients about the use of CAM therapies.[3] Only four of the many oncology massage studies available were cited, giving the doctors a very narrow view of the evidence.

Fellowes et al. performed a meta-analysis of the oncology massage research. Well over a thousand articles, case histories, in vitro studies, animal studies, and human research were found. This lengthy list was pared down to 65 and then ultimately to the ten studies that met their inclusion criteria of randomized, controlled trials that examined the use of two interventions, aromatherapy massage and massage with plain carrier oil, on patients with cancer.[4]

The analysis by Fellowes and his colleagues brought some clarity to the present state of oncology massage research, but it only gives the reader a narrow glimpse into a handful of studies that meet fairly strict criteria. Even though many of the other studies have a small sample size or lack a control group, there is value in examining them. Expanding the inclusion criteria also opens the research process beyond those pursuing graduate degrees, to grassroots practitioners, as well. This approach will give more touch therapists a connection with research.

In this text, trials are presented that show evidence of systematic inquiry. Only hands-on modalities such as Swedish Massage, reflexology, and Reiki are included. Mechanical techniques, such as wrist bands to stimulate acupressure points, or pneumatic cuffs, are not. The patient populations studied represent nearly all aspects of the cancer experience – hospitalization, outpatient status, hospice, and cancer day care. The research comes from diverse parts of the globe – Scotland, Ireland, England, Korea, Japan, Norway, Italy, and the United States.

ISOLATING THE VARIABLES

When researchers set out to explore the effect of an intervention on a patient, they narrow the question down as much as possible. They may ask a question such as: What is the effect of a 10-minute foot massage on fatigue in patients diagnosed with early stage breast cancer? This level of specificity is important.

The reader will notice in the above research question that there are four specific variables: 1) type of intervention – foot massage; 2) length of time – 10 minutes; 3) patient population – early stage breast cancer; and 4) health variable – fatigue. This is the norm within research, to focus sharply on specific aspects of a treatment. By approaching the question in this way, outside influences are minimized. It is not yet known if this is the best way to analyze complementary therapies such as massage. But, since it is the way in which most of the research has been performed up to this point, *Medicine Hands* will recount it in the same way, by isolated variables. We will begin with the two side effects that have received the most research: pain and anxiety.

PAIN

Pain is one of the most feared elements of the cancer experience, and something that affects patients' comfort and quality of life. Providing pain relief is essential in and of itself, but it also can strengthen a person's will to live, thereby improving their chance of survival. Severe pain not only affects the will to live or response to treatment; it may hinder the healing process, or prolong hospitalization. People with chronic pain may be unable to fully participate in life, may sleep poorly, and may find relationships affected.

At best, the management of pain is a complex and inexact science. Despite advances in medications, cancer pain or discomfort related to treatment cannot always be completely managed through analgesics. Cancer pain is inadequately treated for a variety of reasons. Partially this is due to limitations of the drugs, but it is also a consequence of misconceptions by physicians who underprescribe medication for fear of patients developing drug tolerance or addiction. Patients, too, fearing addiction, take less than the prescribed dosage. This fear, however, is unwarranted, as research indicates that cancer patients rarely develop psychological dependence on narcotics.[5] Another reason that contributes to the inadequate control of pain is that people fail to report their pain, believing it is best to be strong and "tough it out."

There is anecdotal evidence to support the idea that combining massage with standard pain medications may help to address the issue of inadequately-treated pain. Some people believe that massage may also allow those wishing to, to use less pain medication. It is not yet known if this is a realistic expectation. Readers will find later in the chapter that the data on the effects of medication use is negligible.

Massage eases pain no longer through deep tissue or myofascial or range of motion techniques, but through understanding and support, communicated through the presence and undivided attention of professional touch...; just placing gentle, attentive, caring hands on the patient is enough.

— PEGGY MAURO, FORMER MASSAGE PROGRAM COORDINATOR, BOULDER COMMUNITY HOSPITAL

*When you are lost in the black valley
of pain, words grow frail and dumb.
To be embraced and held warmly
brings the only shelter and
consolation.*

— JOHN O'DONOHUE, ANAM CARA

Although massage certainly can't replace analgesics, the evidence is fairly strong that it is an effective complement to pain medication. Fellowes et al. cite three studies in their meta-analysis in which pain is reduced. A broader look at the other research also found a variety of bodywork modalities to be effective against pain.

Twenty-five projects examined the effect of systematic touch on pain.[1,6-29] No statistical analysis was performed to compare these studies as was done in Fellowes' meta-analysis. In a meta-analysis, studies must have certain similarities to qualify for statistical analysis. When looked at as a whole, the pain studies are too diverse for comparison. For instance, there is no consistency among the populations studied. Some were groups of chemotherapy patients, others were at the end of life, and still others had finished treatment months previously. A variety of modalities were used, such as Swedish Massage, reflexology, Myofascial Release, Reiki, and Healing Touch. The research designs were numerous as well. Randomized, controlled designed were represented. Some scientists used a crossover design, others had no control group, while some had two arms and others had three. Seldom were the sources of pain differentiated. It was unknown if the pain was muscoloskeletal in origin, a side effect of the cancer, or the result of chemo or surgery.

Despite the many variations in design, sample size, populations, and source of pain, by informally scanning the results, some conclusions can be drawn. And the findings are not vastly different from those that were formally analyzed. The evidence is strong in terms of pain in all but a few studies.[10,27] A wide variety of touch techniques work to decrease pain immediately after the session.

Readers should note that most of the researchers gathered patients' feedback a short time after the massage session. Therefore, it can only be proved at this time that massage works in the short term. Long-term efficacy has not been tested in any significant way. Only a few examinations were made of the long-term side effects. In one, no difference was found between the massage group and the control group when pain was measured three hours and 24 hours after the massage.[29] Another study, this one using Reiki, measured pain seven days following the touch session. Again, no improvement was noted between the massage and control groups.[26] The question of the duration of effect on pain remains to be answered.

ANXIETY

The evidence supporting the use of massage to reduce anxiety is also clear and strong. It can be seen both on clients' faces and in the numbers. Two major meta-analyses of massage, one of massage research in general by Moyers, et al.[30] and one examining research of cancer patients[4], showed that the most consistent effect of massage is the reduction of anxiety. The additional studies included in *Medicine Hands* support this, as well.[9-17,20,21,23,24,27,31,32-35] This is significant despite the fact that there is no consistency in modalities used, length of session, type of cancer patients, or statistical analysis.

Waiting

A young woman, 18 years old, was waiting in the outpatient bone marrow transplant unit. It was her first time in the clinic after being discharged from the hospital. None of the staff had time to tell her what to expect. So there she sat in one of the big chemo chairs, not knowing if the doctor was going to see her or if treatment was going to be started. One of the massage therapists walked over and greeted her, offering a foot massage while the woman waited. Immediately the anxiety drained from her face.

— AUTHOR

Several studies attempted to pinpoint which modalities were most efficacious. Wilkinson[32] and Kite[24] compared aromatherapy massage with regular massage given with almond oil. The evidence wasn't strong enough to come down in favor of one over the other. Both were affective. Fellowes sums it up by stating that "... across these four trials, although greater reductions in anxiety were noted following massage than following no intervention, contradictory evidence exists as to any additional benefit on anxiety conferred by the addition of aromatherapy oils."

Post-White, in a comparison of massage to Healing Touch, found that massage decreased anxiety, Healing Touch did not.[20] Smith found that both massage and the control intervention, a friendly visit, decreased anxiety.[13] Hernandez-Reif[1] compared massage and Progressive Muscle Relaxation. Both were found to be effective.[17]

Clearly, massage has a contribution to make in controlling anxiety. Many questions, however, remain. Does lowered anxiety have a correlation with medication use, improved activities of daily living, or quality of life? How long after a massage do the effects linger? During which parts of the cancer experience is massage most effective – hospitalization? medical procedures? before, during, or after chemotherapy?

Nausea and Vomiting

Antiemetic medications have improved dramatically over the years, and yet nausea, especially delayed nausea, remains a significant problem for cancer patients undergoing treatment, especially chemotherapy. Acute emesis has been more successfully addressed, but the medications are often not effective against delayed nausea, nor are they effective for all patients or all chemos. Dibble et al. found that a third of breast cancer patients in their study were affected by delayed nausea, with days two through four being the worst.[37]

Controlling nausea and vomiting is important for a number of reasons – electrolyte imbalance, dehydration, kidney toxicity, and damage to the esophagus. Vomiting can result in poor nutrition which can lead to fatigue and the inability to rest. Without adequate calorie intake, fat and protein stores are burned, causing muscle wasting. Also, those with a good nutrition status tolerate treatment better.[38]

Controlling nausea during the first treatment of chemotherapy is beneficial because it will reduce anticipatory nausea.[39] This phenomenon is a conditioned response to sights, smells, and tastes that are associated with treatment. Psychological factors, such as anxiety, can also influence anticipatory nausea. If massage reduces anxiety, it is then logical to deduce that it may reduce anticipatory nausea.

Touch practitioners who work with cancer patients will be able to recount many stories of patients suffering from nausea whose experience was magically transformed by massage. However, the scientific research doesn't yet unequivocally support the anecdotal

Anxiety may worsen patients' perception of their physical symptoms or may lead to their overestimating the risks associated with treatment. Because of undertreated psychological symptoms, patients with cancer may not follow through with treatment recommendations or may report a higher severity of physical symptoms.[36]

— Lisa Corbin, MD

evidence. Eleven studies examined the effects of touch techniques on nausea.[8,18,20,21,34,40-45] The results were mixed – so mixed, that no positive trend can be reported.

Corner et al. found no improvement from the application of aromatherapy massage.[34] A minor improvement was noted by Cassileth and Vickers,[21] as was a decrease, albeit statistically insignificant, by Grealish et al. when using reflexology.[18] Dibble et al. (2000) taught patients to hold P6 and St36 for up to three minutes in the morning and as needed throughout the day during the chemo cycle. The acupressure group experienced less intense nausea the first ten days of chemo.[40] Lively's patients had less nausea.[41] However, the strength of this study is diminished by the fact that it was a retrospective study, lacking a randomized, controlled group. A 1984 study by Scott et al. also provided results of decreased frequency, volume, and duration of nausea.[44] One of the weaknesses of this study is its design and the small sample size. Ahles et al. studied bone marrow transplant patients and found that nausea was improved at the beginning of the treatment cycle.[8]

Fellowes and his colleagues[4] only included the studies by Grealish and Ahles in their meta-analysis. Both showed a reduction in nausea but, as was noted above, Grealish found only a statistically insignificant improvement. The sample group in Ahles' study was a highly specific group of patients. Therefore, the results should not be generalized to the general cancer population.

Since Fellowes' analysis in 2004, three new studies have emerged that show the inconclusive state of nausea research. Two of the studies have fair sample sizes, were randomized and controlled, and are well designed and analyzed. In a 2006 study, Dibble taught patients to apply acupressure bilaterally to each P6 point in the morning and when needed during the day. They had significantly less nausea compared to the standard care group and the placebo group that applied pressure to SI3.[43] Yang also found foot reflexology effective in controlling nausea and vomiting for breast cancer patients undergoing chemotherapy.[45] However, Post-White, who compared Healing Touch, massage, presence, and standard care, found that none of the interventions significantly reduced nausea.[20]

What is to be made from this hodge-podge of results? Certainly, nothing cohesive is apparent. Before scientific claims can be made, much more research is needed.

FATIGUE

Fatigue is a universal problem for people with cancer or those undergoing treatment. For many, it is the major troubling symptom and the primary cause of distress.[46] A few new therapies, such as Procrit and Aransep, drugs that increased red blood cell growth, have improved the outlook for some patients. And yet, despite the frequency and severity of this problem, insufficient research has been done on interventions that may improve patients' vigor.

The anecdotal evidence supports the use of massage to ameliorate cancer-related fatigue. For instance, one woman who was dying from liver cancer found that massage was the only thing that gave her the energy to spend time with her family. She was able to shop, take walks, and share meals with them. Another woman who had just finished four rounds of chemotherapy said, "I had so much energy, I went shopping after my massage!" Such stories are common.

And yet, there is a lack of massage research on this topic. The strongest study is by Post-White.[20] A sample of 164 patients receiving chemotherapy were divided into four groups – Swedish Massage, Healing Touch, presence, and standard care. Only the Healing Touch group had a decrease in fatigue. Cassileth and Vickers reported a 41% improvement in fatigue in 1,290 people whose data was examined retrospectively.[21] The studies from Sims,[47] Kite,[24] Ahles,[8] and Yang[45] also produced positive outcomes. Hernandez-Reif examined vigor and found significant improvement.[17]

A variety of modalities were used in the aforementioned studies – Swedish Massage, reflexology, Healing Touch, and aromatherapy massage. An interesting project by Kohara et al.[48] devised an intervention for 20 terminally-ill cancer patients that combined a three-minute foot soak in warm water with lavender oil followed by a ten-minute reflexology treatment with jojoba oil containing lavender. This single-dose treatment resulted in significant improvement in fatigue scores at one hour and four hours. However, the sample size is small and there was no control group for comparison.

These eight studies show a real possibility that massage improves energy levels. The only thing that holds the author back from pronouncing this, is that the number of total studies is too few and the strength of some of the projects is lacking. It is reasonable to expect, however, that touch techniques will be found to improve fatigue, at least in the short term. Further study is needed to examine the question of long-term effects and the effects on those receiving radiation as well as chemotherapy.

INSOMNIA

Improved sleep commonly appears on the massage benefits "top 10" list. Readers will be surprised to know, however, that only five studies have examined massage and the sleep of people with cancer.[9,11,13,23,24] On the surface, it would seem to be an easy thing to measure. But without certain devices which come at a considerable financial cost, it is not possible to directly measure sleep. And so, researchers are left to measure patients' perception of sleep. Often this is unreliable.

The five studies reported in this text did show improvement, except Cawthorne.[9] However, this collection of studies provides no definitive answer. They are too few in number and, with the exception of Kite's,[24] the studies completed to date represent only people who were hospitalized. Generalizing to the wider cancer

Science defines life in its own way, but life is larger than science. Holy things happen that can't be explained or measured – but only witnessed.

— RACHEL NAOMI REMEN, FROM *GRACE IN PRACTICE: CLINICAL APPLICATIONS FOR GRACEFUL PASSAGES*

Technical advances are important but we need to remember the difference between treating disease and treating a patient. Massage is an extension of the time-honored principle of laying on of the hands. Massage therapy can help reduce stress, fears, and pain – all of this without side effects. Whether the mechanism of action of massage is physiologic or psychologic matters not to me. The fact that it makes the patients feel better and allows them to better deal with their illness or treatment is good enough for me. I look forward to the day when this feature is available to all appropriate patients in our hospital.

— ROGER E. ALBERTY, MD,
DIRECTOR, DEPARTMENT OF SURGERY,
ST. VINCENT'S MEDICAL CENTER,
PORTLAND, OREGON

population is impossible at this point. This in no way diminishes the anecdotal evidence, which is plentiful. Cancer patients have said innumerable times, "That was the best sleep I've had since being in the hospital!" or, "I slept so well after my massage."

IMMUNE FUNCTION

There is a saying among researchers that, when paraphrased, says – Just because there is no evidence, doesn't mean it isn't true. This may be the case with the effect of massage on immune function. Oncology massage literature often proclaims that massage therapy fosters immunity. Massage therapists have drawn their own conclusions based on logic. If, as many studies show, psychological distress decreases immune function, then an intervention that decreases stress will improve immunity. Since massage decreases anxiety, it stands to reason that it must benefit the immune system. And while this claim ultimately may turn out to be true, not enough study has been performed to trumpet this as a benefit.

The Touch Research Institute has contributed most of the data on this subject. It has examined the effect of massage on natural killer cell activity and lymphocyte levels among various HIV patients[49,50] and breast cancer patients[1,17] and found improvement in both. The women in both breast cancer projects received a 30-minute massage three times a week for five weeks. The sessions included effleurage, petrissage, and stretching to the head, arms, back, legs, and feet. In the first study, the data of the massage group was compared to that of a control group that received only standard care. The group that received massage showed an increase in NK cells and lymphocytes. The second study piggybacked onto the first. The main change in design was the addition of a third arm to the study in which the use of Progressive Muscle Relaxation (PMR) was compared to massage and standard care. While PMR improved subjects' mood and decreased anxiety, depression, and pain, only the massage group had an improvement in natural killer cell and lymphocyte levels. (NK cells are components of the immune system that play an important role in monitoring and destroying virus-infected cells and new growths and in breaking down tumors as well.)

In their review of research, Hernandez-Reif et al. report a study of breast cancer patients showing that high NK-cell level predicted a lower cancer reoccurrence.[17] How then can practitioners, family, and friends not be hopeful that touch therapies contribute to immunity? Studies from the University of Iowa have been funded to examine this topic further on a group of women with breast cancer and another with cervical cancer. But it will take time before firm conclusions can be drawn. Immunity research can be more complex, costly, and labor intensive than other research, owing to the need for blood draws and saliva collection in order to assay certain biochemical measures.

LYMPHEDEMA

One of the side effects of cancer or its treatment can be lymphedema. In fact, cancer is the most common cause of lymphedema in the U.S. Breast cancer, melanomas, and lymphomas are most commonly associated with lymphedema. But anyone who has had lymph nodes removed and/or radiated in the neck, axilla, or groin, is at risk for lymphedema. Those who have both are at even greater risk. Greater clinical details about this condition are given in Chapter 5. For now, the attention will be on the effectiveness of lymph drainage techniques.

A variety of lymph drainage therapies exist. Dr. Vodder's Manual Lymphatic Drainage (MLD) is probably the best known in North America and Europe, followed by Bruno Chikkly's Lymph Drainage Therapy (LDT). In Australia, the Casley-Smith Method is commonly practiced. These techniques, which are regarded as routine treatment in European hospitals, are considered to be a specialized form of massage that uses a gentle, rhythmic, pumping movement as in MLD, or a "steady, gentle, wave-like motion" as with LDT. Bandaging, compressive garments, exercises, and skin care may also be used in conjunction with lymphatic massage.

Lymphatic drainage techniques have been shown to relieve edema, fibrosis, and the accompanying pain and discomfort. Fibrosis is the process of adhesion or scar tissue formation. These fibrotic adhesions can occur at the site of inflammation, such as radiation causes to the skin and tissue, or around surgical sites.

Research has examined both manual lymphatic drainage techniques and pneumatic compression machines. The use of the latter is questioned. Use of a pneumatic sleeve alone without using lymph drainage therapy may cause further complication, "as the fluid is simply squeezed up to the top of the arm where it can become fibrotic or pool in the upper chest."[51] Manual interventions allow the trunk to be cleared first so that it is ready to receive the excess lymph in the limb. They are advantageous not only in their ability to lower limb swelling but also in improving scar consistency, stimulating revascularization, promoting mobility, and increasing skin elasticity. And, not to be minimized is the human contact, the caring touch that hands-on treatment provides. The sense of being cared for after a traumatic and often disfiguring surgery is immensely healing.

Breast cancer patients are those most often affected by lymphedema. The high rate of incidence and survival make it vital to find effective prevention and management strategies in order that quality of life is maintained. In a review of the incidence of lymphedema, Erickson et al. report that approximately 25% of breast cancer patients develop lymphedema following treatment, and that the prevalence increases over time after radiation therapy. Those who were 15 or more years out from treatment had double the incidence of lymphedema compared with those who are 0–2 years out. Patients who had radiotherapy to the breast only or the the area around the

Additional Resources

- Burt J, White G. *Lymphedema: A Breast Cancer Patient's Guide to Prevention and Healing.* Hunter House Publishers, 1999.

- Földi M, Ströbenreuther R. *Foundations of Manual Lymph Drainage,* 3rd Ed. St. Louis, Missouri: Elsevier, 2005.

- Swirsky J, Nannery DS. *Coping with Lymphedema.* Avery Publishing, 1998.

- International Lymphedema Network – lymphnet.org.

- Lymphovenous Canada – lymphovenous-canada.ca/index.htm.

- breastcancer.org.

So many books have been written on becoming a healer and so many techniques of healing have been developed that people who love some-one with cancer may be concerned that they are not helping in just the "right" way. But we all strengthen the life around us in ways that are uniquely our own. Sometimes we draw on our own life experience and some-times on the deepest instincts of our hearts. And, in the end, it may be simply our commitment alone that has the power to reach across and spark the will to live. When someone's life matters deeply to us, the life in us may speak to the life in them directly and have a far greater healing effect than saying the right words or using the right imagery or the right ritual.

— RACHEL NAOMI REMEN,
MY GRANDFATHER'S BLESSINGS

sternum and clavicles have less incidence of lymphedema than do those radiated in the axilla.[52]

A handful of studies that include the examination of specialized lymphatic drainage techniques have been performed. On the whole, they appear to be effective. But so, too, do compression bandaging, exercises, and education. Anderson et al. found that for minor lymphedema, standard therapy – which consists of customized compression garments, special exercises, skin care, and education about safety precautions – was as effective as adding MLD.[53] McNeeley et al. found that compression bandaging and MLD and bandaging alone were both effective. However, the former was more so.[54] Morgan et al. reported that complex physical therapy (skin care, education, bandaging, exercises and lymphatic massage) decreased arm volume by 50% after a course of treatment.[55] And significant decrease also occurred in Williams' study as a result of MLD.[56]

It is difficult to juxtapose these studies for comparison. Lymphatic drainage therapies lean in a favorable direction and it seems likely that, down the road, they will be declared to be a positive intervention. For now, they qualify for what has become this chapter's mantra: More Research is Needed.

VITAL SIGNS

Vital signs consist of four variables that are used to monitor a person's health status – blood pressure (BP), heart rate (HR), respiration rate (RR), and temperature. Improvement in vital signs is often listed as a benefit of massage but in reality there is minimal research of oncology patients and the results are inconclusive.

The patients in the studies by Post-White,[20] Hadfield,[33] and Wilkie[16] showed a drop in heart rate. (However, Post-White's "presence" group also had decreased HR.) Respirations decreased in Hadfield and Wilkie's group. Interestingly, Post-White's "presence" group showed a slower breathing rate but the massage and Healing Touch groups did not. Aromatherapy massage,[33] massage,[16] and Healing Touch[20] all lowered blood pressure. On the other hand, Olson[26] consistently found no change in HR, BP, or RR as a result of a single Reiki session.

These few studies don't show enough of the puzzle to even hazard a guess at the picture. Touch therapies may turn out to impact vital signs, but then again, the presence of a loved one may be as effective. It must also be asked whether vital signs are an accurate trail marker to be followed. Do lowered BP, HR, and RR always indicate greater relaxation, decreased anxiety, and therefore improved healing? Quattrin et al.[32] questioned this, as well, saying that "'the vital' [sign] parameters did not appear to be a reliable indication because they were subjected to continuous variations on the basis of patients physical, clinical, and emotional conditions." Unless a positive correlation can be made between vital signs and healing, they do not appear to be a useful outcome measure.

MEDICATION USE

The few studies to date have mostly examined the effect of massage on the use of pain medications. While individuals may be able to occasionally decrease their use of analgesics, the group picture doesn't support this practice. Olson found Reiki ineffective,[26] as did Ahles in the use of massage, for bone marrow transplant patients.[8] Wilkie found that massage created a trend toward less analgesic use in her group of hospice patients, but statistically it was not a significant improvement.[16] Only Post-White was able to say conclusively that massage lowered NSAID use over a four-week period for people receiving chemotherapy. Interestingly, the Healing Touch arm of Post-White's study did not improve in NSAID use; only the massage group did.[20]

Lively et al. tracked TPN (total parenteral nutrition) usage in bone marrow transplant patients. TPN, while not a drug, is a costly substance given to those unable to take oral nutrition. If massage decreased the need for TPN, a considerable savings could be realized. Lively reported that their patients indeed did require less TPN, which contributed toward a significant savings.[41]

On the whole, the research performed to date does not hold out great hope that massage will decrease medication use. This is not to say that some individuals won't find this to be true. Many questions remain to be explored. What is clear at this point is that there is little scientific evidence that touch therapies decrease medication use, particularly pain medications.

QUALITY OF LIFE

At the end of the day, less pain, anxiety, and nausea, better sleep and more energy add to quality of life. That is what people with cancer seek. Researchers measure this variable usually with a multidimensional, written questionnaire and sometimes an oral interview. The Rotterdam Symptom Checklist is an example of a tool that has accepted validity for measuring quality of life. Within it are sections that cover psychological distress, physical status, functional status, and global quality of life. Common types of questions revolve around such parts of life as appearance, appetite, constipation, breathing, fear of the future, mood, decreased sexual interest, sleep, and much more.

Interestingly, most of the research that included quality of life as a specific outcome measure was performed with people in palliative or hospice care. This can probably be explained by the fact that in palliative care, maintaining quality of life is the guiding principle. The focus is not on curing the person but on managing physical symptoms and providing emotional support.

The majority of studies involve aromatherapy massage. Wilkinson's study of people in a palliative care center serving both in- and out-patients, is the strongest, owing to the large sample size (87)

If we go all-out for the cure, we could be disappointed, but if we go all-out for peace, there is always healing.

— PETREA KING,
MASSAGE THERAPIST, BUNDANOON,
NEW SOUTH WALES, AUSTRALIA

and the randomized, controlled design. In it, aromatherapy massage (AM) was compared to massage with plain oil. Participants received weekly massages for three weeks. The massage group improved in four of the Rotterdam subscales but not significantly. The AM subjects improved on all subscales except for "severely restricted activities." This led the researchers to conclude that "the addition of essential oil seems to enhance the effect of massage and to improve physical and psychological symptoms, as well as overall quality of life."[32]

Soden et al. also compared AM to massage with plain oil. She and her colleagues were interested in looking at long-term benefits for hospice patients rather than immediate ones. Patients were given weekly massage for four weeks. Their findings showed no significant long-term benefits of either AM or massage with plain oil. However, the researchers fairly pointed out that, "The inevitable tendency of patients with more advanced disease to deteriorate during a six-week period should not be forgotten."[23]

Wilkie and her colleagues explored the use of massage given twice weekly over a two-week period to hospice patients. Massage over this period of time reduced the decline in quality of life and in some instances even improved it.[16] However, no clear results could be pointed to.

Corner et al. studied the quality of life of cancer patients in a rehabilitation setting. Aromatherapy (AM) massage was compared to massage with plain oil and a third group who received only standard care. Massages were administered weekly for eight weeks. In post-massage interviews, 59% of those in the AM group reported improvement in physical symptoms, as did 41% of the massage with plain oil group. Even 33% of the standard care group noted improvements.[34] However, this is to be expected within this group of subjects who were working toward rehabilitation rather than palliation.

Wilcock et al. compared four weekly aromatherapy massages to day care in a palliative day care center. Quality of life improved in both groups. In fact, no statistically significant difference was found between the groups.[57]

Subjects in Kite's study of a series of aromatherapy massage sessions with people attending a cancer support and information center showed a 55% overall increase in quality of life.[24] Wright et al. examined reflexology also with patients attending a cancer support center. Clients perceived a positive impact on functional status, both physical and psychological.[58]

A group of women being treated with radiation received 30-minute Healing Touch (HT) sessions. The control group received mock HT. Both groups showed an increase in physical functioning, but the HT group had improved quality of life scores, specifically for pain, vitality, and physical functioning.[59]

A number of studies researched the effect of touch therapy on quality of life of those nearing the end of life or in palliative care.

Olson examined the use of Reiki with people near the end of life. Sessions were given on days 1 and 4. Improvement occurred in the psychological component. The social and physical variables were slightly benefitted but not significantly.[26] Milligan[55] and Hodgson[56] both examined the use of reflexology on hospice or palliative care clients. The majority of Milligan's patients felt improved quality of life. Less stress and tension was reported, along with an increased ability to cope with their problems. All of Hodgson's participants were improved, even those in the control group who received a placebo reflexology treatment. However, the reflexology group reported greater improvements than did the placebo group. Appetite, breathing, constipation, diarrhea, fears of the future, pain, nausea, sleep, communication, and fatigue were most improved.

Once again, the reader is left with apples and oranges. The studies occurred in a number of settings: outpatient day care, rehab, in-patient hospice, and a cancer support center. Methodologies and research questions differed. What seems fairly clear is that in the short term, the psychological component within the quality of life measure is constantly improved from touch therapies. Physical improvements were also noted in several studies.

The author took note of an interesting phenomenon within this group of studies. Seven of the research projects were done in the U.K., one in Ireland, one in Canada, and only one in the U.S. Does this say something about what is valued in Anglo cultures versus American? Or, perhaps it makes a statement about the level of acceptance of "end of life" in the two cultures. These are intriguing questions to ponder.

Patient Perception

In American hospitals, "patient satisfaction" is consistently evaluated. Some of the oncology massage research has looked at a variable that is related to patient satisfaction, and that is "patient perception" of the service. If health care providers are looking for evidence that people are pleased to receive massage service, there are five studies from which to gather information.[22,32,60,62,63] Those in Wilkinson's study perceived both experimental interventions, aromatherapy massage and massage with plain oil, to be beneficial. Patients felt that both treatments helped them to feel less anxiety, tension, pain, depression, and increased calm.[32] Kelly et al. designed a study that compared two interventions: one, ten minutes of Therapeutic Touch and 20 minutes dialogue; the other, ten minutes of quiet time and 20 minutes dialogue. Their subjects also perceived both interventions to be positive.[62] Milligan's audit of hospice patients found satisfaction with the foot reflexology service.[60] Both Smith's[63] and Post-White's[20] patients perceived more benefit from massage therapy than from the control intervention.

Additional Resources

- Hymel G. *Research Methods for Massage and Holistic Therapies.* St. Louis, MO: Mosby, 2006.

- Menard M. *Making Sense of Research: A Guide to Research Literacy for Complementary Practitioners.* Toronto, Canada: Curties-Overzet Publications, 2003.

- Massage Therapy Foundation: http://www.massagetherapyfoundation.org/researchdb.html. Easy-to-navigate website to conduct research searches.

- Pubmed: http://www.ncbi.nlm.nih.gov/entrez/query.fcgi?DB=pubmed. Another website that is easy to navigate.

- Touch Research Institute: http://www6.miami.edu/touch-research/research.htm.

- www.tracywalton.com: Walton maintains an up-to-date list of oncology massage articles, research reports, and books. (This is not an ordering service.)

This massage has made an unbearable day bearable.

— SUSAN, HOSPITAL PATIENT IN TREATMENT FOR COLON CANCER

OTHER BENEFITS

Many of the benefits of massage are assumed, such as improvement in depression and mood. Depression, common in cancer patients, has been studied mostly as one of many variables in the quality of life questionnaires. Only two studies have specifically isolated depression as an outcome measure: Soden[23] and Hernandez-Reif.[17] Soden compared aromatherapy massage with massage using plain oil. Only the massage group had a significant decrease in depression. Hernandez-Reif's participants, who received basic Swedish Massage, also had an immediate improvement in depression following their massage sessions.

Mood, too, is assumed to improve as a result of massage. Most readers have probably experienced this first-hand. Two studies, Sims[47] and Wilcox[57], indicate that touch therapies show a trend toward mood improvement. Post-White, one of the strongest of all the studies, showed a statistically significant increase in mood as a result of both massage and Healing Touch.[20]

Length of hospital stay has been a much-hoped-for benefit because it would mean a cost saving to insurers. If this could be proved, the thinking goes, then massage would, once again, become standard care in medical centers. There is not enough research yet to fuel hope for this outcome. Menard, in research for her doctoral dissertation, found that her postoperative participants were discharged half a day earlier than the control group. This finding was statistically insignificant.[31] The women who received massage during bone marrow transplantation went home three days sooner than those who did not receive massage, saving the hospital an estimated $1,440 per patient.[40] This study, though, had several methodological weaknesses. Cost savings is such an important influence on health care, that length of stay will hopefully become the subject of more research.

Massage is commonly advocated to promote many of the other side effects of cancer treatment, such as wound healing and scar tissue release, prevention of bedsores, increased range of motion, and improved bowel activity, to list just some. The Info Box on the opposite page lists many others. However, no scientific evidence exists to support these assertions, which is not to say that they aren't true. Many people have experienced improvement for each of these conditions. But therapists must be accurate in how they report the benefits of massage. When speaking about the benefits of massage, therapists could more accurately describe them as "possible" or "potential" benefits.

A Summary of the Potential Benefits of Bodywork for Cancer Patients

1. Moisturizes the skin and prevents problems such as bedsores.
2. Relieves muscle soreness due to prolonged bedrest.
3. Increases circulation. Lymphatic flow is stimulated, which helps in the elimination of waste products; vascular flow is also stimulated, bringing fresh nutrients to the area.
4. Increases range of motion.
5. Increases relaxation.
6. Decreases edema and lymphedema.
7. Sedates or stimulates nervous system, depending on the modality used.
8. Encourages deeper respiration.
9. Improves bowel activity.
10. Increases alertness and mental clarity.
11. Improves sleep.
12. Provides pain relief and reduces the need for pain medication.
13. Decreases symptoms related to chemo and radiation, such as fatigue, nausea, diarrhea, and loss of appetite.
14. Stimulates faster wound healing.
15. Provides faster recovery from anesthesia.
16. Shortens hospital stays.
17. Increases elasticity to scarred areas.
18. Breaks up adhesions associated with scarring.
19. Increases the effectiveness of other treatments, such as pain medication, physical therapy, or a medical procedure.
20. Increases patient's awareness of stress signals.
21. Decreases anxiety and depression.
22. Provides distraction.
23. Provides relief from isolation.
24. Offers meaningful social interaction.
25. Provides a doorway to greater intimacy with family and friends.
26. Provides relief of touch deprivation.
27. Provides a forum for patients to express their feelings.
28. Re-establishes a positive body image.
29. Gives patient a sense of participation in the healing process.
30. Re-builds hope.

Resources

1. Barnett, L. and M. Chambers. *Reiki Energy Medicine*. Rochester, VT: Healing Arts Press, 1996.
2. Gibson, K. *Developing a Hospital-Based Massage Therapy Program*. Self-published. 1994.
3. Nelson, D. *Compassionate Touch*. Barrytown, NY: Station Hill Press, 1994.
4. Ray, B. *The 'Reiki' Factor in The Radiance Technique*. St. Petersburg, FL: Radiance Associates, 1992.
5. Wager, S. *A Doctor's Guide to Therapeutic Touch*. New York: Perigee Books, 1996.

COMPARISON OF MODALITIES

Swedish Massage is the most common modality used in massage studies. Reflexology and aromatherapy massage are the next most often used. Interventions categorized as energy techniques, such as Reiki, Therapeutic Touch, and Healing Touch, have received minimal examination.

Little is known of how the varying disciplines compare in effectiveness. Only a handful of studies have asked the question. Several trials randomized patients to either aromatherapy massage (AM) or massage with a plain carrier oil.[23,32,34] The results are extremely inconclusive except to say that both proved to be beneficial, especially for anxiety. Two different researchers found AM to produce a greater decrease in anxiety than just massage. However, it must be emphasized that the outcomes were very mixed for these two interventions.

Post-White compared massage, Healing Touch (HT), presence, and standard care. Each of the first three interventions was superior to standard care. Both massage and HT improved patients' vital signs, mood, and pain. But massage achieved greater results than Healing Touch in terms of anxiety and use of NSAIDs. Healing Touch, however, decreased fatigue more than did massage.[20]

Cassileth and Vickers examined three different bodywork interventions – full-body massage, light touch, and foot massage. Analysis showed that massage and light touch were slightly better at relieving symptoms than was foot massage. Patients receiving massage or light touch showed an average of 58% improvement in symptoms. Those receiving foot massage had a 50% improvement.[21]

Hodgson looked at the effect of reflexology versus foot massage and reported that all patients experienced increased comfort. However, only 33% of the foot massage group had an increase in quality of life while 100% of the reflexology group improved in this variable.[61]

Several trials compared the use of massage to a non-massage modality. Hernandez-Reif compared Progressive Muscle Relaxation and massage. Massage was found to be more efficacious.[17] Taylor et al. found massage to be of greater benefit than vibrational therapy for a group of women who underwent a laparotomy for removal of possible cancerous lesions.[22]

Nothing conclusive can be claimed about the benefits of one modality over another. The task of examining this has only just begun. Perhaps, at the end of the day, it will be impossible to determine whether one technique is better than another. Too many extenuating factors influence the efficacy of touch therapy – the relationship between client and therapist, the environment that massage occurs in, and the client's expectations, to name just some.[23]

Qualitative Research

Most of the research to date can be categorized as quantitative. Scientists pick an outcome to measure and then count how much or little there is of it. Another type of design, a qualitative one, may hold promise for studying CAM therapies. Qualitative designs rely on the client's subjective experience and on observational data, rather than numbers. They get to the heart of the matter, so to speak.

A handful of qualitative studies have looked at the effect of massage on people with cancer. The information they provide is vastly different than that the quantitative research provides. Billhult and Dahlberg examined the effect of massage received for ten consecutive days on eight women with cancer. They identified a number of themes: 1) The experience of being special; 2) A feeling of greater strength; 3) The creation of a positive relationship with staff members; and 4) Meaningful relief from suffering.[64]

Bredin systematically examined the use of massage on body image issues for three breast cancer patients who had undergone a mastectomy. The six weekly massages revealed experiences that would be no surprise to a massage therapist who works regularly with cancer patients. In addition to improved relaxation and sleep, clients reported emotional healings, such as being able to more easily touch or look at their scar, help in resuming sexual relations, and ability to better cope with their changed self-image.[65]

Dunwoody and her colleagues delivered six aromatherapy massage sessions to 11 people with cancer. A semi-structured group interview was used to uncover themes resulting from the massage sessions. Eight themes emerged, some of which were a feeling of being able to talk freely during the sessions, feeling empowered and involved, and the communication of being cared for through touch.[67]

Massage therapy can play a significant role in reunifying the whole person with themselves and with the human community.[66]

ANNETTE CHAMNESS, CMT

Research Tables

For ease of reference, each study has been distilled down to its bare bones and listed in the following tables. In the preceeding text, the research was organized by quantitative outcomes – fatigue, pain, and nausea, for instance. The Research Tables are organized by modalities – Swedish Massage, acupressure, and reflexology, for example. This will give the reader another perspective from which to examine the research.

The following abbreviations are used in the tables: $\overline{A}$: before; AM: aromatherapy massage; BP: blood pressure; BR: breast; $\overline{c}$: with; CA: cancer; CNS: central nervous system; DBP: diastolic BP; Dx: diagnosis; exper: experimental group; hosp: hospitalized; HR: heart rate; HT: Healing Touch; LE: lymphedema; M: massage; MTh: massage therapist; MLD: manual lymphatic drainage; $\overline{P}$: after; pt: patient; PMR: progressive muscle relaxation; QoL: quality of life; RN: registered nurse; RR: respiration rate; SBP: systolic BP; TPN: total parenteral nutrition; Tx: treatment.

TABLE 3.1 SWEDISH MASSAGE STUDIES

Author/Year	Sample	Intervention	Outcome measures	Results
Sims (1986)	• 6 women receiving RT for BR CA • Crossover design (pts served as own control)	• 10 min slow, stroke back M 3 days consecutive • Control period— 10 min rest	• Symptom distress • Mood • Fatigue	• No signif diff • Trend toward ↓ symptom distress and fatigue, ↑ mood, calmness, vitality from M
Weinrich & Weinrich (1990)	• 28 hosp CA pts • 18 men, 10 women • Randomized to 2 groups	• Group 1 — 10 min FV • Group 2 — 10 min— back M	• Pain	• Males had ↓ in pain • Women no change
Ferrell-Torry & Glick (1993)	• 9 hosp male CA pts experiencing pain • Hospitalized • No control group	• 30 min Swed M to back, neck, feet	• Pain • Anxiety • (HR, RR, BP)	• ↓ pain and anxiety • HR & BP trend toward ↓ • RR ↓ signif
Tope, Hann, Pinkson (1994)	• 104 hosp CA pts • No control group	• Sessions limited to 30 min Common sites: back, shoulders, neck, feet: Swed M & accupresssure • Pts received 2 or more M • Admin by LPN/CMT	• Mood • Tension • Comfort • Sense of isolation	• 99% mentioned relaxation or release of muscle tension • 35% improved mood • 22% assistance in symptom management • 15% felt less isolation
Menard (1995)	• 30 women • Randomized to 2 groups • Posthysterectomy, suspected CA	• Group 1 — standard care • Group 2 — 45 min M beginning 1st day postop continuing until discharge – Swedish M and some acupressure – admin by MTh	• Cortisol level • Systolic BP • Pain • Anxiety • Depression • Use of pain meds • Bowel function • Length of stay	• Group 2 — trend toward improvement in all variables • During 4-wk follow-up, Group 2 had signif ↓ visits to the Dr.
Ahles, Tope, Pinkson, et al. (1999)	• 35 bone marrow transplant pts • Randomized to 2 groups • Control (n=18) • Exper. (n=16)	• Group 1 — standard care • Group 2 — 20 min M of shoulders, head & face c̄ Swed M & acupressure • Up to 9 Ms • Admin by LPN/CMT	• Anxiety • Depression • Fatigue • Nausea • Vital signs (HR, RR, BP) • Use of meds (pain, anxiety, antiemetic)	• M group greater ↓ in distress, fatigue, nausea & anxiety early on • Less anxiety at mid-Tx • Less fatigue at predischarge • Lower DBP • No diff in med use or overall psych symptoms
Bredin (1999)	• 3 BR CA pts who had undergone a mastectomy • Pts distressed about breast loss	• Phase I — in-depth interview • Phase II — 6 M sessions – gentle effleurage – choice of feet, arms, face, or back – admin by author	• Body image issues	• Subjective experiences of the M: – + perception of M – Helped c̄ relaxation – Helped arm on Txed side feel part of the body – Better sleep – Able to look or touch scar more easily – Opened up emotions – Helped to resume sexual relations – Able to cope better c̄ changed self-image

TABLE 3.1 SWEDISH MASSAGE STUDIES *continued*

Author/Year	Sample	Intervention	Outcome measures	Results
Grealish, Lomasney, Whiteman (2000)	• 87 hosp pts • 52 women, 35 men • Served as own control • Primary CA sites varied	• Group 1 — bed rest doing quiet activity • Group 2 — 10 min foot M 3 consec evenings • Admin by RN	• Pain • Nausea • Relaxation • HR	• Group 2 — ↓ pain • Nausea ↓ trend • Relaxation ↑ signif • HR ↓ Groups 1 and 2
Hemphill, Kemp (2000)	• 41 male CA pts undergoing chemo	• Group 1 — 20-min verbal interaction c̄ nurse • Group 2 — 20-min M 3x during a 1 wk period • Admin by nurse MTh	• Pain • Sleep • Symptom distress • Anxiety	• Group 1 — signif improvement in sleep symptom distress, & pain • Anxiety improved in both groups
Wilkie, Kampbell, Cutshall, et al. (2000)	• 29 hospice pts c̄ CA • 20 men, 9 women • Randomly assigned to 2 groups	• Group 1 — standard care • Group 2 — standardarized Swed M, compressions, nerve stroke – Given by LMTs – 30-50 min session – 4 sessions w/in 2 wks	• Pain • QoL • HR • RR • Distress • Morphine use • Longevity	• ↓ pain, HR, RR immed P̄ M • Group 2 ↓ distress and morphine use, but not signif • No signif diff in QoL • Group 1 lived signif longer
Bilhult, Dahlberg (2001)	• 8 female CA pts received M for 10 consecutive days • 75% had BR CA	• Light stroking for 20 min of either hand/forearm or foot/lower leg • Admin to some by healthcare workers with 1-day training; others received from one of the authors	• Qualitative experience of the essential meaning of M in CA care	• M provided: –Meaningful relief from suffering –Positive relations c̄ staff –Experience of being special –Feeling of greater strength –Balance between autonomy & dependence
Cawthorne, Boyle (2001)	• 49 hospice CA pts • Variety of pulmonary tumors • No control group	• M on 2 consecutive evenings • Admin by nurse MTh	• Pain • Anxiety • Nausea • Sleep	• ↓ in pain, anxiety & nausea
Lively, Black, Holiday-Goodman, et al. (2002)	• 31 women c̄ BR & ovarian CA undergoing high-dose chemo & peripheral blood stem cell transplant	• Group 1 — standard Tx • Group 2 — 20-30 min sessions: M to head with focus on SCM & cranial sacral techniques, stillpoint, frontal lift, spheno-basilar compression-decompression, temporal ear-pull; Swed M to leg & thigh • Admin by LMT	• Nausea/vomiting • Length of stay • Cost-effectiveness	• Group 2 — ↓ nausea & TPN use • Length of stay 3 fewer days • Total cost savings per pt $2,850
Smith, Kemp, Hemphill, et al. (2002)	• 41 pts • Randomized to 2 groups • 95% males	• Group 1 — nurse visit • Group 2 — 15-30 min light Swed M • Admin by nurse certified in hosp-based M	• Pain • Sleep • Symptom distress • Anxiety	• Group 2 — ↓ pain and symptom distress, ↓ sleep • Anxiety ↓ in Group 1 • Sleep ↓ in Group 1

TABLE 3.1 SWEDISH MASSAGE STUDIES *continued*

Author/Year	Sample	Intervention	Outcome measures	Results
Lawvere (2002)	• 7 ovarian CA pts hospitalized for chemo • Randomized crossover trial (pts served as own control)	• Group 1 — 30 min rest • Group 2 — Swed M & connective tissue M • Admin by MTh	• Anxiety • Depression • Pain	• Group 2 — anxiety ↓ • Pain & depression drop insignif
Taylor, Galper, Taylor, et al. (2003)	• 105 women • Randomized to 3 groups • Underwent abdominal laparotomy for removal of suspected cancerous lesion, usually ovarian masses	• Group 1— standard care • Group 2—45 min Swed M $\overline{P}$ surgery and at the same time on the following 2 days • Group 3—20 min standardized physiotones therapy and at the same time on the following 2 days	• Pain • Distress	• Group 2 trend toward ↓ in pain and distress on day of surgery • Postop day 2, M trend toward more effective than standard care for distress and better than vibration for pain • Vibration leaned toward ↑ effectiveness over standard care
Toth, Kahn, Walton, et al. (2003)	• 6 hosp pts $\overline{c}$ metastatic or end stage lung or GI CA • Not randomized, convenience sample	• Individualized M 10-60 min (avg 34 min) • Pt offered M every day Pt received 1-9 Ms (avg 3.3)	• Pain • Anxiety • Alertness level	• ↓ in pain • ↑ in anxiety • ↑ in alertness level
Hernandez-Reif, Ironson, Field, et al. (2004)	• 34 women $\overline{c}$ stage I-II BR CA • Randomized to 2 groups	• Group 1—standard care • Group 2—45 min. Swed M/ROM 3x/wk over 5 wks	• Immune function (NK cells, lymphocytes) • Mood measures (dopamine, serotonin) • Anxiety • Depression • Hostility	• M group ↓ anxiety, depression, anger immed $\overline{P}$ M • Long term — M ↓ depression, hostility; ↑ dopamine, serotonin, NK cell, lymphocytes

TABLE 3.2 AROMATHERAPY MASSAGE STUDIES

Author/Year	Sample	Intervention	Outcome measures	Results
Corner, Cawley, Hildebrand (1995)	• 52 pts. $\overline{c}$ a variety of cancers • Randomized to 3 groups • 47 women, 5 men • Some in Tx, others in remission, some in adv stage of illness	• Group 1 — control • Group 2 — 30 min weekly back M for 8 wks using almond oil • Group 3 — 30 min weekly back M for 8 wks using blend of essential oils	• Anxiety • QoL • Depression • Symptom distress	• No diff between M groups • 59% of Group 3, 41% of Group 2, 33% of Group 1 improved in physical symptoms • No change in depression in any groups • Group 3 ↓ in anxiety
Kite, Maher, Anderson, et al. (1998)	• 58 pts at an outpt CA resource center • No control group • Majority were women $\overline{c}$ BR CA receiving RT	• Pt received 6 aromatherapy M sessions roughly 1 wk apart • Sessions tailored to pt	• Anxiety • Depression • Distress • Pain • Insomnia • Fatigue • QoL	• Improvement in all measures

TABLE 3.2 AROMATHERAPY MASSAGE STUDIES *continued*

Author/Year	Sample	Intervention	Outcome measures	Results
Wilkinson, Aldridge, Salmon, et al. (1999)	• 103 pts $\bar{c}$ variety of adv CAs • Randomized to 2 groups • Attending palliative care center as in- or out-pts	• Each group received full body M for 3 consecutive wks • Group 1 — almond oil and 1% Roman chamomile • Group 2 — almond oil	• Anxiety • QoL	• Both groups ↓ anxiety $\bar{P}$ each session • Group 1 improved QoL scores
Hadfield (2001)	• 8 pts. in radiation therapy Tx for brain CA • 7 men, 1 woman • No control group	• Choice of 30 min neck/shoulder, feet or hand M • Choice of lavender or Roman chamomile oil • Session given $\bar{A}$ radiation clinic appt	• Anxiety • Relaxation • Vital signs — HR, RR, BP	• ↓ in all vital signs • No diff in anxiety scores pre- to post-M • In telephone interviews, all pts reported feeling relaxed or less tense

Dunwoody, Smyth, Davidson. (2002)	• 11 CA pts
	• 10 women, 1 man
	• No control group
	• Each pt completed 6 one-hr M sessions
		• Individualized aromatherapy M
		• Oils chosen by pt and practitioner
		• Delivered by RN/aromatherapy MTh
			• A semi-structured group interview was given to uncover themes regarding M sessions	• 8 themes emerged —
				  – ↓ stress
				  – Able to talk freely
				  – AM as a reward
				  – Pts felt empowered and involved
				  – Communication of caring through touch
				  – Feeling of safety to receive sessions in the hosp environment
				  – Reluctant to tell others they were receiving aromatherapy M
				  – Desire to have more than the 6 sessions and to have them more frequently. Effects felt to be accumulative.

Wilcock, Manderson, Weller, et al. (2004)	• 29 day care pts • Randomized to 2 groups • Variety of CAs • Large number of withdrawals, 12 from control, 5 from M group	• Group 1 — standard care • Group 2 — 30 min M to back, neck, shoulders, or hands by qualified aromatherapist using 1% blend of lavender and chamomile in sweet almond oil	• Mood • QoL • Physical symptoms	• No signif diff between groups • All M pts were satisfied $\bar{c}$ the service and wished to continue
Kohara, Miyauchi, Suehiro, et al. (2004)	• 20 terminally ill CA pts • Variety of CAs • No control group	• 3 min footsoak in warm water $\bar{c}$ lavender oil followed by 10 min reflexology Tx $\bar{c}$ jojoba oil containing lavender • Single Tx given by certified aromatherapist	• CA-related fatigue	• Signif ↑ in fatigue • Physical and cognitive subscales signif improved • Improvement shown at 1 and 4 hrs $\bar{P}$ Tx • Affective subscale no signif change

TABLE 3.2 AROMATHERAPY MASSAGE STUDIES *continued*

Author/Year	Sample	Intervention	Outcome measures	Results
Soden, Vincent, Craske (2004)	• 42 hospice pts c̄ adv CA • Randomized to 3 groups • Variety of CAs • Varying levels of pain, sleep difficulties, anxiety, and other symptoms	• Group 1 — standard care • Group 2 — aromatherapy M c̄ carrier oil and 1% dilution of lavender • Group 3 — M c̄ carrier oil • Groups 2 and 3 received 4 weekly, 30 min back M	• Pain • Anxiety • Depression • QoL • Sleep	• No signif benefits in either M group for pain, anxiety, and QoL • Sleep improved in both M groups • Depression ↓ in Group 3 • Addition of lavender did not ↑ the benefit of M

TABLE 3.3 REFLEXOLOGY STUDIES

Author/Year	Sample	Intervention	Outcome measures	Results
Wright, Courtney, Donnelly, et al. (2002)	• Random selection and exam of 47 charts of clients receiving reflexology • Majority receiving or had received chemo, RT, or both • 91% women, 9% men • 60% of clients received 6 or more reflexology Txs • 60% BR CA pts	• Weekly reflexology Txs	• QoL • Identification of common themes related to perceived benefits	• Improvement in 3 QoL indicators: – functional status – impairment – perception of improved health • 34% had sense of relaxation • 30% had enhanced sense of health • 30% had ↑ sleep • 28% had ↑ energy levels • 23% had pain relief • 13% showed no benefits
Milligan, Fanning, Hunter, et al. (2002)	• 20 CA pts attending a support group • 7 men, 13 women • undergoing 6 wk course of Tx	• Individualized foot reflexology session	• QoL • Satisfaction c̄ the service	• ↑ QoL • Satisfaction c̄ service
Stephenson, Dalton, Carlson (2003)	• 36 hosp pts c̄ metastatic CA • Randomized to 2 groups	• Group 1 — standard care • Group 2 — foot reflexology. 2x, 24 hrs apart • Given by certified foot reflexologist	• Pain • Pts beliefs about the use of reflexology to control CA-related pain	• Group 2 — immed P̄ session, ↓ pain • At 3 hrs and 24 hrs, no signif diff between groups • No signif change in beliefs about use of reflexology
Yang (2005)	• 34 BR CA pts undergoing chemo • Randomized to 2 groups	• 40 min foot reflexology each round of chemo • Admin by researcher and 4 assistants	• Nausea • Vomiting • Fatigue	• Improvement in all 3 measures
Quattrin, Zanini, Buchini, et al. (2006)	• 30 hosp pts on Round 2 or 3 of chemo • 11 men, 19 women • 2 groups, not randomized	• 30 min foot reflexology • Admin by trained nursing student	• Anxiety	• ↓ anxiety immed P̄ M

TABLE 3.4 ACUPRESSURE STUDIES

Author/Year	Sample	Intervention	Outcome measures	Results
Dibble, Chapman, Mac, et al. (2000)	• 17 women • Randomized to 2 groups • Undergoing chemo for BR CA	• Group 1 — standard care • Group 2 — pts receive acupressure training — P6 & ST 36. The points were held each morning for up to 3 min & during the day as needed during the chemo cycle (usually 21-28 days)	• Nausea experience • Nausea intensity	• Acupressure group ↓ intensity and experience of nausea the first 10 days of the chemo cycle
Shin, Kim, Shin, et al. (2004)	• Randomized to 2 groups • Postop gastric CA • Receiving 1st cycle of chemo • Each group received antiemetic drugs	• Group 1 — standard care • Group 2 — trained to perform finger acupressure on self for 5 min on P6 3x/day	• Chemo-induced nausea	• Group 2 ↓ in severity of nausea, vomiting; duration of nausea and frequency of vomiting
Dibble, Luce, Cooper, et al. (2006)	• 160 women c̄ BR CA • Randomized to 3 groups • Beginning 2nd or 3rd cyle of chemo • Each group received antiemetic drugs as needed	• Group 1 — standard care • Group 2 — trained to perform finger acupressure each morning for no more than 3 min to P6 bilaterally, and at other times during the day whenever nausea happened • Group 3 — same protocol as Group 2 applied to SI3 (placebo)	• Delayed chemo-induced nausea & vomiting	• Group 2 signif ↓ in amount of vomiting; intensity of nausea • No signif diff between Groups 1 & 3

TABLE 3.5 MYOFASCIAL RELEASE STUDIES

Author/Year	Sample	Intervention	Outcome measures	Results
Crawford, Simpson, Crawford. (1996)	• 12 women Txed for BR CA • Chest wall tenderness due to RT • Unresponsive to anti-inflammatory meds	• Myofascial Release (MFR) 3x/wk for 3-4 wks • Performed by OT trained in MFR	• Pain (chest wall)	• All pts had some ↓ in pain • 67% reported near complete or complete pain relief

TABLE 3.6 STUDIES USING ENERGY TECHNIQUES

Author/Year	Sample	Intervention	Outcome measures	Results
Olson, Hanson. (1997)	• 20 CA volunteers c̄ moderate pain • 18 women, 2 men • Not receiving chemo or RT	• A single Reiki session by a 2nd degree practitioner	• Pain	• 85% had ↓ in pain
Samarel, Fawcett, Davis, et al. (1998)	• 31 women c̄ positive BR CA biopsy scheduled for surgery • Group 1—10 min quiet time and 20 min dialogue • Group 2—10 min Therapeutic Touch and 20 min dialogue	• Touch sessions admin. in pts home w/in 7 days Ā surgery and 24 hrs P̄ hosp discharge. On average, preop sessions given 1.6 days prior and postop sessions given 3.3 days P̄ surgery.	• Anxiety • Mood • Pain	• Group 2 ↓ preop anxiety • No diff on postop measures

TABLE 3.6 STUDIES USING ENERGY TECHNIQUES *continued*

Author/Year	Sample	Intervention	Outcome measures	Results
Olson, Hanson, Michaud. (2003)	• 24 adults c̄ moderate or greater pain • Randomized to 2 groups • 15 women, 9 men • Have not received chemo or RT in past month • In palliative care due to advanced CA • Many close to end of life	• Group 1—standard opoid management and 1.5 hr rest period • Group 2—standard opoid management plus Reiki delivered by Reiki master	• Pain • Vital signs — BP, HR, RR • QoL • Analgesic use	• Group 2—immed. decrease in pain P̄ Reiki • Group 1— improvement in QoL (pyschological component) • No decrease in use of analgesics • No diff. in pain between groups P̄ 7 days
Cook, Guerrerio, Slater (2004)	• 62 women randomized to 2 groups • Newly Dxed BR or gyn CA • Completed no more than 1/3 of radiation Txs	• Group 1—30 min HT. First HT Tx given at about 1/3 point through RT. From then on, HT weekly for 4 wks immed P̄ RT. Last session 4 weeks after RT completed. • Group 2—Mock HT using the same time sequence as Group 1.	QoL	• Group 1 increased QofL, specifically pain, vitality, physical functioning • Group 2 increase in physical role functioning
Kelly, Sullivan, Fawcett, et al. (2004)	• 18 women c̄ early stage BR CA	• Group 1—10 min. TT and 20 min. dialogue • Group 2—10 min. quiet time and 20 min. dialogue • Admin. by a nurse pre- and post-operatively	Perception of interventions	• Pts perceived both interventions as positive

TABLE 3.7 LYMPHEDEMA STUDIES

Author/Year	Sample	Intervention	Outcome measures	Results
Morgan, Mason, et al. (1992)	• 78 women c̄ post-mastectomy LE • Grade 1 LE (n=17), grade 2 LE (n=61) • Lumpectomy (n=20), mastectomy (n=24), radical mastectomy (n=34) • 70 had RT	• Complex physical therapy (skin care, lymphatic M, special exercises, compression bandaging and garments) –Pts received 2 courses of Tx c̄ 1 yr in between –30-45 min lymphatic M 5 days/wk for 4 wks	• Arm volume	• 50% ↓ in arm volume P̄ 1st course • At end of year, 18 pts repeated identical course of Tx, others felt satisfied c̄ their improvement • 50% of remaining LE removed P̄ 2nd course
Andersen, Højris, Erlandsen, et al. (2000)	• 42 women randomly assigned to 2 groups • Txed for early stage BR CA • Unilateral, minor LE of the arm at least 4 months P̄ surgery	• Group 1 (n=22) — Standard therapy (customized compression sleeve, education about LE, exercises, skin care, safety precautions) • Group 2 (n=20) — Same as Group1 plus MLD 8x in 2 wks and education in daily self-M • Admin by Vodder-certified lymphotherapist	• Edema volume P̄ MLD Tx • Edema volume 12 months P̄ MLD Tx	• Both groups signif ↓ in edema • MLD not signif better than standard therapy alone • For minor LE, standard therapy as effective

TABLE 3.7 LYMPHEDEMA STUDIES *continued*

Author/Year	Sample	Intervention	Outcome measures	Results
Williams, Vadgama, Franks, et al. (2002)	• 31 women c̄ unilateral BR CA-related LE • Had LE more than 3 months • Randomized, controlled crossover design, 2 groups • More than 1 yr post-Tx	• Group 1 — 3 wks daily MLD, then 6 wks non-Tx period, followed by 3 wks daily SLD (Simple Lymphatic Drainage — a modified version of MLD) • Group 2—3 wks daily SLD, 6 wks non-Tx period, followed by 3 wks daily MLD • MLD performed by certified Vodder practitioners 45 min daily • SLD performed by patients as a self-care routine 20 min daily	• Arm volume • Dermal thickness • QoL • Symptoms and sensations	• MLD signif ↓ arm volume • SLD non-signif ↓ arm volume • MLD signif ↓ dermal thickness at deltoid only • MLD ↑ emotional functioning, dyspnea, and sleep disturbance • MLD ↑ in pain, discomfort, heaviness, fullness and other sensations
McNeely, Magee, Lees, et al. (2004)	• 45 women c̄ LE • Randomized to 2 groups • LE due to BR CA Tx	• Group 1 — 45 min daily for 4 wks MLD, Mon-Fri c̄ compression bandaging (CB) • Group 2 — CB only	• Arm volume	• Both interventions ↓ LE • MLD/CB showed greater ↓ than CB alone • CB most effective when administered daily for 2 wks

TABLE 3.8   STUDIES THAT COMPARE TECHNIQUES

Author/Year	Sample	Intervention	Outcome measures	Results
Scott, Donahue, Mastrovito, et al. (1983)	• 10 women undergoing highly emetic chemotherapy for ovarian carcinoma • No control (data compared to known clinical responses)	• Pts were coached in progressive relaxation and guided imagery techniques • M consisted of slow-stroke back M for 3 min	• Nausea • Vomiting	• Shorter duration of emetic response • ↓ frequency of vomiting • ↓ intensity • ↓ volume of emesis
Dalton, Toomey, Workman (1988)	• 16 subjects divided into 3 groups	• Pts were instructed to use the following interventions as needed: • Group 1 — standard care • Group 2 — progressive muscle relaxation (PMR) • Group 3 — PMR plus use of distraction (i.e., music) & M were demonstrated	• Pain	• Group 1 had highest pain levels • Groups 2 & 3 had ↓ in pain • No difference in relief between Groups 2 & 3
Smith, Reeder, Daniel, et al. (2003)	• 88 bone marrow transplant pts • 22 men, 60 women • Randomized to 3 groups	• All sessions 30 min • Group 1 — friendly visit (FV) by volunteer • Group 2 — Therapeutic Touch (TT) by RN • Group 3 — Swed M by RN	• Time of Engraftment • Complications (pain, food intake, CNS/neurological, heart, lung, liver, GI, GU, skin, circulation) • Pt perception of benefits	• No diff in engraftment rate • M group ↓ on CNS/neurological complications only • Pt perception of benefits higher for MT v. FV M & TT higher on • comfort rating v. FV

TABLE 3.8 STUDIES THAT COMPARE TECHNIQUES *continued*

Author/Year	Sample	Intervention	Outcome measures	Results
Post-White, Kinney, Savik, et al. (2003)	• 164 CA pts receiving chemo • Randomized to 3 groups • Had pain, nausea, or fatigue rated at 3 or more on a scale of 10 • Variety of CAs — 50% had BR CA	• Crossover design in which pts were their own control • Interventions were standardized, 45 min, provided by RNs certified as MThs or Healing Touch practitioners – Group 1—Swed M – Group 2—Healing Touch – Group 3—Presence	• Outcome measures • Vital signs — BP, RR, HR • Anxiety • Fatigue • Mood disturbance • Pain • Nausea • Medication use • Satisfaction c̄ care	• Groups 1 & 2 ↓ in vitals, mood, pain • Group 1 ↓ in anxiety & 4 wk NSAID use • Group 1 trend ↓ fatigue • Group 2 ↓ in fatigue • No effects on nausea • Group 3 ↓ RR & HR • Overall satisfaction c̄ care not affected. But pts rated more satisfaction c̄ touch interventions than control
Cassileth, Vickers (2004)	• 1,290 in- and out-patients for 3,609 sessions • No control group, retrospective study	• Sessions were 20 min avg duration for inpts, 60 min avg for outpts • Patients could choose from: – Swed M – Light touch M (LT) – Foot massage	• Pain • Fatigue • Stress/anxiety • Nausea • Depression	• Swed M and foot M most commonly given • Swed M and LT M had better results than foot M • Swed M or LT had 58% improvement in presenting symptoms • Foot M had 50% improvement • No signif diff between Swed M and LT • Improvements for inpts did not last • Effects last longer for outpts
Hernandez-Reif, Field, Ironson, et al. (2005)	• 58 women c̄ BR CA stages I-III • Dxed w/in last 3 yrs • 3 mos. P̄ Tx	• Group 1 (n=16)— standard care • Group 2 (n=22)—30 min. Swed M/ROM 3x/wk for 5 wks • Group 3 (n=20)— 30 min. PMR	• Pain • Depression • Anxiety • Anger • Vigor • Immune function (NK cells, lymphocytes) • Norepinephrine • Epinephrine • Dopamine • Serotonin • Cortisol	• Groups 2 & 3 ↓ in depression, anxiety, pain immed P̄ 1st and last session • Group 2 ↓ depression and anger and ↑ vigor by end of study • Group 2 ↓ NK cells, lymphocytes from 1st to last day • Over long term, M was better than PMR; PMR better than standard care

FINAL THOUGHTS

The scientific research has yet to create a clear picture of the effects of massage on oncology patients. It has, though, proved one very valuable point: that massage can safely be given to people at every stage of the cancer experience. Those who still teach that massage is contraindicated for cancer patients can take comfort in the fact that scores of medical centers and clinics around the world have studied massage for this population. Large, well-established agencies and institutions have funded research projects – the National Institutes for Health, the American Massage Therapy Association, the Marie Curie Cancer Centre in Great Britain, and Dartmouth Hitchcock Medical Center in the U.S., to name only a few. This fact conveys an attitude of feasibility and acceptability and is part of the process of reestablishing the idea that touch is vital for all people in all circumstances, especially during treatment for and recovery from cancer.

REFERENCES

1. Hernandez-Reif M, Ironson G, Field T, et al. Breast Cancer Patients Have Improved Immune and Neuroendocrine Functions Following Massage Therapy. *Journal of Psychosomatic Research*. 2004;57:45-52.

2. David Eisenberg in an Editorial on the Institute of Medicine Report on Complementary and Alternative Medicine in the United States – Personal Reflections on Its Content and Implications: *Alternative Therapies*. 2005;11(3):10-14.

3. Weiger WA, Smith M, Boon H, et al. Advising Patients Who Seek Complementary and Alternative Medical Therapies for Cancer. *Annals of Internal Medicine*. 2002;137(11):889-903.

4. Fellowes D, Barnes K, Wilkinson S. Aromatherapy and Massage for Symptom Relief in Patients with Cancer. *The Cochrane Database of Systematic Reviews*. 2004, Issue 3, Art. No.:CD002287.pub2. DOI:10.1002/14651858.CD002287.pub2.

5. Cancer Pain: Treatment Guidelines for Patients. Available at: http://www.cancer.org/downloads/CRI/NCCN_Pain_II.pdf. Accessed November 22, 2006.

6. Dalton J, Toomey T, Workman M. Pain Relief for Cancer Patients. *Cancer Nursing*. 1988;11(6):322-28.

7. Tope DM, Hann DM, Pinkson B. Massage therapy: An old intervention comes of age. *Quality of Life – A Nursing Challenge*. 1994;3:14-18.

8. Ahles TA, Tope DM, Pinkson B, et al. Massage Therapy for Patients Undergoing Autologous Bone Marrow Transplantation. *Journal of Pain and Symptom Management*. 1999;18(3):157-63.

9.   Cawthorne L, Boyle DA. Massage as Cancer Nursing Therapeutic: Impact on Symptom Distress During Hospitalization. (Abstract of podium session, 2001 Oncology Nursing Society 26th Annual Congress, San Diego, CA). *Oncology Nursing Forum*. 2001;28(2):324-5.

10   Ferrell-Torry AT, Glick OJ. The use of therapeutic massage as a nursing intervention to modify anxiety and the perception of cancer pain. *Cancer Nursing*. 1993;16:93-101.

11. Hemphill L, Kemp J. Implementing a therapeutic massage program in a tertiary and ambulatory care VA setting. *Nursing Clinics of North America*. 2000;35(2):489-97.

12. Lawvere, S. The effect of massage therapy in ovarian cancer patients in Massage Therapy. *The Evidence for Practice*. St. Louis, MO: Mosby/Harcourt, 2002.

13. Smith MC, Kemp J, Hemphill L, et al. Outcomes of Therapeutic Massage for Hospitalized Cancer Patients. *Journal of Nursing Scholarship*. 2002;34(3):25762.

14. Stephenson NL, Weinrich SP, Tavakoli AS. The effects of foot reflexology on anxiety and pain in patients with breast and lung cancer. *Oncology Nursing Forum*. 2000;27(1):67-72.

15. Toth M, Kahn J, Walton T, et al. Therapeutic Massage Intervention for Hospitalized Patients with Cancer. *Alternative and Complementary Therapies*. June 2003: 117-124.

16. Wilkie DJ, Kampbell J, Cutshall S, et al. Effects of Massage on Pain Intensity, Analgesics and Quality of Life in Patients with Cancer Pain. *The Hospice Journal*. 2000;15(3):31-53.

17. Hernandez-Reif M, Field T, Ironson G, et al. Natural Killer Cells and Lymphocytes Increase in Women with Breast Cancer Following Massage Therapy. *International Journal of Neuroscience*. 2005;115:495-510.

18. Grealish L, Lomasney A, Whiteman B. Foot Massage: A Nursing Intervention to Modify the Distressing Symptoms of Pain and Nausea in Patients Hospitalized with Cancer. *Cancer Nursing*. 2000;23(3):237-43.

19. Weinrich SP, Weinrich MC. The effect of massage on pain in cancer patients. *Applied Nursing Research*. 1990;3(4):140-145.

20. Post-White J, Kinney ME, Savik K, et al. Therapeutic Massage and Healing Touch Improve Symptoms in Cancer. *Integrative Cancer Therapies*. 2003;2(4);332-44.

21. Cassileth BR, Vickers AJ. Massage Therapy for Symptom Control: Outcome Study at a Major Cancer Center. *Journal of Pain and Symptom Management*. 2004;28(3):244-249.

22   Taylor AG, Galper DL, Taylor P, et al. Massage for Postoperative Pain and Distress. *The Journal of Alternative and Complementary Medicine*. 2003;9(1):77-89.

23. Soden K, Vincent K, Craske S. A Randomized Controlled Trial of Aromatherapy Massage in a Hospice Setting. *Palliative Medicine*. 2004;18:87-92.

24. Kite SM, Maher EJ, Anderson K, et al. Development of an Aromatherapy Service at a Cancer Centre. *Palliative Medicine*. 1998;12:171-180.

25. Olson K, Hanson J. Using Reiki to Manage Pain: A Preliminary Report. *Cancer Prevention and Control*. 1997;1(2):108-113.

26. Olson K, Hanson J, Michaud M. A Phase II Trial of Reiki for the Management of Pain in Advanced Cancer Patients. *Journal of Pain and Symptom Management*. 2003;26(2):990-997.

27. Samarel N, Fawcett J, Davis MM, et al. Effects of Dialogue and Therapeutic Touch on Preoperative and Postoperative Experiences of Breast Cancer Surgery: An Exploratory Study. *Oncology Nursing Forum*. 1998;25(8):1369-1376.

28. Crawford J. Myofascial Release Provides Symptomatic Relief from Chest Wall Tenderness Occasionally Seen Following Lumpectomy and Radiation in Breast Cancer Patients. *International Journal of Oncology, Biology, and Physics*. 1996;34(5):1188-1189.

29. Stephenson N, Dalton JA, Carlson J. The Effect of Foot Reflexology on Pain in Patients with Metastatic Cancer. *Applied Nursing Research*. 2003;16(4):284-86.

30. Moyers CA, Rounds J, Hannum JW. A Meta-Analysis of Massage Therapy Research. *Psychological Bulletin*. 2004;130(1):3-18.

31. Menard M. The Effect of Therapeutic Massage on Post-Surgical Outcomes. Doctoral dissertation, University of Virginia. 1995.

32. Wilkinson S, Aldridge J, Salmon I, et al. An Evaluation of Aromatherapy Massage in Palliative Care. *Palliative Medicine*. 1999;13:409-17.

33. Hadfield N. The Role of Aromatherapy Massage in Reducing Anxiety in Patients with Malignant Brain Tumors. *International Journal of Palliative Nursing*. 2001;7(6):279-85.

34. Corner J, Cawley N, Hildebrand S. An Evaluation of the Use of Massage and Essential Oils on the Wellbeing of Cancer Patients. *International Journal of Palliative Nursing*. 1995;1(2):67-73.

35. Quattrin R, Zanini A, Buchini S, et al. Use of Reflexology Foot Massage to Reduce Anxiety in Hospitalized Cancer Patients in Chemotherapy Treatment: Method and Outcomes. *Journal of Nursing Management*. 2006;14(2):96-105.

36. Corbin L. Safety and Efficacy of Massage Therapy for Patients with Cancer. *Cancer Control*. 2005;12(3):158-164.

37. Corbin L. Delayed Chemotherapy-Induced Nausea in Women Treated for Breast Cancer. *Oncology Nursing Forum*. 2003;30(2):40-47.

38. Bender CM, McDaniel RW, Murphy-Ende K, et al. Chemotherapy-Induced Nausea and Vomiting. *Clinical Journal of Oncology Nursing*. 2002;6(2):94-102.

39. Arakawa S. Relaxation to Reduce Nausea, Vomiting, and Anxiety Induced by Chemotherapy in Japanese Patients. *Cancer Nursing*. 1997;20(5):342-49.

40. Dibble SL, Chapman J, Mack KA, et al. Acupressure for Nausea: Results of a Pilot Study. *Oncology Nursing Forum*. 2000;27(1):41-47.

41. Lively BT, Black CD, Holiday-Goodman M, et al. Massage therapy for chemotherapy-induced emesis, in *Massage Therapy: The Evidence for Practice*. St. Louis, MO: Mosby/Harcourt, 2002.

42. Scott D, Donahue D, Mastrovito R, et al. The Antiemetic Effect of Clinical Relaxation: Report of an Exploratory Pilot Study. *Journal of Psychosocial Oncology*. 1983;1(1):71-83.

43. Dibble S, Luce J, Cooper BA, et al. Acupressure for Delayed Chemotherapy Induced Nausea and Vomiting: A Randomized Clinical Trial. 2006. (Submitted for publication.)

44. Shin, Y, Kim T, Shin M, et al. Effect of Acupressure on Nausea and Vomiting During Chemotherapy Cycle for Korean Postoperative Stomach Cancer Patients. *Cancer Nursing*. 2004;27(4):267-74.

45. Yang JH. The Effects of Foot Reflexology on Nausea, Vomiting and Fatigue of Breast Cancer Patients Undergoing Chemotherapy. *Taehan Kanho Hakhoe Chi*. 2005;35(1):177-85.

46. Holley SK. Evaluating Patient Distress from Cancer-Related Fatigue: An Instrument Development Study. *Oncology Nursing Forum*. 2000;27(9):1425-1431.)

47. Sims S. Slow Stroke Back Massage for Cancer Patients. *Nursing Times*. 1986;82(13):47-50.

48. Kohara H, Miyauchi T, Suehiro Y, et al. Combined Modality Treatment of Aromatherapy, Footsoak, and Reflexology Relieves Fatigue in Patients with Cancer. *Journal of Palliative Medicine*. 2004;7(6):791-96.

49. Ironson G, Field T, Scafidi F, et al. Massage Therapy Is Associated with Enhancement of the Immune System's Cytotoxic Capacity. *International Journal of Neuroscience*. 1996;84:205-18.

50. Diego M, Field T, Hernandez-Reif M, et al. HIV Adolescents Show Improved Immune Function Following Massage Therapy. *International Journal of Neuroscience*. 2001;106:35-45.

51. Harris R. An Introduction to Manual Lymphatic Drainage: The Vodder Method. *Massage Therapy Journal*. 1992;31(1):55-66.

52. Erickson VS, Pearson ML, Ganz PA, et al. Arm Edema in Breast Cancer Patients. *Journal of the National Cancer Institute*. 2001;93(2):96-111.

53. Anderson L, Højris I, Erlandsen M, et al. Treatment of Breast-Cancer-Related Lymphedema With or Without Manual Lymphatic Drainage. *Acta Oncologica*. 2000;39(3):399-405.

54. McNeely ML, Magee DJ, Lees AW, et al. The Addition of Manual Lymph Drainage to Compression Therapy for Breast Cancer Related Lymphedema: A Randomized Controlled Trial. *Breast Cancer Research and Treatment*. 2004;86:95-106.

55. Morgan RG, Casley-Smith JR, Mason MR, et al. Complex Physical Therapy for the Lymphoedematous Arm. *Journal of Hand Surgery*. 1992;17B:437-441.

56. Williams AF, Vadgame A, Franks PJ, et al. A Randomized Controlled Crossover Study of Manual Lymphatic Drainage Therapy in Women with Breast Cancer-Related Lymphoedema. *European Journal of Cancer Care*. 2002;11:254-261.

57. Wilcock A, Manderson C, Weller R, et al. Does Aromatherapy Massage Benefit Patients with Cancer Attending a Specialist Palliative Care Day Centre? *Palliative Medicine*. 2004;18:287-90.

58. Wright S, Courtney U, Donnelly C, et al. Clients' Perceptions of the Benefits of Reflexology on Their Quality of Life. *Complementary Therapies in Nursing and Midwifery*. 2002;8:69-76.

59. Loveland Cook CA, Guerrerio JF, Slater VE. Healing Touch and Quality of Life in Women Recieiving Radiation Treatment for Cancer: A Randomized Controlled Trial. *Alternative Therapies*. 2004;10(3):34-40.

60. Milligan M, Fanning M, Hunter S, et al. Reflexology Audit: Patient Satisfaction, Impact on Quality of Life and Availability in Scottish Hospices. *International Journal of Palliative Nursing*. 2002;8(10):489-96.

61. Hodgson H. Does Reflexology Impact on Cancer Patients' Quality of Life? *Nursing Standard*. 2000;14(31):33-38.

62. Kelly AE, Sullivan P, Fawcett J, et al. Therapeutic Touch, Quiet Time, and Dialogue: Perceptions of Women with Breast Cancer. *Oncology Nursing Forum*. 2004;31(3):625-631.

63. Smith MC, Reeder F, Daniel L, et al. Outcomes of Touch Therapies During Bone Marrow Transplant. *Alternative Therapies in Health and Medicine*. 2003;9(1):40-48.

64. Billhult N, Dahlberg K. A Meaningful Relief From Suffering: Experiences of Massage in Cancer Care. *Cancer Nursing*. 2001;24(3):180-84.

65. Bredin M. Mastectomy, Body Image and Therapeutic Massage: A Qualitative Study of Women's Experience. *Journal of Advanced Nursing*. 1999;29(5):1113-20.

66. Chamness A. Massage Therapy and Persons Living with Cancer. *Massage Therapy Journal*. 1993;Sept:53-65.

67. Dunwoody L, Smyth A, Davidson R. Cancer Patients' Experiences and Evaluations of Aromatherapy Massage in Pallliative Care. *International Journal of Palliative Nursing*. 2002;8(10):497-504.

Chapter 4

Inching Forward

The Need for a Less Demanding Approach

The act of massage unites heaven and earth, spirit and matter, divine and mundane.

— AUTHOR

Massage can produce results that are truly sublime. Paul was coaxed back to life after months of treatment for tonsil cancer. For Christa, massage was a ray of light in an otherwise dark world. "It made life worth living." Lois felt whole again despite never being cured of the disease. For Jackie, foot massage received during chemo restored her confidence in the goodness of humankind. Rosemarie felt the sacredness of being in church.

At other times, especially if the massage is given with too much vigor, unfavorable outcomes can occur. Sue encountered a bodyworker who mistakenly thought a deep massage following four rounds of chemotherapy would help to eliminate the accumulation of toxins. Instead it sent Sue to bed for three days with flu-like symptoms. It was six months before she dared try another massage. Following treatment for breast cancer, Sonia returned to her weekly massage sessions. After the very first massage, she developed lymphedema from the use of overly vigorous pressure on the quadrant of the body in which lymph nodes had been removed. Ralph sought out non-painful, comforting massage after undergoing surgery for prostate cancer. He knew that his body had been traumatized by the medical procedure and he wanted to resensitize it. Instead, the practitioner was overly zealous. The first time she put her hands on him, the discomfort was so intense, Ralph almost punched her.

During cancer treatment and the recovery period, which may be a year or longer, the body needs its resources to heal instead of coping with unnecessary stressors, such as vigorous exercise or deep massage. The experience of cancer treatment can be extremely demanding on all levels – physical, emotional, mental, and spiritual. All parts of a person's life are affected. Preparing family meals becomes a huge task. Work hours, socializing, shopping, and exercise are reduced or temporarily eliminated. Energy is sapped by worry about finances, family members, and the future. Patients put one foot in front of the other with the goal of just getting through treatment.

Much of the time, it is not the disease that saps energy or damages the body, it is the side effects from surgery, radiation, and/or chemotherapy. Blood counts, immune function, lymphatic drainage, digestion, and organ vitality are all affected and take time to improve. Therefore, people who have undergone cancer treatment require bodywork that is less demanding. It is the purpose of this chapter to explain why bodywork sessions must be gentler and how this can be accomplished. Central to this is the concept of "inching forward."

WHY BE LESS DEMANDING

There is no physiological evidence as to the demand massage places on the body of someone who has undergone cancer treatment. We must, therefore, remind ourselves of what is known about deeper massage and its general effects on the body and then extrapolate about its effect on the person with cancer. Forceful massage stimulates the sympathetic nervous system, causing the heart rate to accelerate, blood vessels to constrict, blood pressure to elevate, and the gastrointestinal system to become depressed. These physiological activities which are associated with the "fight or flight" response are also a reaction to constant anxiety and trauma, such as accompany the cancer experience.

The long periods of stress that accompany "fight or flight" have been shown to raise cortisol levels, slow wound healing, increase susceptibility to infections, interrupt sleep patterns, result in pervasive anxiety and/or depression, and disrupt eating and elimination patterns, resulting in poor nutrition. People recovering from cancer treatment do not need the added stress that vigorous or deep massage places on the entire being.

Many of the consequences of cancer treatment are visible to both the patient and practitioner – fatigue, nausea, easy bruising, incisions, or hair loss. Underlying these visible side effects, however, are assaults to the body that cannot be seen. Chief among these are the demands chemotherapy and radiation place on the body's major organs,

Brushing my teeth and having my feet massaged are the only two nice things that have been done to my body since being in the hospital for cancer treatment.

— BERNICE, PORTLAND, OREGON

Darlene

Darlene was a long-time massage consumer. When she was diagnosed with breast cancer, Darlene thought massage would provide a welcome relief from the side effects of chemotherapy. But after just two sessions, she quit. The massage sessions, unadjusted for her new body, caused severe pain and fatigue for days following the massage. A year later Darlene tentatively decided to try massage again at an oncology massage clinic. Knowing about her prior unpleasant experience, the therapist approached this hesitant client with great mindfulness, hoping to regain Darlene's trust in massage. In the follow-up phone call the next day, Darlene gave an unequivocal thumbs up! She enthusiastically told the therapist that she had the energy to go shopping that evening and slept better than she had in months.

— AUTHOR

Too often I want to be heroic and create earth-shattering effects, fearing that small accomplishments are not enough.

— AUTHOR

---

especially the heart, lungs, kidneys, liver, and gastrointestinal system. Not only is the body unable to function at peak efficiency; permanent damage sometimes occurs. Lois, for instance, underwent radiation for Hodgkin's Disease. Included in the field of treatment were her heart, lungs, breasts, and spine. As a result, Lois was left with congestive heart failure, scarred lungs, breast cancer secondary to the treatment for lymphoma, and kyphosis, all of which required adjustments to her massage sessions.

The organs of detoxification, including the circulatory and lymphatic system, become overextended as the body metabolizes not only the drugs but the debris from dying cancer cells and other cells affected by the treatments. This cellular debris overloads lymph nodes which are part of the body's filtration system. Additionally, during treatment, patients are more sedentary. Muscular action is the prime stimulator of the lymphatic system and venous return. The lack of it causes lymph and blood flow to stagnate, much like sediment in a pond. Poor circulation contributes to poor oxygenation and the buildup of cell waste products – hence a lack of energy. A demanding massage can then stir up the proverbial sediment, overwhelming the systems involved in detoxification. Readers may have had the experience when taking a lymphatic massage class of feeling unwell following practice sessions. Imagine the response of a body that has undergone cancer treatment.

The person affected by cancer treatment needs the restorative action of the parasympathetic response, which slows heart rate, dilates blood vessels, and increases intestinal perstalsis and gland activity. Long, slow, undemanding strokes, such as effleurage, initiates these rejuvenating, parasympathetic reactions; so do undemanding modalities such as Reiki, Jin Shin Do, or Breema. It makes sense to avoid stirring up the waste products. This spares the client from experiencing flu-like symptoms for days following the massage. A focus on being supportive and nurturing creates many beneficial outcomes – physical energy increases, people feel whole and lovable, and pain and anxiety lessen, just to name a few.

We can also look at the anecdotal evidence for support. A wealth of examples offer proof for the need to be undemanding when working with this population. For example, a hospital massage student once massaged a 31-year-old man who was being prepared for a bone marrow transplant. Willie was very fit and his blood counts were all good; his nurse gave the green light for whatever the patient wanted in terms of pressure or length of session. Even though the massage student tempered the pressure, and despite the fact that the massage strokes felt comfortable to Willie at the time, he woke later that night in significant pain, which he attributed to the massage. From that point on, Willie was wary of massage and never again accepted our offer of a session during his hospital stay.

Another client who came for massage during chemotherapy always felt flu-like symptoms following his sessions. It wasn't until he had received several massages that he and the therapist realized that his nauseous sensations were a direct side effect of the bodywork session.

A third patient, someone who had recently been admitted to hospice, requested deep bodywork from the massage therapist. The practitioner sensed that this woman was not a candidate for vigorous bodywork and was, with some effort, able to convince the patient that light acupressure would be more appropriate. As in the first example, the bodywork felt good to the patient in the moment, but later the woman admitted that even the light pressure had caused her discomfort at the end of the day.

In the above stories, the discomfort experienced by patients was not primarily the result of the person's cancer but mainly was caused by the side effects from treatment. These are the predominant issues. The type of cancer is not, by and large, an issue, except at the end of life when the disease is affecting the body's functioning. Whether a client was diagnosed with stage 4 breast cancer, multiple myeloma, non-Hodgkin's lymphoma, or stage 2 kidney cancer is not as relevant to the massage plan as the cancer treatments they have received.

Most patients receive their cancer treatments from allopathic practitioners. Information about these treatments will be presented first. While the toxicity of these interventions is well-known, readers must also remember that alternative treatments, such as herbs, also create a demand on the body and may require gentler bodywork. Brief coverage of the side effects of alternative treatments will follow the section on conventional cancer treatments.

SIDE EFFECTS OF CONVENTIONAL CANCER TREATMENTS

Despite all of the new therapies touted in the media, surgery, radiation, and chemotherapy are still the staples of conventional oncology treatments. These three therapies are often used in conjunction with each other. One patient, such as a metastatic lung cancer patient, might receive all three interventions: surgery to remove the lobe of the lung containing the tumor, followed by chemotherapy and then radiation. Another patient whose disease has not spread, may just be treated by surgery; a third, such as a man with prostate cancer, may receive radiation followed by drugs to lower his testosterone level. The treatment decisions made by the patient and doctor are based on a complex set of factors, such as general health, age, the degree to which the cancer has spread, patient beliefs, family expectations, and even the level of health insurance coverage.

Cancer treatments are used with a number of intentions. The primary goal of treatment is the cure or long-term complete remission of the disease. However, a cure is not always possible, in which case the disease can sometimes be managed as a chronic condition, or as controlled partial remission. Even when the medical team believes that it is no longer possible to cure the cancer, treatment is often continued in order to give patients the best possible chance. Chemo and radiation can often stop or slow the growth of the disease for the time being. Having that time can be important to patients and their

*Deep massage is like **shouting** to the body. Comfort-oriented touch is like whispering to it.*

— BRIDGET KINGSTON,
MASSAGE THERAPIST,
SAN FRANCISCO, CALIFORNIA

Esther

Esther is a perfect example of the power inherent in taking charge and having hope. Five months after being diagnosed with pancreatic cancer, which often causes death within several months, she started weekly Reiki sessions. Esther lived another year after starting those sessions, mostly on hope generated by the pursuit of potential treatments. The day Esther lost hope was apparent; she arrived for her Reiki session greatly fatigued and dispirited, the sparkle gone from her eyes. That morning her doctor had told her nothing else could be done, that she was wasting her time to continue searching.

— AUTHOR

Healing does not take place in the fast lane.

— ANONYMOUS

families. A sense of hope is fostered by continuing treatments, and the power of hope cannot be underestimated.

Surgery, radiation, and chemotherapy may also be employed as rehabilitative or palliative measures. Palliative measures are used to control the cancer and improve the quality of life. For instance, radiation or chemo may be given to reduce the size of a tumor that is causing pain or obstructing a vital organ. Palliative surgery may be performed in the case of a large tumor that is impinging on other organs. It also may be used to prevent the development of a calamitous problem, such as obstruction of the superior vena cava or the collapse of a vertebra due to spinal metastases. Surgery also is performed for rehabilitative reasons, such as breast or facial reconstruction, skin grafts following resections for melanoma, or the fashioning of a neobladder out of the lower portion of the bowel after surgery to remove the bladder.

In the following sections, the three main cancer treatments will be dissected so that the reader can more fully understand the clinical reasons for using a less demanding massage approach with the person treated for cancer. Also touched upon are lesser known allopathic treatments and alternative therapies. The treatments for cancer are complex and could fill an entire book. Only generalities are presented here. It is not possible to present information on all of the various diagnostic scans cancer patients may receive or the many differing medications they may be prescribed. Other more detailed material is available from oncology nursing texts, cancer society brochures, or on the internet.

SURGERY

Surgery is sometimes performed in the pursuit of curing cancer or reducing a mass prior to chemotherapy to make this treatment more effective. Or, it may be part of a palliative action in which the tumor or part of it is removed to make the person more comfortable, as in the case of a mass impinging upon a nerve. Surgery is performed to reconstruct damaged parts of the body, such breast reconstruction. There are both long- and short-term side effects that occur from surgery that bodyworkers must be aware of.

If desired, low impact bodywork can begin immediately after surgery. But for the first several weeks, the body is repairing blood and lymphatic vessels damaged from the incision. During this time, the patient needs to be "pieced back together" rather than enduring another invasive intervention, such as a vigorous massage.

Patients who have had surgery are at risk for thromboembolic disorders, commonly referred to as blood clots. This is especially true of surgeries that entail larger amounts of blood involvement, such as an abdominal or thoracic surgery. Injury to the lining of veins from catheters also contributes to the risk. Persons with cancer are more likely to develop postoperative thrombophlebitis than a person without cancer. Most likely this is due to emboli that have formed from the combining of platelets, cancer cells, fibrin, and other constituents of the blood. The potential for clot development is a reason to moderate any touch therapies given to the postoperative client. Surgery to replace a hip or knee are accompanied by the same clot potential. Joint replacements amongst cancer patients may be the result of long-term prednisone use or bone fragility related to radiation therapy. More information is given in Chapter 5 on the risk for thromboembolic disorders.

Cancer patients often have lymph nodes removed, either to excise the cancer or as part of the diagnostic process. Lymph node removal, particularly from the neck, axilla, or groin, puts the person at risk for lymphedema for the remainder of their life. Detailed information is given in future chapters to guide massage therapists when working with those at risk for lymphedema.

Because the direction in health care is toward more outpatient procedures and shorter hospital stays, surgery patients are not allowed to linger in the hospital any longer than necessary. Women are often discharged one day after a mastectomy, a colon cancer patient can be sent home a day or two after having part of the bowel removed, and a man who has had a prostatectomy can be discharged in a similar amount of time. This trend means a greater reliance on home care, requiring family and friends to deal with drains, dressings, colostomies, feeding tubes, and catheters. Greater mindfulness must be brought to these situations so as to avoid displacing the device or causing discomfort to the client.

Other information regarding surgical patients is found in Chapter 5.

RADIATION

Approximately 60% of those with cancer will receive radiation therapy at some point. Unlike chemotherapy, which is a systemic intervention, radiation therapy is a localized treatment to a well-defined area (with the exception of total body irradiation, or TBI, which is used in a very small number of specialized circumstances). It may be used alone or in conjunction with surgery or chemotherapy. Radiation is used for a variety of reasons – to eliminate the disease, to shrink the tumor prior to surgery so that the procedure is less invasive, and to kill rogue cells following surgery. In addition, radiation therapy is administered to control the cancer's growth and spread, allowing the person to live for a time symptom free; to improve a patient's quality of life by diminishing symptoms caused by the advance of the disease; or to shrink a growth that is obstructing a vital area of the body such as the GI tract, a major blood vessel, or the kidneys, or is compressing the spine.

Radiation destroys the ability of cancer cells to grow and multiply by damaging the cell's DNA. Cells that divide rapidly, such as cancer cells, are more sensitive to radiation than are slowly dividing or resting cells. Poorly differentiated cells, too, are more sensitive, as are well-oxygenated cells, both of which are qualities of cancerous cells.[1]

Side Effects of Surgery

Short-term side effects:
- risk for thrombus
- depression of immune system
- tenderness at incisional site

Long-term side effects:
- risk of lymphedema due to nodal dissection
- adhesions and scarring
- numbness or hypersensitivity in the vicinity of the surgical site
- body image issues
- unconscious guarding of the surgical or procedural site

Adapted from work by Charlotte Versagi.

Delivery of radiation can occur in many ways. Below, the two most common ways, external beam and internal implants, will be discussed. Both methods require the massage therapist to adjust the session, but external beam has a particularly long list of reasons to be less demanding.

EXTERNAL BEAM RADIATION

The method familiar to most readers is external beam radiation. This form of treatment delivers a beam of radiation to a localized area from a machine that is positioned at a distance from the body. The radiologist maps out a field of treatment in which the beam of radiation is directed at the tumor from a number of different angles, often three to five. These angles, as well as the intensity of the beam and radiation dosage, target the center of the tumor or tumors and attempt to minimize the radiation damage to surrounding healthy tissue.

The actual treatment takes only a few minutes, but time is spent beforehand carefully positioning the patient on the treatment table so that healthy tissue is not accidentally irradiated. This process is generally repeated in a variable number of treatments. For example, in certain types of breast cancer, the radiation treatments may be given five days a week, often for 6–8 weeks. Other conditions will require different radiation schedules. Palliative treatment to areas affected by bone metastases are often given at a higher dose for only a few treatments. These treatments are often highly effective at relieving neurological pain caused by tumor growth. The stem cell transplant patient being treated with total body irradiation (TBI), will receive treatment twice a day for several days.

The most noticeable effect of radiation is to the skin in the treated area. The skin may become very dry and look red, irritated, sunburned, or tanned. Severely affected areas may even develop blisters or peel and weep, particularly in skin folds such as the axilla and groin. Usually the skin will be appear to be recovered within several weeks after the end of treatments; however, it may remain tender and delicate for longer periods. It should always be treated with the utmost tenderness. Joachim Zuther, author of *Lymphedema Management: The Comprehensive Guide for Practitioners*, recommends that post-radiation patients pat the affected area dry after bathing rather than toweling dry. Rubbing can cause further breakdown of the skin.[2] In some people, the treated skin remains permanently darker and the tissue beneath is hardened, owing to the acute inflammation inflicted on the area. Put quite simply, radiation causes a "welding" of the tissues as scar tissue replaces a portion of the healthy tissue and tumor. In Chapter 5, further details are given about the damage inflicted by radiation therapy to the skin and neighboring tissues.

As with chemotherapy, radiation affects not only tumor cells, but also normal cells, including all tissue in the path of the beam. External beam radiation enters the body at the specified location plotted out by the technicians and scatters somewhat when it enters the body. Nearby tissues are affected and the radiation exits on the opposite side of the body. All tissue along that pathway will be affected, including healthy tissue in the path of the beam and the areas of scatter. Bones in the field of treatment can lose their integrity, becoming fragile. The functioning of major organs, such as the heart and lungs, can become diminished due to scarring. If the neck, axilla, or groin are part of the irradiated area, lymphatic and circulatory system functioning can be severely damaged due to scarring and adhesions in the nodal clusters and capillary beds.

It is important to remember that the beam has an exit point as well as an entry, which means that skin on opposite sides of the body will be affected. The ability of radiation to pass through the body is the reason that radiation departments are often in the basement of the hospital. A lead-lined room must be built to contain the radiation; otherwise it passes through everything in the surrounding area.

Common short-term side effects of external beam radiation:

- fatigue (consistent with all radiation therapy sites)
- nausea, vomiting and diarrhea (primarily if digestive system is in the field of treatment)
- skin tenderness or fragility at treatment site (both beam entry and exit areas)
- risk of lymphedema if RT to neck, axilla, or groin
- low blood counts, especially if sternum or ilium are part of field of treatment
- dysfunction of glands and organs in field of treatment (i.e., decreased or absent saliva production for oral or neck areas of treatment)

Common long-term side effects of external beam radiation:

- skin can be fragile for years, as well as hypersensitive to heat, cold, and pressure
- bones in the field of treatment may become more fragile
- scarring and adhesions to all tissue in field of treatment
- tendons may be less pliable
- joints may be less resilient and more arthritic
- permanently darkened skin in the area of treatment
- secondary cancers from the RT
- damage to major organs and glands in field of treatment (i.e., permanent damage to saliva production)
- risk of lymphedema if RT to neck, axilla, or groin

Adapted from work by Charlotte Versagi

Blood counts are sometimes affected if the sternum or ilium are in the field of treatment. These are the two biggest bone marrow producing areas. Healthy bone marrow goes on to become the various components of blood. Irradiated bone marrow can cause a short-term deficiency in the blood counts, causing immune deficiency, fatigue due to anemia, and potential for bruising or bleeding.

When given externally, the radiation does not cause the body to become radioactive. It is completely safe to be in contact with clients as they go through the period of radiation therapy. The only time that patients may be radioactive is if they are undergoing internal forms of radiation. This will be covered in the next section.

Additional Resources

- American Cancer Society
  www.cancer.org

- Canadian Cancer Society
  www.cancer.ca

- Cancer Backup (Europe)
  www.cancerbackup.org.uk

- Dollinger M, Tempero M,
  Rosenbaum E, et al. *Everyone's Guide
  to Cancer Therapy*, 4th ed. Andrews
  McNeel Publishing, 2002.

INTERNAL FORMS OF RADIATION

Another way to deliver radiation is internally via implants, injections, or orally-taken radioactive substances. These methods of delivery are used less often than external beam radiation and have vastly different side effects. One form of internal radiation is brachytherapy, which is administered through radioactive implants. Brachytherapy can be administered in both inpatient and outpatient settings, depending on the type of implant which is used. The radiation is delivered directly into or adjacent to the tumor via the implants. These devices come in a variety of shapes and sizes. Some are the shape of a grain of rice, others are like a ribbon, wire, tube, needle, or cone.

Some gynecological cancers are treated with surgically implanted catheters into which a radioactive source is placed. These are temporarily placed near tumors for several days while the patient remains in the hospital. The patient is not radioactive, but the source is. Visitors and nursing personnel must limit their time in these rooms and remain behind mobile, lead shields as much as possible, due to the radioactive levels.

Prostate cancer is often treated with brachytherapy in the form of small, permanent radioactive implants that are about the size of rice grains. This is done primarily as an outpatient procedure. The amount of radiation released is low level and localized. Typically these patients can resume normal activities with selected cautions and restrictions, such as limiting the amount of time that young children can sit on the patient's lap, or wearing a condom during sexual intercourse. The institution which implants the radioactive seeds will give patients an information sheet with explicit instructions regarding safety.

Many other cancers are treated with these main types of brachytherapy. For inpatient procedures, the radiation source is either removed before discharge or the patient's level of residual radioactivity is judged to be within nationally recognized safe levels. It is safe for most practitioners to be around clients who are not hospitalized during this time. However, pregnant therapists should check with the client's radiologist to be certain it is safe for them to be in the presence of the person with radioactive implants.

Thyroid cancer is sometimes treated with an oral dose of radioactive iodine. This procedure creates systemic radioactivity in the patient. Often, the procedure is done on an inpatient basis but is sometimes performed in an outpatient clinic. Either way, strict limits are placed on the amount of distance the patient must remain from others, even for personnel providing care. During her confinement, Janet wrote to a friend, "For the next week, I will be home and radioactive. I get to look at the cat through a glass door. He is quarantined from me and I am sure he has no idea why." During these same days, the massage therapist, too, is restricted from working with the client.

The side effects of internal radiation therapy are different than with external beam therapy. Scarring, adhesions, and burns are not caused by implants or ingestion of radioactive substances. The major complaint of people receiving internal radiation is fatigue. The therapist's main job, then, is to match the energy of the bodywork session to the energy of the client.

CHEMOTHERAPY

In oncology parlance, the term "chemotherapy" refers to drugs given to kill, slow, or stop the growth of cancer cells. More specifically, these medications are classified as antitumor or antineoplastic drugs. Antitumor agents are given for many reasons: to reduce the size of large, bulky tumors before surgery; to increase the sensitivity of the cancer to other therapy, such as radiation; to treat cancers that can metastasize; or to treat tumors that may not have spread but are, for some reason, inoperable or not in locations where radiation is advisable. These drugs are usually given intravenously but some are administered in tablet form and some via injection.

Other groups of pharmaceuticals, such as antidepressants, narcotics, and antifungals, antivirals, and antibiotics, are used to manage the side effects of the antitumor medications. A patient may, for example, be on Arimidex and Cytoxan to kill the cancer, Ambien to sleep, Procrit to support red blood cell growth, prednisone for mood, appetite, and pain, Zoloft for depression, and Zofran for nausea. All of these drugs place a demand on the body, particularly the liver and other organs of detoxification.

Chemotherapy is given in an assortment of combinations and on a variety of schedules. It may be weekly for six weeks or every third week for 18 weeks. One condition that commonly derails the schedule is neutropenia, insufficient white blood cells. Outpatients whose white blood cell count is below 2.0 (the norm is around 5–10) on the day of chemotherapy, may have their treatment delayed until the count rises. Usually this takes a week. Other factors may slow the treatment timetable, such as excessive diarrhea and vomiting, fatigue, or impaired mental status.

When the lengthy list of side effects caused by cancer treatments is studied, it becomes very clear why bodywork, or other manual interventions, should be done in a gentle and measured way. Chemotherapy, for instance, commonly results in the following short-term side effects, each of which requires the therapist to be less demanding in their approach:

- fatigue
- immunosuppression
- easy bruising or bleeding
- sensitive or fragile skin
- nausea, vomiting, and diarrhea
- peripheral neuropathy
- pain
- edema
- pain medications

Betty

To my amazement, when I arrived at my first radiation appointment – with more than a bit of anxiety – there was a sign in the dressing room announcing free massages every Thursday after radiation treatment! I signed up immediately and on that first Thursday was ushered into a quiet room with soft music and a warmed bed. I felt transported to another realm, soothed and extraordinarily well-cared for. Maybe if I'd had weekly massages like this for most of my working life, I wouldn't have even walked down the cancer path. I feel extremely grateful and fortunate to have been the recipient of the thoughtful, gentle, but powerful gifts of this oncology massage therapist and cannot recommend the treatment highly enough – especially for those going through time of health challenges.

— BETTY, DENVER, COLORADO

- constipation
- anxiety, depression, emotional volatility
- insomnia

Other consequences of chemotherapy can be long-term. They include:

- peripheral neuropathy
- anxiety and depression
- insomnia
- bone fragility (due to osteoporosis)
- reproductive system damage (i.e., early menopause or infertility)
- joint and muscular pain
- permanent damage to specific organs
- skin discoloration or sensitivity
- memory deficits ("chemo brain")

ANTINEOPLASTIC (ANTITUMOR) DRUGS

Different antitumor drugs and different combinations of drugs are used for each type of cancer and work by various means. Often, two or more drugs are used. Some chemotherapies act on the cells' DNA, some inhibit cell division, while others change the hormonal environment. By and large, these drugs are designed to attack fast-growing cells. The intended target is tumor cells, but other fast-growing cells get caught in the cross fire, such as the skin, hair, nails, the lining of the digestive tract, and bone marrow (cells that create red blood cells, white blood cells, and platelets.)

The list of drugs used to kill tumors is very long, too long for a massage therapist to try to memorize. Even oncology nurses who work around these medications daily do not know all of the drugs and their side effects. Just as there are hundreds of types of cancer, there are hundreds of chemotherapeutic agents, each with their own effect. Indeed, side effects experienced by a person depend on many individual factors, such as dose of chemo, combination of types of chemo and other treatments, a person's physical resiliency, and other undefined factors that all contribute to the type and degree of each side effect. Rather than learning the names and side effects of each type of chemotherapy, a therapist will do her best to become knowledgeable of the side effects common to chemotherapies. In general, the side effects are as follows:

> ### The Goodness of Humankind
>
> I once sat next to a woman on a flight to San Francisco who revealed that she had received chemotherapy for cancer. The clinic where she had been given treatment had a massage therapist who rubbed patients' feet as they received their IV medications. My seat mate raved about how glorious it was. I asked if she could describe why the foot massage was so wonderful. It was difficult for her to put into words except to say that it restored her confidence in the goodness of humankind.
>
> — AUTHOR

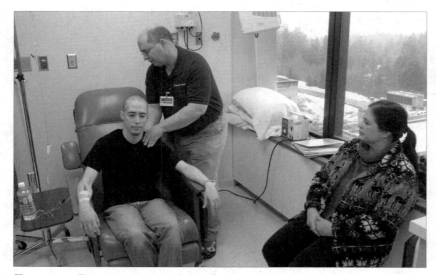

Figure 4.1 Patient receives chemotherapy and massage at the same time.
Photograph by David J. Lawton

Skin and hair: Dryness, sensitive to touch some days, breaks in skin, petechiae (red or purple dots under the skin); alopecia (loss of hair).

Blood: Myelosuppression (lowers platelet, white blood cell, and red blood cell counts)

Gastrointestinal (GI) tract: Nausea, vomiting, diarrhea, loss of appetite.

Musculoskeletal system: Fatigue, malaise, weakness, aches in joints.

Nervous system: Certain chemotherapy agents cause peripheral neuropathy in the hands and feet. Patients may have burning sensation, intermittent shock-like pain, a sensation of "pins and needles," a "crawling" feeling, tingling, or simply a complete lack of feeling.

Psychological: Depression, confusion, forgetfulness or short-term memory impairment (named as "chemo brain" by patients).

ANALGESICS

Analgesics are medications given to reduce and control pain. The type administered depends on a number of factors, such as the severity and the location of the pain. Narcotics are the strongest medications used: opiates such as morphine, codeine and heroin, and synthetics such as oxycodone, oxymorphone, fentanyl and methadone. Other

After the poking and prodding during my treatment, the gentleness of the massage made me feel human again.

— KATHY RAWLINS,
SAN FRANCISCO, CALIFORNIA

Gloving and Chemotherapy

Antitumor drugs are known for their toxicity. Less well-known is the fact that chemotherapies are, in and of themselves, cancer-causing agents. This makes massage therapists wonder if they should protect themselves when working with chemotherapy patients. Generally, antitumor drugs are eliminated through urine and feces, which poses no threat to massage therapists who are in skin-to-skin contact with a patient undertaking chemotherapy. Only two drugs are known to eliminate through the skin. One, Thiotepa, is the drug for which gloving within 24 hours is a clear necessity. This is based on nursing practice. However, therapists will rarely encounter this medication, so gloving for it becomes a moot point.

The other drug that have been suggested as a candidate for gloving, because it eliminates through the skin to some extent, is cyclophosphamide, also known as Cytoxan.[3-7] Many cancer patients receive this medication. But there is no strong evidence to mandate gloving when massaging clients on this drug. One study showed that health care workers can be exposed to a minute amount of cyclophosphamide 16–24 hours following infusion.[3] Based on animal data, this would only account for an extra 1–2 cases of cancer per million workers a year,[4] an insignificant risk on the whole.

The scant research that has been done on this topic points to two helpful pieces of information. Cyclophosphamide is not immediately secreted through the skin. Therefore, massage can be safely given during chemo infusion without gloves. Second, cyclophosphamide excretion in the urine peaks 12–18 hours after infusion.[5] This provides some evidence that 24 hours is an adequate amount of time to allow the cyclophosphamide to leave the body and that massage can also be given without gloves after that.

On the other hand, comprehensive information on skin excretion and other routes of worker exposure are not readily available or known, so there is an element of uncertainty about massage and gloving. It is important that practitioners be at ease when giving massage. If donning gloves gives them peace of mind, they should not hesitate to wear them. It makes little or no difference to the patient whether the practitioner is gloved or ungloved.

Between the morphine and this foot massage, I'm in heaven!

— BERNARD, PHOENIX, ARIZONA
BONE MARROW TRANSPLANT PATIENT

pain medications include steroids, NSAIDS (nonsteroidal anti-inflammatory drugs), aspirin, ibuprofen, and acetaminophen. Sometimes these work better than narcotics for certain types of cancer pain. They may also be prescribed along with narcotics. Some antidepressants and anticonvulsants are used for pain, usually for neurological discomforts.

Narcotics: One of the most common misconceptions about narcotics is that they cause addiction. While narcotics used over time do create physical tolerance and physical dependence, these are totally distinct from addiction, which is defined by the World Health Organization as "compulsive use of drugs for nonmedical reasons; it is characterized by a craving for mood-altering drug effects, not pain relief."[8] One of the primary benefits of narcotic pain relievers is that the dose can be steadily increased as physical tolerance develops. The majority of cancer pain can be well managed with the careful monitoring of a combination of narcotic and non-narcotic analgesics. Some people who have had chronic cancer for a long period require relatively high doses of narcotic pain relievers. Such people should never be treated or thought of as "addicts."

Narcotics can be given through various "routes" – e.g., orally, intravenously, rectally, or via skin patch. Side effects of narcotics may include lethargy and the depression of functions such as breathing and peristaltic bowel activity. Side effects that may relate to massage include:

Central Nervous System (CNS): Drowsiness, dizziness, confusion, sedation, euphoria, headache

GI: Nausea, vomiting, cramps, constipation. Constipation is the result of decreased perstalsis in the bowel and lowered intestinal secretions, which cause a dry stool

---

Nancy

Chemotherapy was a nightmare for Nancy the first time around. She suffered from nausea, diarrhea, fatigue, sleeplessness, drastic hair and weight loss, and was unable to work. When the breast cancer reoccurred a few years later, she sought out Reiki treatments in hopes of easing the side effects of the chemo regimen. Nancy's plan was to go for chemotherapy after work on Thursday and spend the next three days recovering in time to return to work on Monday.

Reiki practitioner Phil Morgan would arrive at Nancy's house every Thursday at 5:30, just as she was coming home from the outpatient clinic. Nancy would lie down on the bed and within 30 minutes of starting the session she was asleep. Phil always gave special attention to the liver, kidneys, thymus, and adrenals. Two hours later he would quietly let himself out. Nancy would sleep through most of Friday and Saturday, wake up late Sunday morning and spend the day puttering around the house. By Monday morning she was ready for work. The Reiki sessions reduced or alleviated all of the side effects that plagued her the first time. Even the hair loss was much less.

The power of these hands-on treatments was made clear one week when Phil had to leave town and was unable to find a replacement. When she arrived home on Thursday evening after the chemo appointment, Nancy went to bed as usual but could not sleep. The entire weekend she was nauseous and unable to sleep. Not surprisingly, Nancy did not make it to work that Monday morning. Needless to say, she and Phil never missed another session.

— AUTHOR

Genitourinary (GU): Decreased libido, urinary retention

Respiratory: Depresses breathing, dries secretions, lessens dyspnea

Skin: Rashes, profuse sweating, itching

Non-steroidal anti-inflammatories: These drugs have mild pain-relieving, anti-inflammatory, and fever-reducing effects. This category includes both non-narcotic analgesics such as aspirin, and non-steroidal anti-inflammatory drugs (NSAIDS) such as Celebrex, ibuprofen, and naproxen. Commonly they cause the following side effects:

Blood: Easy bruising

GI: Stomach upset, bleeding, ulcers

Skin: Rashes

Steroids: The most common steroidal drugs prescribed to cancer patients are prednisone and dexamethasone (Decadron), which have a multitude of uses. At higher doses, steroids function as an antineoplastic. Given in lower doses, a steroid acts as a pain medication because of its anti-inflammatory action. It is used to suppress the immune system in certain leukemias in which a lower lymphocyte count is desired. It may be employed to affect hormone levels, because many cancers arise in tissues that are dependent on hormones, such as breast, uterine, or thyroid cancers. Appetite is also improved on this drug. Prednisone and dexamethasone have many side effects which have implications for bodywork:

Blood: Low platelets, immunosuppression (especially susceptible to fungal infections)

Cardiovascular (CV): More susceptible to hypertension, thrombophlebitis, embolisms, tachycardia

GI: Can cause diarrhea, nausea, abdominal distention, increased appetite

Psychological: Mood changes, euphoria, depression, emotional volatility

Skeletal: Steroids cause calcium to be leached from bones. High dose or long-term use can cause osteoporosis. These patients may need hip and knee replacements more often than normal and their bones may fracture more easily

Skin: Can become parchment-like, wounds heal poorly, petechiae, flushed, sweaty

Other: People on large doses of steroids may not sleep well. They may be very talkative, which they are not able to control. Water retention is common due to electrolyte imbalances.

When I was on prednisone, I was so tired. The most I slept was three hours at a time. Massage gave me a chance to rest.

— EILEEN DOLAN,
PORTLAND, OREGON

ANTICOAGULANTS

The purpose of anticoagulants is to prevent blood clots from forming or to assist in dissolving them. People with cancer are put on these drugs if they have a history of blood clots. These drugs are also known to be effective in reducing tumor formation. The side effects include:

Blood: Low platelets, easy bruising

CNS: Fever

GI: Diarrhea

Skin: Rashes, wheals, severe itching, petechiae

ANTIDEPRESSANTS

Antidepressants are given to cancer patients for psychological and physical reasons. Because depression can amplify the perception of pain, by reducing depression, pain is also lessened. These drugs also help to control a variety of other physical discomforts, such as insomnia and the tingling or burning pain from nerve injury. As with other forms of treatment, these drugs can cause side effects:

CNS: Drowsiness, dizziness

CV: Orthostatic hypotension (causes dizziness when standing up too quickly), tachycardia, hypertension, palpitations

GI Tract: Dry mouth, constipation

Other: Blurred vision

ANTIEMETICS

This group of drugs is used to control nausea and vomiting. Some of them accomplish this by blocking neurotransmitter receptors for serotonin and dopamine. Drugs from other categories are also used to control nausea or are used in conjunction with antiemetics. For example, the steroidal medication Decadron, cannabinoids such as marijuana and Marinol, Ativan, and antihistamines such as Benadryl and Dramamine, are used to quell nausea. Some of the newer antiemetics such as Kytril, Zofran, Aloxi, and Emend have very few

Figure 4.2 The massage therapist continues her ministrations while the nurse attends to the patient's IV catheter.

Photograph by Don Hamilton

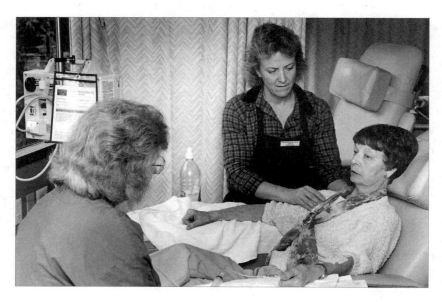

side effects for most people and have tremendous ability to control nausea and vomiting when used in combination with other antiemetics.

Musculoskeletal (MS): Sedation

Other: Distorted perception

ANTIMICROBIALS

Immune suppression is common in people receiving many types of chemotherapy (and biotherapy). At this time, the person is in danger from many organisms that would not bother a person with a healthy immune system. Bacteria, fungi, and viruses are found everywhere and many varieties live on our skin, in our mouths, genitals, and intestinal tract. Indeed, many within the intestinal tract assist in digestion.

When the immune system is suppressed or a person must take antibiotics, a frequent occurrence among those receiving chemo, the normal organisms become opportunistic and get into the blood, the lungs, the urinary tract or the skin. For example, almost everyone carries some form of herpes virus (especially the type which creates cold sores) and/or the varicella virus (responsible for chicken pox and shingles). It is not uncommon for a person who is immune suppressed for any reason to have cold sore or shingles outbreaks.

Three common antimicrobial agents are antibiotics, antifungals, and antivirals. They have similar side effects:

Blood: Some antivirals lower all of the blood cell counts

CNS: Headaches, weakness, dizziness, fever, confusion

Therapists Ask

Q *When is the best time to give massage in relation to chemotherapy?*

A Bodywork can safely be given before, during, or after chemotherapy. When given before, patients find that the anticipatory nausea is quelled. Massage can replace anticipatory nausea with anticipatory pleasure. This is the thinking of Dr. Judy Schmidt in Missoula, Montana. The first person her new patients meet is Sue, a full-time massage therapist in the chemo clinic. By initially associating chemotherapy with massage, patients look forward to coming to the clinic instead of dreading it.

Some people prefer to have massage given while receiving chemotherapy. It provides a relaxing distraction when endless hours must be spent waiting in the outpatient clinic - waiting for drugs to drip into veins, waiting to see the doctor, or waiting for lab results. And, as was seen in a handful of studies, massage, given during chemotherapy, reduces nausea, vomiting, and diarrhea. Touch therapy given during chemotherapy usually focuses on the hands, feet, and lower legs because these are the most accessible parts of the body. But shoulders, neck, and the head are also easy to reach. Sessions are given to a clothed patient sitting in a lounge-type chair.

Some massage clients prefer to receive their sessions immediately after leaving the chemo infusion clinic. This was true of Jane who would drive from her treatment to the massage therapist's office, receive a gentle full-body session and then go home to her four-year-old. Those sessions worked miracles for Jane. Rather than needing to go to bed for several days after infusion, she was able to remain in the flow of family life and take care of her active preschooler.

GI: Nausea, vomiting, diarrhea, anorexia

MS: Fatigue

Skin: Rash, itching

DIURETICS

Diuretics are given to decrease fluid volume retained in the body, by increasing urine output. Most act by increasing the excretion of sodium and chloride, which causes water to follow through osmosis. These drugs may be needed by cancer patients with ascites, fluid build-up related to hormonal changes, chemotherapy, or pulmonary edema.

Blood: Electrolyte imbalance, dehydration, neutropenia, leukopenia, thrombocytopenia

CV: Orthostatic hypotension, dizziness

GI: Nausea

GU: Renal failure

MS: Cramps, stiffness

Skin: Rash, itching

COLONY-STIMULATING GROWTH FACTORS

These medications are used by cancer patients to stimulate the production of white blood cells, red blood cells, and platelets. Blood cells are greatly affected by chemotherapy and sometimes radiation. Hematopoietic drugs bring the blood counts back up more quickly. Without this assistance, patients often must go off their treatment schedule until the white blood cell count in particular reaches a certain level (usually around 2.0 for outpatients). The closer they can stay to the established schedule, the more effective the treatments are. Other hematopoietic drugs increase red blood cell production, which decreases the fatigue associated with poor oxygenation. The growth factors Neupogen and Leukine also are given to trigger the production of stem cells and move them into the blood stream prior to harvesting the cells for a stem-cell transplant. Colony-stimulating growth factors are known for one main side effect:

Skeletal: Deep bone pain

HORMONAL AGENTS

A number of cancers are influenced by hormones. For example, excess estrogen is one of the driving forces behind certain breast cancers, and testosterone is a contributor to prostate cancer. Hormonal medications are given to diminish or block the action of the hormones that feed cancers. For instance, prostate cancer patients are sometimes prescribed estrogen to block the effect of testosterone. The side effects involve:

Reproductive system: Early-onset menopause in women. This can cause hot flashes, insomnia, emotional disturbance, and the other

INFO BOX

Common colony-stimulating growth factors:

- Epogen, Aransep, or Procrit (red blood cells)

- Leukine (various white blood cells)

- Neumega (platelets)

- Neupogen or Neulasta (neutrophils)

INFO BOX

Common hormonal agents for breast and prostate cancer:

- Arimidex – breast
- bicalutamide (Casodex) – prostate
- corticosteroids – breast and prostate
- diethylstilbesterol (DES) – breast and prostate
- finasteride (Proscar) – prostate
- Herceptin - breast
- letrozole (Femara) – breast
- lupron – prostate
- tamoxifen – breast

symptoms typical of menopause. Men who are given female hormones undergo a slight feminizing process in their bodies.

Other: Body image can be an issue for men undergoing hormone therapy

OSTEOGENIC DRUGS

A variety of conditions can weaken the bones of cancer patients. For example, bone fragility can be caused by bone cancer or metastatic spread to bone, certain chemotherapies, radiation to the bone, or hormonal imbalances. Hormones can be disrupted by the sudden onset of menopause, radiation to the reproductive organs, surgical removal of the reproductive organs, or hormone therapies designed to reduce the level of certain hormones, such as estrogen and testosterone. These drugs work by preventing bone loss; some also create bone growth. The common side effects include:

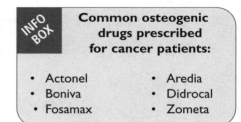

Common osteogenic drugs prescribed for cancer patients:

- Actonel
- Boniva
- Fosamax
- Aredia
- Didrocal
- Zometa

CV: Hypertension

GI: Abdominal pain, anorexia, nausea, constipation, diarrhea, esophageal ulcers (oral formulations)

MS: Bone, joint, and muscle pain, osteonecrosis of the jaw

Other: Fever

BIOTHERAPIES

Biotherapies, sometimes referred to as immunotherapies, are emerging as the fourth main type of cancer treatment. Although this treatment is not nearly as widespread as chemotherapy, radiation, and surgery, it is growing rapidly. Basically, these modalities stimulate immune function, which plays an important role in destroying aberrant cells such as tumor cells. Agents that readers may be aware of include interferon, interleukins, of which there are many, and monoclonal antibodies.

Interferon is a natural part of immune surveillance, recognizing dangerous cells such as pre-cancerous ones, and destroying them. It is activated by the immune system to signal neighboring cells and in turn trigger the resistance mechanism that activates other immune cells. Interleukins, too, are naturally-produced proteins of the immune system. One type, interleukin-2, causes the immune system's T-cells to multiply and perform a variety of functions, including killing cancer cells. Interleukin-2 may also be able to activate natural killer cells which are known to kill tumor cells.[9]

Monoclonal antibodies (MoAbs) are produced by fusing antibody-producing cells and tumor cells. The antibody recognizes specific antigens found on malignant cells and mounts an immune response to the tumor. Two well-known MoAbs are Rituxan, which is given for B cell lymphoma, and Herceptin, an effective agent for certain type of breast cancer that overexpresses a receptor on the cell surface called HER2/neu.[10]

Each of these therapies stimulates the immune system in a unique way; however, the side effects have much in common. All of the agents are toxic. In general, they cause flu-like symptoms, such as fever, chills, fatigue, muscle and joint aches, GI problems, and headaches. Anorexia, neutropenia, and thrombocytopenia also can be present. In addition, interleukins can be responsible for fluid retention; pulmonary, cardiac, and renal toxicity; skin changes, such as rashes, itching, dryness, and erythema; as well as confusion, depression, hallucinations, and paranoia.[9,10] At this point in the chapter, it will be evident to readers that the side effects of biotherapies will also require less vigorous bodywork.

Other immunotherapies are being researched – tumor vaccines and gene therapy, for instance. These cutting-edge treatments are still a thing of the future. Not enough is yet known to generalize about their side effects.

THE DEMAND OF ALTERNATIVE TREATMENTS

Allopathic cancer care can be harsh, invasive, and toxic. This reality drives many patients to look for a cure that seems more gentle and humane. Cancer patients read about, or are told about, alternative methods that may potentially cure cancer and/or support their immune system, detoxify them, or help in other ways in their fight against cancer. A majority of cancer patients seek out alternative treatments such as herbs, supplements, special diets, prayer, bodywork, acupuncture and many other less conventional treatments. Occasionally, people forego mainstream medicine altogether and bank their hopes solely on alternative methods.

Unfortunately, most cancer patients use alternative treatments by self-diagnosing and self-prescribing. If they aren't sleeping, patients will go to the health food store to find an herb that helps with insomnia. Some will see a detox kit and purchase it, thinking that since chemotherapy is now over, they should proactively try to cleanse their body. They consume a variety of substances or try the idea of the day, all without telling their physician or being monitored in any way.

There is a perception by many patients and their practitioners, including some massage therapists, that natural interventions are benign. While many alternative therapies can be benign if used correctly, many interventions can be harmful. They can interact with conventional treatments, they can overload the lymphatic system or detoxification system, and they can cause negative effects.

Bodyworkers should take seriously the side effects created by alternative therapies. Patients should be encouraged to tell their medical doctors what they are taking, as well as seeking medical advice from a qualified naturopathic physician. The alternative therapies patients take may impact the massage session, and patients often do not report to anyone that they are taking these treatments. But it makes no difference whether the fatigue is from radiation

INFO BOX

Integration of Complementary Modalities

Bodyworkers often integrate complementary modalities into their sessions. Aromatherapy, sound, and hot rocks are examples. The concept of less demand must be applied toward these disciplines, as well. Each can impose a level of demand on the person that is fragile from cancer treatment.

Just as with the application of touch, begin with a milder form of the modality. In aromatherapy this could mean the use of Roman chamomile or lavender instead of peppermint, which is a more stimulating essential oil. When using hot rocks, begin with a moderate temperature that is soothing to the body. Remove the rocks after a shorter time.

therapy, a raw foods diet, or graviola, a South American herb. The same adjustments must be made to the massage sessions. Just as with conventional allopathic treatments, the focus, when working with people using alternative therapies, should be on building health, not tearing it down with heavy-handed bodywork. Touch sessions should be a low-impact experience that leaves the client feeling energized, relaxed, and in touch with their body.[11]

PSYCHOLOGICAL DEMANDS OF TREATMENT

To this point, the material has dwelled on the physical side effects of cancer interventions. Equally important are the psychological repercussions. Patients undergo a variety of medical and surgical procedures as part of diagnosing or monitoring the disease. These, along with the treatments for cancer, can be invasive. So, it is no surprise that clients are protective of all or part of their body. Touch practitioners must contact the cancer survivors' body with supreme tenderness and mindfulness so as to help dissipate the fear that has unconsciously lodged in the body. Massage should never re-traumatize the person.

For readers who are not familiar with what cancer patients go through, imagine some of their treatments. Visualize being left alone in a lead-lined room, lying on a stainless steel table while the technicians operate the machinery that is over your head with remote controls because it is too dangerous for them to be in the room. Imagine repeating this every day for 35 days. Try to envision IVs being placed in your arm each time you are given chemotherapy. See yourself having radioactive dye injected into your veins or your neck being awkwardly positioned for 40 minutes while a diagnostic scan is performed. Imagine that your head is locked in a mask that insures there will be no movement while radiation is beamed into your brain, or that your jaw was removed because of tongue cancer, or that your bowels empty into a bag attached to the outside of your body, or that your hair has fallen out. It is no wonder that people with cancer develop post-traumatic stress disorder (PTSD) or, at the least, feel traumatized by these invasive treatments.

The health care providers who must deliver these treatments do their best to be sensitive, but there is an inherent intrusiveness that affects most patients. Touch therapy is one of the best ways to heal the insults to the body, mind, and spirit. In order to accomplish this, practitioners must be willing to set aside their agenda, to move more slowly and more gently into the relationship, with an emphasis on building trust. The body must be cradled and embraced, coaxed and coddled. The overall sense is of "being" with the client rather than "doing" something to them. Enough poking and prodding has occurred already.

Like anyone who has suffered a physical or psychological trauma, cancer patients may be disconnected from their body or the part of the body that has been treated. They may be unaware of how their body

The patient's body must be touched with hands of peace, whispered to, reverently anointed, or handled as if it is a delicate flower.

— AUTHOR

Massage can be an instrument to help people touch deeper places in themselves.

— AUTHOR

feels, including pain levels or areas of holding, and therefore unable to give the massage therapist accurate feedback. Barb, for example, had filled out her intake without noting that she had undergone any kind of surgery. Upon beginning abdominal massage, the therapist noticed a medium-sized scar on the right, lower part of her belly. The therapist slowly and gently touched the scar, asking about its origin. In response, the client gasped with a look of surprise. She had totally blocked out the surgery because the experience was so terrible. When the scar was touched in the massage session, the attending surgeon's face had spontaneously loomed into Barb's mind, causing her alarmed response.

This story illustrates the importance of respecting the emotional story contained within the tissue. For the cancer survivor it may be a story of fear, anger, sadness or even bravery and holding strong in the face of adversity. It is vital to stay within safe emotional boundaries of the client, never trying to coerce them to move ahead with the work until they are ready. Even then, always ask permission and get continual feedback so that the pace is comfortable. Work gently so as to establish an environment of trust with the client. This is important as people with cancer try to regain their wholeness after treatment.

The emotions from cancer treatment can still be locked in the body years later. Sandy, a massage therapist in an oncology massage class, had an emotional reaction when her partner placed a gentle hand on Sandy's sternum as part of a class exercise. Three years before, she had undergone a very painful diagnostic procedure in that area. Until that moment, Sandy had not realized that there was still trauma associated with it.

Jill, another massage therapist attending an oncology massage training, experienced the power of gentle touch. Eight years prior, she had been treated for non-Hodgkins lymphoma. One of the diagnostic exams was a bone marrow biopsy in the hip. Even though Jill had had a great deal of bodywork since then, there was still pain in her hip from the procedure. But, during a gentle touch exercise, Jill released the pain. She described how it rose up to meet the therapist's hands which were neutral and without ambition. The pain was replaced by the wonderful sensations of being touched without an agenda.

When first beginning to work with people living with cancer, err on the side of caution. Go slowly. Do too little rather than too much. Take care on all levels – physical, emotional, and mental. Fears must be honored, physical injuries embraced, and beliefs listened to.

THE EFFECTS OF THE DISEASE PROCESS

Certainly not to be overlooked when deciding on a massage plan are the side effects from the disease itself. Some side effects of cancer are the same as those caused by the treatments, while others are unique to the disease process. Practitioners working with people who are recovering from treatment and showing a decrease in symptoms, can slowly inch forward in the level of demand. However, clients whose disease is worsening will not be candidates for the "inching forward" concept. Instead, therapists will most likely maintain a gentle to moderate level of demand with no attempt to to increase the pressure of strokes.

Following is a list of conditions related to the disease process that will force therapists to reduce the level of demand:

- ascites
- bone metastases
- cachexia
- easy bruising or bleeding
- edema
- fatigue
- osteoporosis
- pain
- risk of clot formation
- thrombocytopenia
- tumor site

HOW TO BE LESS DEMANDING

When performing body-centered therapies with an oncology client, practitioners must make adjustments in three main categories:

1. The level of demand (both physical and psychological)

2. Avoidance of certain sites on the body

3. Positioning

A number of adjustments may be necessary so that the bodywork session is less demanding:

- Decreasing the pressure
- Slowing the speed of the strokes
- Handling the body with great mindfulness
- Decreasing the duration of the sessions
- Changing modalities
- Letting go of the intention to "fix" the client in favor of just "being"
- Giving the sessions at the client's home

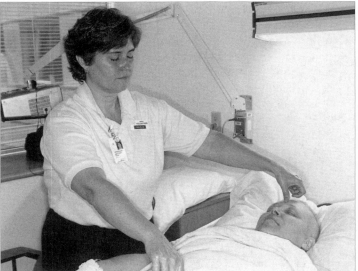

Figure 4.3 Fragile patient receives Polarity Therapy, an undemanding modality.

Generally, not all of these variables need to be changed for each client. Patients require individual adjustments and the modifications might change from week to week. For instance, Alan was very fatigued and depressed during radiation treatment. The two adjustments he consistently needed were a decrease in pressure and slowing the speed of the strokes. One week near the end of his radiation, Alan was so deeply distraught, that he could barely relax enough to lie down. That session ended abruptly as Alan bolted off of the table, unable to lie still for a moment longer.

The majority of oncology patients who are in treatment always require less pressure and slower strokes. By doing this, it is possible to administer nearly any touch technique, even those normally thought of as vigorous, such as trigger-point therapies. Most people also need us to handle the body with exquisite mindfulness. Even then, cancer clients are often brought to tears as the trauma dissipates from their bodies. Lois always cried at the beginning as the therapist's hands lightly cradled her face. Betsy had finished treatment for breast cancer a month previous. Just the placing of the practitioner's hands mindfully onto the treated arm brought a big breath. When asked about that breath, Betsy quietly started to cry and said, "When you touch me, I'm afraid. I was handled so roughly throughout my treatment."

One of the best ways for therapists to lessen the demand is to let go of any intention to fix the person beneath their hands. When practitioners want to "fix," that expectation places a demand on the client, a goal that implies success or failure. And, as Rachel Naomi Remen points out, "There is distance between ourselves and whatever or whomever we are fixing. Fixing is a form of judgment."[12] To be present with people is enough, to embrace their bodies and psyches just as they are. People change when they are received in this way.

GAUGING THE LEVEL OF DEMAND

The side effects of chemotherapy and especially radiation can linger over the long term, forcing bodyworkers to adjust the level of demand for many months and sometimes more than a year.

Gauging the level of demand of massage on a cancer client's body is difficult for both the client and the therapist. Patients who have received massage prior to being diagnosed with and treated for cancer mistakenly believe they can tolerate the same type of bodywork sessions as before. That is never the case, ever. Ever! Even the most robust of clients find that they must modify their activities as they are going through treatment and recovering from it. The most common adjustment to the massage session will be the use of a soothing, nurturing pressure rather than a deep or vigorous one.

The concept central to this chapter is that of "inching forward" with the level of demand. Begin the first session with the idea of creating a baseline. Engage in superficial contact, focusing on no more than the surface layer of muscles. If the person is fragile, use a level of touch that focuses only on the skin. For the first session after the start of treatment, even if client and therapist have worked together for

Beatrice

Beatrice had never had a massage and was hesitant to accept my offer of a foot massage as she received chemotherapy. With her daughter's encouragement, she agreed to try. However, I left for a moment and when I returned, Beatrice had changed her mind and no longer wanted to try the massage. Three weeks before, she'd had her big toe on the right foot amputated from diabetic complications. I was guessing that this was what was worrying her. "How about if I massage the other foot and the opposite hand since it doesn't have a catheter in it?" I suggested. She agreed to this. Beatrice enjoyed the massage so much that when I finished the one foot and hand, she asked to have the treated foot massaged, as well.

— AUTHOR

years, perform the entire massage at an undemanding level, resisting the client's urging for deeper pressure or the therapist's need to do more. Concentrate on restfulness, tranquility, and ease. There should be no attempt to dig deep or fix musculoskeletal problems. Interestingly, even when the massage is gentle, with no specific agenda, amazing clinical outcomes occur. The research is fairly clear about the effect of massage on pain and anxiety. Both of those variables show significant improvement immediately following touch sessions. Anecdotal evidence also suggests that systematic touch can help some people sleep better, temporarily decrease fevers, decrease nausea, improve bowel function, and decrease fatigue. Deep effortful bodywork is not necessary to achieve profound results.

Massage school education trains therapists to ask clients if the pressure they are using is comfortable. While this is a necessary question, it is not an adequate measurement for the therapist. The feedback that a cancer client gives in the moment is not always an indication of what is appropriate. Time and again clients have told stories of how wonderful a massage felt while they were receiving it, only to be in pain or feel flu-ish that evening or the next morning. Granted, this discomfort is temporary and causes no long-term damage, but it can create an aversion to massage, such as occurred with Willie who was mentioned earlier in the chapter (page 60).

Lymphedema, however, is the exception to this rule of "it's only temporary." When lymphedema is triggered, which can happen because of overly vigorous massage, it can cause long-term side effects.

Remembering that many of the side effects of treatment cannot be seen on the surface, the therapist must use other guideposts in order to gauge the appropriate level of demand. **Appearance often cannot be used to gauge the level of demand because patients often appear amazingly healthy.** In fact, bodyworkers must be cautious not to read too much into a client's bright facade. The following three areas can assist the therapist in gauging the level of demand. However, the best course of action is still to inch forward.

Other demands on the body. The body may already be overtaxed from the other interventions and activities. For instance, perhaps the client is zealously trying to regain her health and has increased her level of exercise, is receiving acupuncture, and is taking supplements prescribed by a naturopath to cleanse the liver. Perhaps she is in the process of returning to work after months away or has been packing and lifting heavy boxes in order to move to a new house. Heavy, or even moderate, massage during these times would be ill-advised.

Exercise level. This can tell a practitioner a great deal about how much the body can tolerate. However, do not assume that if the client is able to walk several miles or is back in the gym, that it means the massage does not need to be moderated. It still does need to be given in a restrained manner. (Inch forward!)

Length of time in treatment. The person who has had cancer treatment for years will be less able to tolerate a robust massage.

> ### Paul
>
> I recently saw a lung cancer hospice patient at his home. Paul is a sedentary 70-year-old who is on oxygen. The first session I massaged him in a sitting position focusing on his head and neck, shoulders, hands and feet. A week later he requested that I do some more work with him laying on his hospital bed. He took off his shirt and I again massaged his feet, lower legs, added the arms and back and did head and shoulder work. It was all very gentle.
>
> I was devastated to learn from Paul that he had a lot of muscle aches for two days after the massage session. However, he wants me back and would like to try the bed again but I am feeling a little gun shy.
>
> — JEAN VANETTEN, LMT, ROCHESTER, NEW YORK

Patients who have leanings toward complementary modalities may request that the massage therapist assist them in detoxification of the body. Helping a client detoxify following cancer treatment is an appropriate goal, but it should come after other things have been accomplished. Confidence in the body must be regained, the trauma of undergoing medical treatment dissipated, wholeness reestablished. The "new normal" must be discovered. All of this may take months or more. Detoxification regimens place demand on the entire body, a body that is still processing the consequences of chemotherapy, radiation, or surgery. Wait until the client is well-recovered from the obvious side effects of treatment, such as fatigue and immuno-suppression, and is no longer on a long list of medications.

FINAL THOUGHTS

After wading through this chapter with its long lists of side effects, readers may be feeling that they shouldn't work with cancer patients for fear they will break. That was surely not the purpose. The goal was twofold: 1) to make therapists aware of how taxing the various parts of cancer treatment are on the entire person, body, heart, and soul; and 2) to convey that nearly all cancer patients can receive some sort of touch therapy if certain adjustments are made, particularly if the level of demand is decreased. Skilled touch can be given at every stage of the cancer experience: during hospitalization, during the pre- or post-op period, in the out-patient clinic, during chemotherapy and radiation, during recovery at home, remission or cure, and in the end stages of life. Not only are physical needs addressed, but emotional, social, and spiritual ones are, as well.

It is true that cancer and cancer treatment limit the massage choices. But within those limits, there are many rich and creative possibilities for touch. [13]

— TRACY WALTON, LMT,
CAMBRIDGE, MASSACHUSETTS

Acknowledgment: Parts of this chapter previously appeared in Bodywork for Cancer Patients: The Need for a Less-Demanding Approach. *Massage and Bodywork*. June/July 2005, pp 16–26.

Examples of touch techniques that can be given with minimal or no change (ideal during treatment):

Bowen Technique
Compassionate Touch ®
Cranialsacral therapies
Healing Touch

Jin Shin Jyutsu ®
Polarity Therapy
Reiki
Therapeutic Touch

Examples of touch techniques that can be used during treatment and recovery, but only if the level of demand is greatly reduced:

Acupressure
Aston-Patterning ®
Ayurvedic Massage
Bindegewebmassage
Lomilomi (gentle strokes only)
Lymph drainage therapies
Fascial release

Myotherapy
Neuromuscular Therapy
Russian Massage
Seated Chair Massage
Swedish Massage
Trigger Point Therapy
Zero Balancing ®

Examples of deep bodywork modalities that call for a lengthy waiting period before administering:

Hellerwork
Lomilomi
Pfrimmer Deep Muscle Therapy ®

Rolfing ®
Thai Massage

REFERENCES

1. Iwamoto R. *Radiation Therapy in Oncology Massage*, 4th Ed. St. Louis, MO: Mosby, 2001.

2. Zuther J. *Lymphedema Management: The Comprehensive Guide for Practitioners*. Thieme. 2005. New York, NY: Thieme Medical Publishers.

3. Fransman W, Vermrulen R, Krombout H. Occupational Dermal Exposure to Cyclophosphamide in Dutch Hospitals: A Pilot Study. *Annals of Occupational Hygiene*. 2004;48(3):237-244.

4. Sessink PJM, Bos PB. Drugs Hazardous to Healthcare Workers – Evaluation Methods for Monitoring Occupational Exposure to Cytostatic Drugs. *Drug Safety*, 1999;April 20 (4):347-359.

5. Hirst M, Mills DG, Tse S, et al. Occupational Exposure to Cyclophosphamide. *The Lancet*. January 28, 1984. pp.186-188.

6. Duncan JH, Colvin OM, Fenselau C. Mass Spectrometric Study of the Distribution of Cyclophosphamide in Humans. *Toxicology and Applied Pharmacology*. 1973;24:317-323.

7. Madsen ES, Larsen H. Excretions of Mutagens in Sweat from Humans Treated with Anti-Neoplastic Drugs. *Cancer Letters*. 1988;40:199-202.

8. Tolerance, Physical Dependence and Addiction. Available at: http://www.whocancerpain.wisc.edu/eng/11_3/tpda.html. Accessed June 30, 2006.

9. Immunotherapy: Interleukin-2. Available at: http://www.melanomacenter.org/treatment/interleukin.html. Accessed June 30, 2006.

10. Monoclonal Antibodies. Available at: http://www.meds.com/immunotherapy/monoclonal_antibodies.html. Accessed June 30, 2006.

11. Weizer K, N.D. Interview with author on January 30, 2006.

12. Remen R. In the Service of Life. *Noetic Sciences Review*. Spring 1996. pp.24-25.

13. Walton T. Clinical Thinking and Cancer. *Massage Therapy Journal*. Fall 2000. pp.68-80.

Chapter 5

First Do
No Harm

Adjusting for Common Side
Effects of Cancer Treatment

Bodyworkers commonly believe that the type of cancer is the most important factor when planning a massage session. In reality, it is the treatments that are most influential. There are hundreds of types of cancer, each of which can manifest in unique ways depending upon the individual. To try to categorize massage adjustments by the disease would be time-consuming and inefficient. It is easier to become familiar with the general side effects of chemotherapy, radiation, and surgery.

By making the right adjustments, massage can be given at nearly every stage of cancer treatment. Not only can it be given, it should be given. Skilled touch provides comfort, connection, or distraction. It offers support during medical procedures or can be an expression of affection. Fatigue can be alleviated or wholeness regained.

No matter the purpose, the prime goal that must underlie the administration of all massage, especially during and after treatment is this: First Do No Harm. Therapists generally believe that if their intention is positive, no harm can come to clients. Trusting that one's good intention will keep patients safe is not always enough. Many cancer patients have been inadvertently harmed by well-intentioned therapists. A compassionate, well-intentioned heart

Decades of nurturing instinct came through your hands, especially in those last 10 minutes. I did not have a chance to give you a long enough hug to express my thanks. Thank you for creating an environment that makes being an expressive human being feel safe and normal.

MICHAEL, WHO USED MASSAGE IN
PREPARATION FOR SURGERY
FOR A BRAIN TUMOR

must be combined with clinical knowledge in order to create a safe environment.

Massage is something that many people with cancer look forward to because it makes them forget their disease for a short time. It is something that reminds them that they can still participate in normal activities. Those who have been through cancer treatment must, however, find their "new normal." Sometimes this new normal is temporary, lasting through the treatment and recovery period. Often, the new normal is permanent, activities must be reduced, ROM never quite returns, or job schedules must be less demanding. A new normal must also be established for bodywork sessions. Clients will no longer be able to tolerate the same level of vigor during treatment. Some will fully recover, while others will require long-term adjustments.

Most importantly, ALL people with cancer, in treatment for cancer, or recovering from cancer, can receive touch therapy of some kind. The only group of patients who must temporarily suspend bodywork sessions are those who are receiving radiation therapy that makes them radioactive. However, this is a minute percentage of patients and the suspension is usually for a few days to a week. Otherwise, with the right adjustments to the session, everyone with a history of cancer can enjoy the benefits of massage.

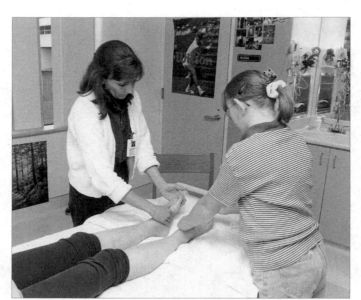

Figure 5.1 Massage can be given at every stage of the cancer experience by family or professional.

The previous chapter explained the clinical reasons for reducing the level of demand on people in treatment or recovering from it. This chapter is an extension of the previous one and expands into the topic of safety. A safe massage plan revolves mainly around the side effects of chemotherapy, radiation, and surgery. Except near the end of life, the disease itself does not require major adjustments to the bodywork sessions.

The massage adjustments in this chapter are organized around three categories. The first, **pressure**, is a vital part of lessening the demand and is the most important adjustment in terms of safety. Too much pressure or vigor can leave people feeling fatigued, nauseated, or in pain. Heavy pressure often feels comfortable at the time of the massage. It is later in the day that the client feels unwell. Therapists must realize the importance of this fact. This piece of information has been placed in various chapters throughout the book because it is so crucial.

Another frequent adjustment is **site** restrictions, perhaps due to an incision, central IV catheter, or skin condition. Thirdly, adjustments are often needed in **positioning**. For example, a person with lung cancer may be unable to lie face down on the massage table or may need the head elevated because of breathing difficulties. Breast cancer patients invariably must lie on their sides for months after surgery. The

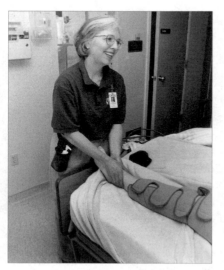

Figure 5.2 With the right adjustments, everyone with cancer can enjoy the benefits of massage.

Figures 5.1 and 5.2 by Don Hamilton

Massaging Feet and Telling Stories

Massaging someone's feet in the infusion room lends itself more to the sharing of stories than to the rubbing of one's extremities. It's as if when the movement of hands on feet begins, the cover of the book opens and the relating of life unfolds.

I have found time and time again that both the receiver and the giver initially connect with touch; however, the opportunity to connect at a much deeper level almost always presents itself. There is safety in touching the feet. And the position of the therapist and patient, face-to-face and eye-to-eye, affords the means to communicate in a multifaceted way. With the exception of asking a couple of leading questions, I spend little time talking and open my ears and heart to what is about to transpire.

Although each story is as unique as the person telling it, there seems to be a pattern in the lives that we share with each other. Important family members and friends and their influence on the person's cancer experience are mentioned: who has stayed and who has left because the experience was either a new opportunity or a fearful obstruction; what it was like to be "hit" with a cancer diagnosis; or, what meaning is unfolding for this person diagnosed with cancer.

The practice for me becomes one of being present. I spend so much of my life rushing around, planning projects, talking to people. To sit in the presence of another, telling me their intimate and unique story, becomes a sacred experience. It is an honor to receive the gift of sharing this special life experience. And then I realize that we are in this dance of giving and receiving, touching each other in ways that words cannot. For me, massaging feet is one of my favorite ways to open the cover of a new book, a new story, a new adventure.

— JAMIE DAMICO, RN, CMT,
FLORISSANT, CO

brain cancer patient who is dizzy may need extra assistance getting off and on the table and in dressing and undressing. Extra time and effort is needed from the therapist to ensure clients are comfortable on the table. People often need permission or encouragement to try positions other than the typical prone and supine options. Some will need to stay in their recliner or wheelchair. Others will find that massage chairs are impossible because of radiation burns on the chest or breathing difficulties.

In the following pages, information will be presented about specific conditions that are associated with cancer or its treatment and how to safely administer bodywork without doing harm. Some side effects are temporary, others can last a life time. The side effects are listed in alphabetical order. This in no way represents the severity or frequency of various conditions. They are presented in this way for ease of referencing. If the list were given in order of most important conditions to least

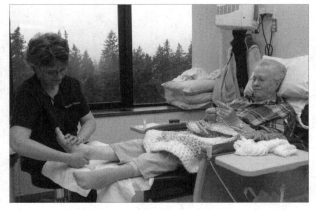

Figure 5.3 Knitting, massage and chemo.

Photograph by David J. Lawton

important, the top three would be neutropenia, thrombocytopenia, and thromboembolic disorders. Not every side effect is given in this chapter because the number of them is too great.

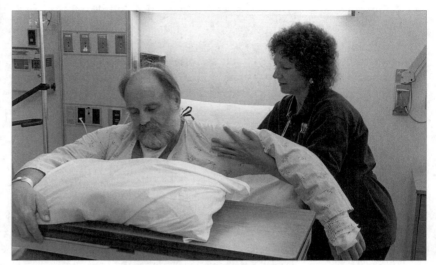

Figure 5.4 Positioning is one of the adjustments that must often be made.   Photograph by Don Hamilton

ALOPECIA

When she put her hands on my head, I felt like God was touching me.

CATHERINE, BREAST CANCER CLIENT, WASHINGTON, DC

Alopecia is the medical term for loss of hair, a frequent side effect of certain chemotherapies or radiation to the head. Chemo patients lose their hair because the anti-tumor drugs are toxic to hair cells on the scalp. The shaft becomes brittle, causing the hair to break off. This is not a dangerous condition but is psychologically distressing for some, especially women. For many, this is the worst aspect of treatment.

When a person has a host of conditions that prevent bodywork to the whole body or that prevent firm pressure, the head is an area that is nearly always safe to massage. Therapists should be respectful of patients' desire to keep the head covered. Offer to massage the scalp, but never push the idea onto the patient. Patients who do experience head massage generally come to love it. The wig, scarf, or colorful hat then comes off quickly, sometimes with wild abandon.

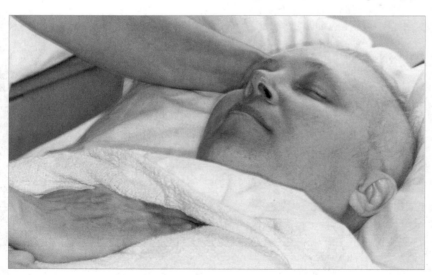

Figure 5.5 The head can almost always be safely massaged.

Photograph by Don Hamilton

Massage Adjustments

Pressure:
- The scalp is sensitive at times, requiring practitioners to be mindful of pressure. Patients complain of itching, burning, and tingling sensations.

Site:
- At first, the head may be off-limits for some patients without hair, usually because of shyness. Once they have experienced their first scalp massage, a comfortable rapport develops between therapist and client.

Other:
- Massage to the head of someone losing their hair will yield clumps of hair. Place a towel or pillow case under the head to remove the hair after the massage. Remember, too, that the hair on the entire body will fall, not just the head hair. During this time, give the touch session without lubricant.

ANEMIA

Red blood cells, the component of blood that delivers oxygen to tissues, can be affected by chemotherapy, radiation, and sometimes by certain cancers, especially leukemia. A drop in red blood cells is referred to as anemia. The main side effects are fatigue, shortness of breath, and chills. One function of red blood cells is the conservation of heat. This is why the person chills easily when the RBCs are in short supply. The level of demand must be lowered for several reasons.

Massage Adjustments

Pressure:
- Fatigue

- Inability of the vital organs to function at peak levels

Other:
- Keep plenty of clean blankets handy in case clients are chilled.

ANOREXIA-CACHEXIA SYNDROME

People in treatment for cancer or in the advanced stage of the disease can become nutritionally depleted in a couple of ways. Anorexia is the loss of appetite. Cachexia, a state of wasting and malnutrition, includes anorexia and metabolic changes triggered by the disease. Anorexia can occur because of the effect of the treatments on GI functioning, taste or metabolic changes, anxiety about the cancer, pain, or fatigue. One way that the disease process can trigger cachexia is through the release of cytokines, small chemical messengers which accompany inflammation. The metabolic rate rises and the breakdown of protein increases, including in skeletal muscle. Wasting, weight loss, fatigue, immunosuppression, and the inability to perform daily activities of living occur.[1,2]

...tell the client who is completely bald that she is beautiful, in some way. Compliment her beautiful eyes or cheekbones or the shape of her head; find something wonderful to say about her choice of wig. These patients are, understandably, very aware of their personal sense of beauty and are often quite upset about this part of their care.

— CHARLOTTE VERSAGI,
LMT, ROYAL OAKS, MICHIGAN

Massage Adjustments

Pressure: • Fatigue, loss of body mass, and immunosuppression all require a less demanding approach.

• The use of broad strokes is often better for people who have undergone severe weight loss rather than an acupressure style of bodywork.

Site: • Be especially mindful of thinning skin over bony prominences or areas in which the skin shows evidence of decubitus ulceration.

Positioning: • Change of position is one of the most effective ways of maintaining the health of the skin. Even if it is time-consuming and requires extra effort, encourage repositioning.

BONE FRAGILITY

The bones of a cancer patient can become fragile for a number of reasons – bone metastases, osteoporosis due to steroid use or chemotherapy (usually for breast, ovarian, or prostate cancers), and radiation to the bone. No matter the cause, the adjustments to the massage plan will be the same. Mindfulness about pressure will always be needed and sometimes adjustments to positioning or avoidance of the fragile areas. This is needed because the bone lacks the normal strength and is vulnerable to breaking. Certain bones, such as the humerus, femur, and spinal column, may be reinforced with rods.

Fragile bones may or may not be accompanied by pain. In the middle stages of the disease, bone metastases especially may feel like a deep ache. Muscular guarding of the fragile area further adds to the discomfort of the bone pain. As the disease advances, the pain can be difficult to tolerate and people may prefer not to be touched.

There is nothing stronger in the world than tenderness.

— HAN SUYIN

Massage Adjustments

Pressure: • Some patients with fragile bones can benefit from and tolerate light to moderate pressure that is controlled and mindful.

• Therapists should work only with soft tissue, mindful not to compress the skeletal system.

• People with mild to moderate bone fragility may be able to tolerate gentle ROM exercises performed slowly and with great mindfulness, avoiding extreme positions.

Site: • Areas of severe fragility may cause pain to the client, especially in the case of advanced bone metastases. Clients may prefer that these areas be avoided.

• Avoid pressure in areas of bony prominence.

Positioning: • Spinal metastases may require positioning adjustments. Some patients can be positioned on their side. Others may need to be log-rolled when changing positions.

• Avoid extreme positions that unduly strain an area with fragile bones. For example, the person with pelvic mets should not receive extreme stretching of the lower extremities.

INFO BOX

Patterns of Metastatic Spread Related to Bone

Breast and prostate cancer account for approximately 80% of bone metastases.[3] Awareness of this condition is important as the affected bones are vulnerable to breaking and cannot tolerate vigorous bodywork.

Breast: thoracic spine/ribs/pelvis/ humerus/upper femur

Prostate: hips/spine/femur/ribs

Lung: spine/skull/ribs/scapula/other bones

Other primary cancers that may have bone spread: thyroid, kidney

Less frequent spread to bone: colon, stomach, pancreatic, testicular, liver, melanoma, esophageal

BREATHING DIFFICULTY

Breathing difficulty can be brought on by tumors or fluid in the lungs, ascites, medications, pneumonia, or radiation to the lungs, to name just some. Positioning will be one of the major adjustments to the massage session.

Fear and anxiety can also cause shortness of breath or rapid breathing, and vice versa. Touch is extremely helpful during such times. Something as simple as holding the patient's feet or head can relax the breath.

Massage Adjustments

Pressure: • The person who is having difficulty breathing needs a gentle, sedating pressure.

Positioning: • Lying prone (and for some, even supine) will increase the breathing difficulty.

• For some, side-lying will be manageable.

• Those with severe shortness of breath or coughing should be positioned on their back with the head and/or upper body elevated.

In Desperation

I have nursed for many years on bone marrow transplant units in several large, urban teaching hospitals. One very dear patient, a young man in his 30's, had undergone an allogeneic transplant and had developed a number of complications. As my night shift evolved, his ability to breathe was decreasing, and his anxiety level was extremely high. We had tried a number of different interventions including a face mask that delivered 60% oxygen. Nothing would coax his oxygen level above 90%, which was lower than we wanted it to be. In desperation, while standing at his feet, I began instinctively to massage them. I saw him visibly relax. But even better, I also watched his oxygen level stabilize to the safe range. As long as I massaged his feet, his breathing remained calm and even.

— MARY JANE SHANNON, RN, SYRACUSE, NEW YORK

*Once safe practice guidelines for a
given client are clear, corroborated by
the client's medical staff and
understood by all, the therapist is
released from the fear and confusion
about massage and cancer. Once
liberated, they are free to focus on
the quality of their own presence.
They are free, as well, to approach
the client's body with reverence for
its multiple strengths. A massage
therapist is in a unique position,
within the sacred medium of physical
contact, to witness the client in all of
their wholeness.*[5]

— TRACY WALTON, LMT,
CAMBRIDGE, MASSACHUSETTS

CONSTIPATION

Constipation may seem trivial when compared to some of the permanent side effects caused by cancer treatments, but it can make or break a patient's quality of life. Narcotic pain medications and certain chemotherapies are the common culprits, resulting in sluggish bowels. Other causes can be tumor obstruction in the bowel, compression on the intestinal or spinal nerves, pressure from ascites, and dehydration.

Many interventions can contribute to healthy bowels: sufficient water intake, good nutrition, stool softeners, laxatives, and exercise. Massage also can assist in keeping the bowels moving, especially when the cause is sluggishness. A group of 15 British hospice patients attending a day-care center had fair success in using a self-care routine. They were taught to do self abdominal massage for use at home. All of the people had less abdominal distension and flatulence after one week of practicing the technique. Five patients felt that their bowel function had become more normal within four weeks time. Three others reported theirs to be more normal after six weeks. (The remaining seven clients dropped out of the project prior to its ending.)

There are times, however, when abdominal massage is inadvisable. The following are contraindications for abdominal massage:

- known or suspected abdominal obstruction

- large abdominal tumor

- presently receiving radiation to the abdomen or is within six weeks of the end of treatment

- recent abdominal surgery[4]

Even when the abdomen should be avoided, the remainder of the body can be massaged. The general relaxation of massage will still be beneficial.

Attention to this problem is best given from the start of treatment rather than after the bowels have already become sluggish. The practitioner can give whatever abdominal massage is part of her bodywork tradition and teach the client or a family member to do a twice daily self-routine. This routine could be a simple Swedish one in the direction of peristaltic flow, or attention to the digestive zones on the hands and feet.

Massage Adjustments

Pressure: • Adjust pressure to the client's comfort.

Site: • At times constipation can be so severe that the person cannot tolerate any touch to the area.

• When touch is intolerable to the abdomen, bodywork can be given to reflex zones instead, or as Polarity Therapy above and below the belly.

Positioning: • The person who is in discomfort from constipation may not want to change positions at all, happy to remain in a supine position for the entire session.

Other: • Diet, water consumption, and exercise play a big role, as well. The bodyworker might encourage the person in treatment to consult with a nutritional expert in oncology-related matters.

EDEMA

Edema is the accumulation of fluid between cells. In cancer patients it can be the result of many different factors – nutrition, renal or cardiac dysfunction, inactivity, blood clot, and tumor growth are possible causes. Certain medications, inflammation, or electrolyte imbalance also can contribute to edema. (This condition is not to be confused with lymphedema, which is often the result of lymph node removal or radiation to certain clusters of nodes. Lymphedema is characterized by the presence of protein in the fluid. This subject is covered in detail beginning on page 96.)

Edematous tissues are puffy and fragile. The skin integrity may be poor due to being overstretched, thereby increasing the chance of a pressure sore or skin breakdown. People with edema often have reduced blood flow, which further aids skin breakdown.[6]

Since massage during cancer treatment is focused on comfort, people with edema can often receive some type of touch therapy, such as light lotioning to the legs. This is usually true even for patients with renal or cardiac insufficiency. The key is to not place an extra demand on these systems. This can be accomplished with non-forceful pressure and by shortening the length of the session.

Edema is sometimes a by-product of infection or a blood clot. When this is the case, therapists are cautioned against the use of touch therapies that involve movement or pressure. Swelling due to obstructions, such as a tumor, would also preclude the use of any type of touch that moves fluid. Techniques such as Reiki that do not use pressure or stroking have been safely substituted in these cases. However, only perform touch therapies with the doctor's or other health care practitioner's permission. Bodyworkers who give massage in a medical center that is particularly conservative might be wise to avoid administering any type of touch therapy to an edematous site caused by infection or clots. This will avoid the perception of wrong-

INFO BOX

Additional Resources

• Curties D. *Massage Therapy and Cancer*, 2nd Ed. Toronto, Ontario, Canada: Curties-Overzet Publications, 2007.

• Guided Imagery for Cancer Patients www.healthjourneys.com.

• Edited by Mackereth P, Carter A. *Massage and Bodywork – Adapting Therapies for Cancer Care*. Churchill Livingstone, 2006.

• Kuner S, Orsborn CM, Quigley L, et al. *Speak the Language of Healing: Living with Breast Cancer without Going to War*. Conari Press, 1999.

• Lorde A. *The Cancer Journals*. Aunt Lute Books, 1980.

• Persad R. *Massage Therapy and Medications*. Curties-Overzet Publications, 2001.

• Wible J. *Pharmacology for Massage Therapy*. Lippincott Williams and Wilkins, 2005.

doing should any problem arise. Instead, focus on the hands, shoulders, face, and head, if these areas are unaffected.

The guidelines listed below are intended for use with edema. Later on in this chapter, the phenomenon of lymphedema is discussed. With a few exceptions, the guidelines are similar. However, the two types of edema have very different causes and outcomes and call for separate discussion.

Massage Adjustments

Pressure:
- Use a light effleurage or light rhythmical compressions with the palm, massaging toward the heart.

- Edematous tissues are fragile. Use only the amount of pressure required for lotioning.

- The skin in the swollen area may also have poor integrity if the edema is a chronic condition. Avoid touch to any areas that are not intact.

- Reduced duration may be necessary to prevent overloading major organ systems.

- A limb with edema due to a blood clot (or suspected clot) should not be massaged with any stroking motions. Resting the hands gently on the limb is the only allowable touch.

Site:
- Begin massaging at the most proximal section of the limb (the upper arm or thigh), then move down to the next section (the forearm or lower leg), and then do the hand or foot. Massaging in this sequence allows the area upstream to empty, thereby creating space for the fluid that will drain from the lower regions.

- Give attention to the joints, as fluid pools there. Passive ROM exercises could be used to assist the movement of fluid through the elbow.

- Limbs with obstruction or infection-related edema should be avoided. Resting the hands on the limb or using energy modalities may be substituted with staff approval.

- A limb with edema due to a blood clot should be avoided.

Positioning:
- Elevate affected limbs

- Be mindful of placing the person in a side-lying position on an edematous limb as it may be uncomfortable. Additionally, the weight of the body may create an occlusion, especially in the upper body.

I had expected the heavy-handed, "chop chop" massage seen in the movies. I was pleasantly surprised to receive such light, supportive touch.

— KAREN, +200 DAYS SINCE BONE MARROW TRANSPLANTATION

FATIGUE

Fatigue is the most common and distressing symptom associated with cancer and its treatments. Cancer-related fatigue can occur for varying reasons, most of which are related to treatment. It may be due to a low red blood cell count, a side effect of chemotherapy and sometimes radiation, organ toxicity, or an over-burdened lymphatic system. Some medications can contribute to fatigue, decreased activity creates lethargy, and then there are a host of psychological variables that bring a person's energy down, such as fear, hopelessness, or feeling out of control. All in all, it significantly lowers quality of life. Many peoples' vigor does return but it always takes at least a number of months and sometimes years. Others never again regain their full energy due to permanent side effects of treatment.

There are new medications or medical interventions to remedy many of the side effects of treatment, but no standardized treatments exist for the problem of fatigue. Possibly massage therapy has an important role to play in this area. Currently, only a small amount of scientific evidence exists to indicate that massage has a positive effect on fatigue, but clients frequently report increased energy following bodywork sessions. They report being able to run errands, shop, exercise, and spend time with family. Bodywork that is demanding should be avoided until the patient's energy returns to normal or near normal. One way to gauge this is by the amount of exercise, house or yard work the person is able to do compared to pre-treatment.

Massage Adjustments

Pressure: • Use light to moderate pressure throughout treatment phase.

• As the patient recovers, slowly inch forward with the pressure.

Positioning: • Severely fatigued clients may tolerate only minimal repositioning.

Other: • Severe fatigue may require shorter sessions.

HAND AND FOOT SYNDROME

Hand-foot syndrome (HSF) is a skin reaction, usually on the palms of the hand and sometimes on the soles of the feet, that is caused by certain chemotherapies, such as Doxil, Xeloda, and 5FU. Hand-foot syndrome is not to be confused with peripheral neuropathy. HFS is characterized by skin that is red, swollen, blistered, cracked, tender, or painful and can be accompanied by numbness or tingling. These side effects are the result of small amounts of the drug leaking from capillaries in the palms of the hands or soles of the feet.[7] Mild HFS is

After my massage at the oncology clinic, I felt energized and productive that evening and on into the next day. This surprised me because in the past, I have felt "wiped out" by massage.

CHERYL, BREAST CANCER CLIENT,
PORTLAND, OREGON

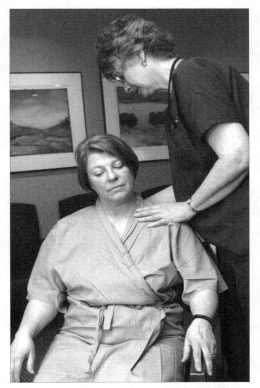

Figure 5.6 Massage that is undemanding often improves a client's energy.
Photograph by David J. Lawton

not particularly problematic. In its severe form, however, it is extremely painful when walking or using the hands. Breakdown of the skin causes easy entrance for the microorganisms that cause infections.[8]

Massage Adjustments

Pressure: • If HFS is mild, gentle pressure is usually tolerated.

• Patients will tolerate massage to the hands and feet after the first round of the chemotherapy, but after two or three rounds, those areas should be avoided.

Site: • DO NOT massage areas that are moderately or severely affected. The skin is too fragile.

• DO NOT apply heat. It too increases drug leakage. Also, friction increases the amount of drug leakage.

Positioning: • Elevation of the affected area may provide some relief.

Now I know what the hands of an angel feel like.

— FRANK, BONE MARROW
TRANSPLANT PATIENT,
PORTLAND, OREGON

HERPES, SHINGLES, AND CHICKENPOX

These three diseases are caused by the same family of viruses and are a serious event to someone with cancer. Varicella, the virus responsible for shingles and chickenpox, can disseminate to the liver, spleen, central nervous system, GI tract, bone marrow, and lymph nodes. Herpes and varicella are viruses that remain dormant in the body and become reactivated during times of immunosuppression, which is common for those with cancer.

Massage Adjustments

Site: • Shingles eruptions occur predominantly on the torso. The safest and most comfortable course of action is to give massage on the extremities until the skin lesions have healed and the scabs have disappeared. Shingles can be very painful even for months after the lesions have healed.

• Avoid areas with lesions.

Other • When either of these viruses is present, glove, even if the infection is far from the area being massaged.

LYMPHEDEMA

No group of patients is affected by lymphedema more than people treated for cancer. Although lymphedema can be caused by congenital influences, surgery for conditions other than cancer, or be the result of trauma, cancer treatment is one of the most common causes. Lymph nodes removed from or radiated in the neck, axilla, or groin are the main cause, although it can also arise when lymphatic channels are obstructed by a tumor or surgery damages the pathways.

The lymphatic system has been likened to a sewage treatment plant with the lymph nodes acting as the filtering system for plasma protein molecules, fats, cellular debris, and bacteria and virus. If the lymph nodes have been removed or damaged by radiation, the "sewage" contained in that part of the lymphatic system goes unfiltered or is poorly filtered. Movement through the system also occurs more slowly, creating a back-up into the affected quadrant. This back-up of excess fluid and protein is lymphedema. Unfiltered protein is one of the problematic aspects of lymphedema and sets it apart from "edema." Left unfiltered, excess protein causes tissues to thicken and become fibrotic. Lymph then stagnates, providing a medium for bacterial growth which in turn increases the risk of infection.

Proteins are recycled from the vascular system through the lymphatics. During cancer treatment, the protein load dramatically increases due to cellular breakdown. This breakdown includes tumor cells that have been killed off by treatments and other cells from the body affected by chemo or radiation. The lining of the GI tract is a good example of non-tumor cells that break down during treatment. This explains why a patient who is at risk for lymphedema will sometimes develop it during chemotherapy. The by-products of chemo overload the lymphatic system.

Key to safe practice with these clients is understanding the direction in which the superficial lymphatic fluid drains. In people whose lymphatic system is intact, lymph converges toward two main groups of nodes, the axillary and inguinal. As shown in Figure 5.6, two main watersheds divide the body into quadrants. If some of the nodes in a quadrant have been removed and/or damaged by radiation therapy, the capacity of the lymphatic system is lessened in that quadrant. The combination of surgical removal AND radiotherapy further decreases the lymphatic transport capacity of the affected quadrant and increases the possibility of lymphedema.

A third watershed is present just above the clavicles. It drains lymph from the neck and head. Removal of nodes from the main clusters in the neck, or radiation to this area, can create lymphedema in the neck or head. This might occur as a result of such cancers as tonsil, tongue, or sinus.

Many events can trigger lymphedema. Insect bites, overuse, and airplane flights are prime examples. Overly vigorous massage, too, can trigger lymphedema or exacerbate an existing case of it. Deep, or even moderate, bodywork can cause hyperemia which is characterized by reddening of the skin. The affected quadrant of a person whose lymphatic capacity has been diminished cannot always handle the greater fluid volume created by hyperemia. Vigorous massage can also initiate the inflammatory process which triggers the release of histamines. Histamines cause fluid to migrate to the area, further burdening a compromised lymphatic system.[9]

Therapists Ask

Q What is the difference between edema and lymphedema?

A Edema is the accumulation of fluid between the cells and is the sign of an underlying condition, such as congestive heart failure or hormonal imbalance. Joachim Zuther, one of the leading Manual Lymph Drainage educators, defines lymphedema as "protein-rich edema."[8] It is the excess protein and cellular debris that differentiate lymphedema from edema.

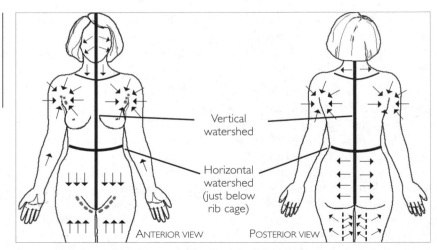

Figure 5.7 Two main watersheds divide the body into quadrants. In people whose lymphatics are undamaged, most of the superficial lymph drains toward the axillary or inguinal nodal clusters. Lymph from the head and neck drain toward a third watershed just above the clavicles.

Sentinel Node Biopsy

Years ago surgeons removed all of a person's lymph nodes when performing a mastectomy. Therapists who massage breast cancer patients treated in the 1970's or even the 80's, will encounter this situation. These patients are at increased risk for lymphedema compared to present-day clients who more and more often have a sentinel node biopsy. In this procedure, instead of removing nodes without clinical evidence for the need, just one or two nodes are taken. This is done by injecting a radioisotope accompanied with dye into the region. The surgeon is able to see on a monitor where the dye travels to first. It is this node and usually the next that are sent to pathology for viewing. If the cancer has not spread to the sentinel node, the others are spared from dissection, leaving the patient's lymphatic system in a healthier condition.

Not only does inflammation increase the fluid load, it can also increase the protein load. Proteins include not only those recycled from the vascular system, but also proteins from cellular breakdown, such as occurs when a tumor is being killed by chemotherapy or radiation. Non-tumor cells, such as the lining of the GI tract, also become part of the protein load. The lymphatic system of a person with diminished transport capacity will be pushed to the limit and perhaps beyond by the increased protein load. One of the problems related to excess proteins in the tissue is that of increased collagen production by fibroblasts. This goes on to create hardening or sclerosis of the edematous tissue. Drainage of the extremity is then further complicated.

It is those who are being treated on an outpatient basis, such as in the radiation oncology department, or clients who finished their treatment years ago, that present the most complicated scenario for massage practitioners. Unfortunately, there is no way to know which of the individual patients who are at risk for lymphedema will develop an occurrence of it. Many go their entire life without an incident. Others constantly have residual fluid which waxes and wanes in the affected limb. Some teeter unknowingly on the brink of lymphedema until a certain confluence of events overloads the lymphatic system. For one breast cancer patient it was the strain of moving from one house to another, followed by an out-of-town guest for a week, which caused her to become "run-down," and the final straw was moving buckets of rocks while landscaping the new front yard. These events increased the burden on the patient's lymphatic system, a system that could no longer handle such an overload.

The statistics regarding lymphedema occurrence vary widely. Breast cancer patients are most commonly affected. The range for them has been reported to be as few as 5% to as high as 40%.[11,12] However, the lymph nodes of many other cancer patients are either surgically removed or radiated, also putting them at risk. The person treated for a head and neck cancer may have the nodes in the neck dissected or radiated. The axillary nodes of a lung cancer patient may be affected by treatment or the inguinal nodes of a colon or ovarian cancer patient. It is vital to ask all people with a history of cancer treatment if they have had lymph nodes removed or treated with radiotherapy. It is difficult to know statistically just how many people develop lymphedema because it can manifest many years after treatment has occurred.

There is no curing or reversing lymphedema, only constant monitoring and management. Not only are people at increased risk for infection in the affected limb; their body image can be affected, as well as activities of daily living. The excess fluid creates heaviness in the limb which can cause discomfort, joint pain, loss of mobility, and postural problems. Once a person has had an occurrence of lymphedema, future episodes may happen more easily and take longer to vanish. This is because the muscular pumping units called lymphangions wear out as they continually pump against the resistance caused by the excess fluid. It could be compared to the fatigue caused by swimming upstream.

The management of lymphedema is a complex situation and requires a great deal of training. Only practitioners with lengthy, supervised training, such as occurs with Manual Lymphatic Drainage or Lymph Drainage Therapy, should attempt to manage a person's lymphedema. Touch practitioners without training in lymphedema management should refer clients to a specialist. The rehabilitation departments of many hospitals have practitioners such as physical and occupational therapists who are extensively trained to work with those who have lymphedema.

When massage clients are under care for lymphedema, confer with their lymphatic practitioner about adjustments that should be made to relaxation or therapeutic massage sessions. Often lymphedema

INFO BOX

Advice for people at risk for lymphedema

Avoid the following:
- muscle strain
- direct heat such as hot tub, sauna, or a heating pad on the affected side
- cuts
- insect bites and stings
- injections
- sunburn
- blood pressure taken on the affected side
- tight garments or jewelry on the affected side
- positions that occlude lymphatic flow, such as static positions
- flying without a compression garment on the affected limb

Bev

I'd been through surgery, chemotherapy and radiation. My "treatment" was over; doctors said my long-term survival looked good. But the lymphedema in my left arm was not better; the puffiness, heaviness and discomfort nagged me constantly. The doctors were empathetic but had little to offer in the area of treatment or advice. The physical therapist prescribed exercises that brought minimal relief. Saddened by the prospect of living my life in discomfort I continued to search for answers. After hours of searching the internet, I learned specialized massage therapy could facilitate lymphatic drainage in areas with lymphedema. Unfamiliar with treatment, my medical team could offer me no referral. Not until almost nine months post-surgery did I, through a friend, find a massage therapist trained in lymphedema.

My expectations for massage therapy were not high; I'd been repeatedly told by my doctors that there was little that could be done to relieve the symptoms brought about by the lymphedema in my left arm. However, massage treatments rapidly brought me remarkable relief, both physically and mentally.

Weekly lymphatic massage treatments minimized my lymphedema symptoms. Gone was the persistent puffy, heavy and aching feeling in my left arm. There was also significant improvement in the range of motion lost in my left arm as a result of tight, inflexible scar tissue. The mental funk that I had been sliding into lifted. The healing was holistic. Massage therapy gave me back my quality of life.

— BEV, ANCHORAGE, ALASKA

A Day at the Spa

A spa day is a popular treat for cancer patients, particularly women. With the right adjustments, this can be a wonderful day of healing. Without them, the spa experience can overwhelm someone with limited energy.

Usually, a day at the spa includes a handful of treatments. An example is a facial, body wrap, massage, and steam room. When a person is in treatment or recovery from cancer, they should be guided by the staff to choose services from the menu that will be less taxing. Good choices would be a pedicure, energy balancing session, a tepid body wrap, and a facial. Limiting the number of choices to three would be a reasonable starting place.

specialists prefer that their patients wait until the swelling is under control before they receive massage; or, they may request that the patient receive no massage in the affected quadrant. The requests of the lymphedema specialist supersede the desires of the massage practitioner. Lymphedema is a serious condition. Controlling it is a higher priority than relaxation massage.

Giving relaxation or therapeutic massage to the person with lymphedema, or at risk for it, can be complicated. In order not to initiate or exacerbate lymphedema, the safest course is to avoid bodywork to the affected quadrant that causes reddening of the skin.[10] This does not mean that massage to the area is contraindicated. Bodywork should be given to the treated side. The key is to use a pressure that does not redden the skin.

Even if people at risk for lymphedema have never had an incident, they remain vulnerable indefinitely. There is no safety window. Lymphedema can begin at any time. The literature recounts many stories of people whose lymphedema did not occur until years after treatment. One reason for this may be that as people age, lymph nodes atrophy, which diminishes the capacity of the lymphatic system.

The following adjustments are intended to give therapists basic guidance in the administration of relaxation massage or therapeutic bodywork to people at risk for lymphedema. Those wishing to be part of a client's lymphedema management team need additional training.

Massage Adjustments

Pressure:
- If the person is at risk for lymphedema, use a level of pressure on the affected quadrant that does not redden the skin. Administer fascial release or trigger point techniques in a slow, controlled way that does not redden the skin.

- Do not perform light, feathery strokes. These stimulate the movement of lymph.

- Do not perform exaggerated stretches or twists in the affected area.

- Therapists who are unsure or untrained in massaging someone with lymphedema should only rest the hands on the affected quadrant until guidance has been received by a lymphedema specialist. The remainder of the body can be massaged with adjustments relative to the person's general health.

Site:
- Massage the untreated side first. If it is the patient's first massage, be gentle, even with the untreated side, in order to gain their trust.

- Stroke only toward the heart on the treated limb. This is the direction that lymph is trying to flow – toward the heart. (See Figure 5.8)

- Massage segments of the limb sequentially using a proximal to distal order. For instance, begin with the shoulder, then upper arm, elbow, forearm, and hand. End with long strokes that connect the entire limb.

- Limit the amount of time to no more than a few minutes in the affected quadrant. This will ensure that the area is not overworked. Even gentle work can overburden the lymphatic system by moving too much lymph. Remember, the quadrant is more than just the limb!

- Do NOT aim strokes at areas of nodal involvement. (See Figure 5.9.) Holds, however, are safe and beneficial to perform.

- Keep strokes lateral on the affected upper arm or leg.

- If the affected quadrant is in the upper body, massage the back with strokes that move down past the rib cage. (See Figure 5.10.) The rib cage is the demarcation line between the upper and lower quadrants. The opposite is true if the lower quadrants are affected. Extending the strokes up past the rib cage, with the patient's permission, would be helpful because the lymph nodes in the upper body are undamaged.

- With patients at risk for lymphedema in the upper quadrants, strokes that travel lateral to medial and proximal to distal on the back are best. (See Figure 5.10.)

Positioning:
- Do not allow an affected arm to hang off of the massage table or be occluded by the position in a massage chair.

- Do not position the patient side-lying on a limb with lymphedema.

CHAPTER 5
FIRST DO NO HARM:
ADJUSTING FOR COMMON
SIDE EFFECTS OF CANCER
TREATMENT
101

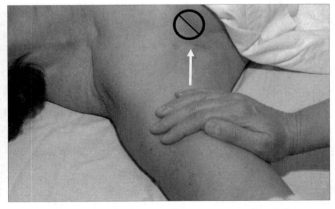

Figure 5.8 Stroke only toward the heart on the treated limb.

*Figure 5.9 Do **NOT** aim strokes at areas of nodal involvement.*

Figures 5.8 and 5.9 by Don Hamilton

Other:

- Educate clients and patients beforehand so that they understand why light pressure is being used. Most people will not fuss about the lighter pressure if they understand the reasoning.

- The person at risk for lymphedema can still have firm pressure in the non-treated quadrants, assuming that their general health is sufficient. When told this, most people accept the limitations on the affected side. For instance, someone treated for breast cancer can have deeper massage below the rib cage – i.e., to the gluteals, hamstrings, or quadratus lumborum. Someone at risk for lymphedema in the lower quadrants can have firmer pressure in the shoulders, scapula, and around the thoracic spine.[3]

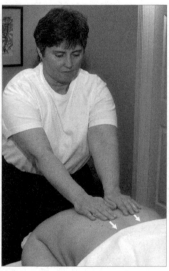

Figure 5.10 When upper quadrants are at risk for lymphedema, extend strokes on the back down past the bottom of the rib cage.

Photographs 5.10 and 5.11 by Don Hamilton

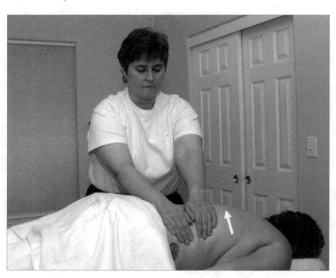

Figure 5.11 For those at risk for lympedema in the upper quadrants, strokes that travel lateral to medial and proximal to distal on the back are best.

MEDICAL DEVICES

Massage sessions can be impacted by a number of medical devices. Commonly, people receiving chemotherapy have venous access devices placed in the chest or arm. Surgical patients can have drains and collection bags attached to their bodies.

VENOUS ACCESS DEVICES

Many patients who are on chemotherapy will have a central IV catheter, also known as a central line. These lines, which can be permanent or temporary, are extremely helpful to the patient who must have many blood draws, rounds of chemo, or injections. Most often central lines are on the right side of the chest. The tubing is inserted into either the subclavian vein or the internal jugular vein and then threaded down into the superior vena cava, positioning the catheter tip just above the right atrium of the heart. These types of central lines – also referred to by their inventors' names, Hickman, Groshong, Bard, or Quinton – protrude from the body and have several inches of tubing that extend out. Central lines can also protrude from the arm. These are known as PICC lines (or peripherally inserted central catheters). The tip is located just above the heart but the initial insertion site is in one of the veins in the arm. Increasing numbers of people are being discharged from the hospital with these catheters. With PICC lines, massage of the arm and chest should be avoided.

Another type of central IV is a port-a-cath. It is inserted under the skin and has no external openings. Ports can be placed anywhere but are most often placed on the right side of the chest for anatomical reasons. There are several advantages to this type of central venous catheter: less risk of infection, and less restrictive for the physically active person.

Catheters also may be placed in the inguinal area, especially to deliver chemotherapy around the liver. Inguinal catheters are used for hospitalized patients and usually are left in for only a handful of days. Because they put the patient at an even higher risk for a blood clot, it is best to avoid massaging the leg on the catheterized side.

Areas of the body that contain venous access devices should be avoided during bodywork and no pressure should be applied to the general area containing the catheter. A good rule of thumb is to stay 3-4" away from the device. There are a number of reasons for this. The device, such as the one in Figure 5.12, is prone to infection. Avoiding the area will reduce the chance of introducing bacteria into the incision where the device has been placed. Passing over the central line can cause the patient discomfort or could potentially displace the device.

Practitioners must be aware of the risk of blood clots related to these catheters. They should familiarize themselves with the signs of a potential blood clot (refer to the section on thromboembolic disorders on pages 119–122). Most often the clot occurs in the arm or chest. The safest course of action is to maintain a gentle pressure to the arm of the catheterized side. Some patients who have central lines are also on low doses of blood thinners, usually coumadin, to help prevent clot formation. Even when the dose of coumadin is low, these people are nonetheless prone to more easy bruising or bleeding.

CHAPTER 5
FIRST DO NO HARM:
ADJUSTING FOR COMMON
SIDE EFFECTS OF CANCER
TREATMENT
103

One of my patients always needs Ativan to calm her down before I start chemotherapy. Today, because of the massage, I didn't have to do that.

— Amy, RN,
Oregon Health and
Science University

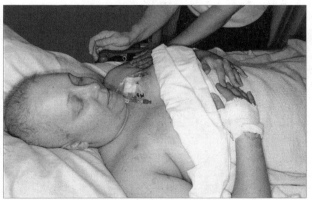

Figure 5.12 A central IV catheter can be seen on the left side of this patient's chest.

Photograph by Don Hamilton

*May I be embraced by the
presence of the holy;*

*May I be centered in thought,
word, and deed;*

*May I be open to this day of joy
and thanksgiving;*

*May I give the gift of love to
others in all that I do and
may I be open to receive love
from others;*

May I walk in my own path;

*May I be physically, mentally,
and spiritually strong so that
I may truly be present to the
world around me;*

*May I be open to the Spirit of
Life whose roots uphold me
and whose wings set me free.*

— DR. MELISSA L. BUCHAN

DRAINS, PUMPS, AND SHUNTS

Drains may be present following surgery to remove excess fluid, the accumulation of which causes discomfort. Therapists should know where the internal portions of the drain are located, avoiding pressure to the entire area. Also, refrain from massage strokes that displace the tissue containing the drain. These devices are very temporary and are removed as soon as the surgical wound has stopped draining fluid.

Pumps for chemotherapy, which are approximately the size of a tape measure, may be placed in the abdominal fascia to deliver medications on a continuous basis. Analgesics and chemotherapy are sometimes administered this way. Practitioners should be aware that commonly these devices have tubing that travels internally to the large veins of the liver. Knowledge of the device's location and destination will help the therapist avoid pressure along the entire pathway. If the client is not certain of the location of both the pump or access device and the catheter (tubing) pathway, either avoid the general area or perform only energetic techniques in the vicinity.

Pain medication is sometimes delivered into the cerebrospinal fluid via an abdominal pump attached to a catheter with its tip implanted into the spinal column. This is known as intrathecal pain management. The catheter itself travels from the location of the pump laterally and posteriorly to the lumbar spine. As with other catheter lines, do not massage along the pathway of the device.

Other devices requiring caution include Ommaya reservoirs, devices implanted into the front of the head. Chemotherapy can be administered through this device into nasal cavities, the brain, and the cerebrospinal fluid. Shunts are tubes which allow fluid to drain from one portion of the body to another. They can be placed in the head to remove excess fluid from the brain, in turn moving the fluid down to the abdomen for reabsorption. Both shunts and Ommaya reservoirs require both health care provider permission and great mindfulness when massaging the head and neck.[13]

COLLECTION BAGS

Patients who have undergone surgery to remove tumors from intestines, kidneys or bladder may require temporary or permanent openings in the abdomen or lumbar areas to drain stool, urine or, infrequently, bile. These openings are called "ostomies." The urine, stool or bile are collected in pouches which are attached to the skin by a special ring of material with adhesive backing.

Ostomies are named by the site which they drain; for example, nephrostomies are surgical openings which allow urine to drain from the kidney via a catheter to the lumbar area of the lower back, and colostomies drain from the affected area of the large intestine to the lower abdomen.

When massage is provided to a person with any type of drainage or collection bag, great care should be taken in the vicinity of the appliance and bag so that the adhesive remains intact. While most are very durable, some patients have difficulty maintaining the integrity of the connection between skin and the appliance and any pressure in the vicinity of the ostomy could dislodge the appliance. Poor adhesion of the appliance allows caustic or acidic material (stool, bile or urine) to contact the skin, causing breakdown in the area of the ostomy.

Some patients require urinary catheterization because of surgical or tumor damage to nerves which provide bladder control. Indwelling urinary catheters are generally well secured, and most people who must live with the catheters are able to help the therapist understand safe positioning for the drainage bag.

CHAPTER 5
FIRST DO NO HARM:
ADJUSTING FOR COMMON
SIDE EFFECTS OF CANCER
TREATMENT
105

Massage Adjustments

Pressure:
- In the general area of the device, massage gently so as not to disturb it.

- Central lines put people at increased risk for blood clots in the area of the device. Gentle pressure will ensure that any potential clots are not dislodged.

Site:
- Stay several inches away from medical devices.

- Energy work such as Therapeutic Touch or Reiki can be done over the area of the site, working without direct skin contact.

Positioning:
- Give patients permission right from the start to position in side-lying instead of prone, or to not move at all.

- If positioning is restricted because of these devices, the person will most likely be unable to lie prone. Usually, your client will be able to tell you what position is the most comfortable. If your client has an ostomy and collection bag, he or she will be able to tell you how durable the connection is and what measures are needed to protect it.

- To pad around a port, place a folded wash cloth or hand towel next to the proximal border.

- To pad the external central line (this is the IV with "rabbit ears"), place a hand towel under the device between it and the chest wall.

Oh, yeah… It's spa day! It's so nice to see a uniform come into the room to give instead of take.

— Patient exclamation upon seeing the hospital massage therapist

Nausea, Vomiting, and Diarrhea

A quiet session of bodywork can help diminish nausea, a common side effect of chemotherapy, radiation, or anesthesia. Clients who have never had a gentle massage may decline the offer of bodywork, thinking that it will be too stimulating and add to their discomfort. For some people who don't feel well, being touched seems too much

*Giving massage to another is a form
of communication in which the
hands do much of the talking.*

— TEDI DUNN AND MARIAN
WILLIAMS, *MASSAGE THERAPY
GUIDELINES FOR
HOSPITAL AND HOME CARE*

to bear. Techniques given to the feet are the easiest. Clients do not
have to move; plus, a small area of the body is being touched, which
is less demanding.

Nauseated patients may have an emesis basin at their side. If it is
necessary to move the basin at any time, glove the hand that will be
in contact with the basin and then rewash the hands after ungloving.
This will protect the practitioner from coming into contact with any
infectious agents as well as any toxic chemicals.

Massage Adjustments

Pressure:
- Avoid pressure or force that creates movement.

- Vigorous rocking should be avoided. Sometimes a very
  subtle rocking is tolerated well but care must be
  exercised with any rhythmic motion.

Positioning:
- Self-limiting.

- Patients may prefer to stay in one position, usually
  supine.

Other:
- Keep a receptacle, such as a waste basket, handy in case
  the person is nauseous during the session.

- Easy access to the bathroom is helpful, as well.

NEUTROPENIA (IMMUNOSUPPRESSION)

Neutropenia is a condition in which the level of white blood cells,
specifically neutrophils, is reduced. The result is suppression of
the immune system. Neutrophils are the first line of defense against
bacterial infection. Therefore, they are especially important for cancer
patients and are "the single most important predisposing factor to
infection."[14] The importance of infection cannot be overstated. It is a
common cause of death for those with cancer.

A number of cancer-related influences can contribute to
immunosuppression: chemotherapy and other medications such as
prednisone, and radiation, particularly to the sternum, pelvis, or long
bones. The disease itself can be the cause of immunosuppression, most
notably with leukemias, lymphomas, and multiple myeloma. Age, too,
can lower the level of immunity. The drop is not as dramatic as that
caused by cancer treatment, but it is still an influence.

The normal level of white blood cells (WBCs) is between 4,500
and 10,000 per cubic millimeter. These numbers are most often
denoted as 4.5–10 (normal values may vary, depending on the
laboratory), with the zeros dropped off to make the numbers more
manageable.

Most often immunosuppression occurs as a side effect of
chemotherapy, which works by killing off fast-growing cells, such as
tumor cells. However, other fast-growing cells, skin, hair, and the bone

marrow stem cells which make white cells, red cells, and platelets also are damaged by chemotherapies. Often, the white blood cell count of a person undergoing chemotherapy will drop below 1.0. During this time they are extremely susceptible to colds, flu, herpes, and fungal and yeast infections.

More than 60% of patients who are neutropenic will experience an infection. The starting places can be in areas of skin that has lost it integrity, such as the open, weeping skin caused by radiation damage. Patients who receive IV therapy, biopsies, or catheter placement are at risk for bacteria or other microbes entering the procedure site. Long-term central venous catheters also create a high risk for infection. Once a colony of organisms invades, they migrate more easily through the body of a person affected by cancer treatment. This is the result of the mucosal layer being damaged by chemotherapy and radiation, which allows the infectious agents to migrate more easily.[15]

High-dose chemotherapy, such as precedes a stem cell transplant, compromises the immune system severely. White blood cell counts drop as low as .1 during this time and patients are at significant risk of lethal infection. Even fresh food and flowers are not allowed because of the bacteria and fungus on them. Generally, the white count starts to increase a couple of weeks or so after the high-dose chemo. It takes months, and for some people even years, before the low end of the normal range is achieved. For a more detailed explanation of the bone marrow or stem cell transplantation procedure, see the Info Box on pages 108–109.

Radiation, particularly to the sternum and ilium, can also cause blood cells to be damaged. The reason for this is that these two areas are the big producers of bone marrow. Bone marrow goes on to become the various components of blood. Generally, if it occurs at all, neutropenia caused by radiation tends to be less severe than that resulting from chemotherapy.

Certain cancers, such as leukemia and non-Hodgkins lymphoma, are connected with immune dysfunction. While leukemia patients can have plenty of white blood cells, the cells do not function normally. This is true of lymphomas as well. Lymphocytes are plentiful, but they are damaged and function poorly.

Immunosuppressed patients have a greater susceptibility to bacterial pneumonia and fungal infections. And herpes, shingles, cytomegalovirus and Epstein-Barr virus are more easily reactivated. A suppressed immune system causes a variety of other complications besides the risk for infection. Patients may be affected by malaise, fatigue, and fever. And, as the years advance, they are at increased risk for other malignancies.

Fever is the main symptom of an infection. In massage school, students were strongly advised not to massage someone with a fever. That is true if massage is defined as a circulatory event that

Continued on page 110

CHAPTER 5
FIRST DO NO HARM:
ADJUSTING FOR COMMON
SIDE EFFECTS OF CANCER
TREATMENT
107

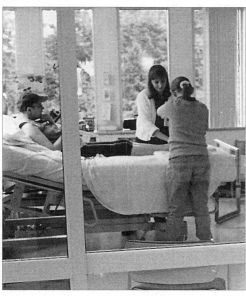

Figure 5.13 Bone marrow transplant patient receives massage from a professional therapist and the patient's 11-year-old daughter.

Photograph by Don Hamilton

Bone Marrow Transplantation

Bone marrow transplantation (BMT) is the process of transplanting the cells which create all blood cells, including those that make up the immune system, in order to eradicate certain cancers. These cells are called "hematopoietic stem cells." They are the primordial cells that transform into the various components of blood and can be found in bone marrow or circulating in the blood stream.

The BMT is primarily used for systemic cancers such as leukemias, lymphomas, or multiple myeloma. In children, other diseases in addition to the leukemias and lymphomas are sometimes treated with BMT – neuroblastoma, Wilm's tumor, aplastic anemia, sickle cell disease, and severe combined immune deficiency, among others. The process of BMT allows the patient to receive a high dosage of chemotherapy which is sometimes combined with total body irradiation (TBI) in order to increase the likelihood of curing the person's disease or causing long-term remission of incurable diseases such as multiple myeloma.

There are two common types of transplantation. In autologous procedures, the patient donates his/her own cells prior to transplant. Allogeneic transplants involve the cells of a donor such as a sibling whose tissue matches that of the patient as closely as possible. The sort of transplant used is dependent upon the type of disease, its level of advancement, age, general health condition, and donor availability.

Stem cell transplantation is not a surgical procedure like an organ transplant. The actual transfer of new stem cells to a patient takes place in the patient's room and has the appearance of a blood transfusion. In one to three weeks, the infused cells migrate back to the bone marrow where they grow into red blood cells, white blood cells, and platelets. This treatment "rescues" the individual's immune system, shortening the time of immunosuppression and supplying a new start to the patient's immune system.

Patient's Experience of BMT

The effects of high dose chemotherapy, especially with the addition of TBI, are severe. For all intents and purposes, the person's ability to make white cells, red cells, and platelets is destroyed until the newly infused stem cells are fully functioning. During this period, the patient's blood cell counts drop precipitiously. The white blood cell count drops to .1 (normal range is 4.5–10) and platelet levels are often at 6 or lower (normal range is 150–400). At this time, the patient is in a highly precarious position. Infections common to a normal individual could kill a BMT patient. The risk of bleeding due to low platelets is so severe that people aren't allowed to brush their teeth in case the gums bleed. Anemia (low red cell count) may contribute to feelings of fatigue, shortness of breath, or malaise.

A number of other side effects occur affecting multiple organ systems. The severity of these side effects varies widely. The kidneys and liver may go into failure, and the heart and lungs can become toxic. Many patients who have allogeneic transplants suffer from some degree of graft-versus-host-disease (GVHD). The donor's new stem cells (the graft) see the body (the host) as an enemy and attack it. GVHD can affect the skin, GI tract, and liver, resulting in skin rashes or discoloration, nausea, vomiting and diarrhea, inability to absorb nutrients, and liver dysfunction. Even massage lotion will not absorb into the skin of some people with GVHD.

CHAPTER 5
FIRST DO NO HARM:
ADJUSTING FOR COMMON
SIDE EFFECTS OF CANCER
TREATMENT
109

Patient's Experience of BMT, continued

Stem cell transplantation is an isolating experience for patients, due to the need to protect them from infectious agents during immunosuppression. Emotional problems can arise during this time. Further contributing to mood shifts are drug reactions or the person's lack of preparation for the physical and emotional intensity of the treatment. Anxiety and depression are common. Nurses in BMT units often find that during this period they supply as much emotional support as medication.

Patients are discharged when the blood counts have returned to certain levels, generally 15–30 days after transplant. Those receiving "allo" transplants must remain within 20–30 minutes from the hospital for an extended period of time, usually 80–100 days. A medical crisis can develop quickly for stem cell recipients, particularly those receiving another person's stem cells, and they must be able to get to the hospital rapidly. Recovery from a BMT is lengthy. For those who have the undergone allogeneic procedure, recovery may take up to two years or more. Those who have undergone an autologons transplant recover more quickly.

Massage Therapy and BMT Patients

Massage is highly beneficial before, during, and after stem cell transplantation, but it must be performed with great mindfulness and care, especially during and following the transplant. Nurses are very protective of their neutropenic and thrombocytopenic patients because of low immunity and the risk of bleeding or bruising. Good handwashing before working with any of these patients cannot be overemphasized. The greatest danger is from infection, and good handwashing is the best protection against transmitting microbes.

A bruise for one these individuals is potentially a serious event. The touch therapist must use only the amount of pressure required to spread the lotion or apply non-invasive modalities, such as Reiki, Polarity Therapy, or cranialsacral therapies. Besides the risk for bruising and bleeding, organ toxicity, fatigue, nausea, and a number of other complications demand the use of light pressure.

Following discharge from the hospital, massage therapists can continue administering bodywork that is non-demanding. If the individual wants firmer pressure, the practitioner should inch forward over a long period of time, perhaps a year or more, as the patient's energy returns. Most people experience fatigue for an extended period. For those who have had allogeneic transplants, GVHD can continue for years. This can have a profound effect on many organ systems, especially the skin. People who are years out from their transplant still have bouts that cause a scleroderma-like hardening of the skin and GI problems.

Practitioners are perhaps reading this section and wondering if it is advisable to massage people affected by such grave complications. Absolutely! It is one of the few pleasant sensations patients experience, especially while in the hospital. Massage gives people something to look forward to during the long days of semi-isolation. Gentle, systematic touch can reduce anxiety, pain, fatigue, nausea, and neutropenic fevers. One woman told her therapist that massage gave her the will to live. The power of touch to help people feel connected to each other in a caring way is very profound and cannot be underestimated.

manipulates soft tissue, which is the usual meaning in pathology texts or massage school. However, when massage is defined as any form of systematic touch, those with a fever can receive bodywork techniques that are very still and do not use any pressure, such as Healing Touch.

Massage Adjustments

Pressure:
- The person who is immunosuppressed usually doesn't feel well and may have a fever. Use light pressure so as not to be demanding on the body.

Site:
- Avoid touching skin that is not intact because of the risk for infection. Open areas become a portal of entry for infectious organisms.

- Stay alert to the possibility of a fungal infection under the nails of the feet. Glove if a fungus is present.

Other:
- Thorough handwashing is extremely important for preventing infection in the patient. It is necessary to do the handwashing just before touching the client and after the room has been set-up. Hands should be dried on disposable paper towels rather than re-usable cloth towels.

- Therapists who are sick, or on the verge of illness, should postpone sessions with immunocompromised people. Wait until the major symptoms of the illness have passed, to avoid worrying the patient. They can be very fearful of those who are coughing or blowing their nose.

- Clean massage equipment thoroughly, including the lotion bottle.

- Do not set lotion bottles, pillows, blankets, or other massage equipment on the floor.

- Do not use lubricant containers that require dipping into the jar. Organisms could be passed from client to client.

- As with clean linen each time, blankets or beach towels used for warmth should be freshly laundered.

- Massage is beneficial during this time because patients often feel socially isolated due to the fear of infection.[6]

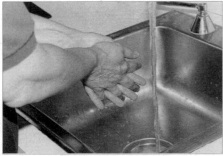
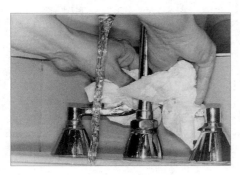

Figures 5.14 and 5.15 Thorough handwashing is extremely important.
Photographs by Don Hamilton

PAIN

Pain is one of the most feared parts of the cancer experience. And it is a realistic fear. Approximately one-third of those in treatment report pain and at least two-thirds with advanced disease report pain.[16,17]

"Complex" best describes this topic. Pain in a person with cancer can be the result of a tumor compressing a nerve, joint pain due to chemotherapy, muscular pain from anxiety, or incisional pain following surgery. Deep bone pain can accompany bone metastases or it can be a side effect of the growth factor Neupogen. The muscles of the chest wall, irradiated because of breast cancer, may be bound down, causing pain on movement. The weight of an arm with lymphedema may pull the shoulder down, resulting in chronic pain. Or perhaps a client's pain has nothing to do with cancer, but is, instead, related to arthritis or an old sports injury.

Other pain can be a signal that the cancer has returned or spread. Familiarity with the side effects of treatment and the diseases is one step in sorting through the various pains a cancer client may present with. Particularly important is understanding the patterns of metastatic spread. One of the common side effects of bone metastasis is pain. The reader can refer back to the section on bone fragility, pages 90–91, to review this information.

Cancer patients can have pain for three main reasons: 1) the tumor, 2) the treatment, or 3) other issues, such as a muscle strain or emotional stress and anxiety. In order to act from a safe place when presented with a complaint of pain, the therapist must try to ascertain which category the pain belongs to, before trying to address it. Massage has limitations and cannot be expected to relieve all pain, nor is it safe to try to address all pain.

Most cancer pain is the result of pressure by the tumor on tissue and nerves. Generally, bodyworkers can do nothing to directly relieve this kind of pain. For instance, pain caused from a tumor obstructing the bowel or impinging a nerve cannot be improved with massage. Heroic measures are completely unjustified and uncalled for with this category of pain. Imagine that a client with multiple myeloma presents with a sore lower back. If the bodyworker jumps to the conclusion that the sore back is muscular in nature and tries to fix it without knowing the source of the pain, serious consequences can occur. Multiple myeloma occurs in the bones and can weaken them. Patients have been known to have fractures from massage that is too vigorous. Indeed, those with multiple myeloma can break ribs simply by sneezing.

However, tumor pain can result in musculoskeletal guarding. When this is the case, massage can be effective in creating general overall relaxation. This sometimes makes the tumor pain more tolerable.

It is obvious by now that some treatment-related pain can be addressed through bodywork. For example, radiated tissue that has become welded together can, through careful touch therapy, be returned to its former level of comfort and function. The same is true of incisional pain or adhesions as a result of surgery. Normal sensation tends to return more quickly when massage is performed on feet affected by peripheral neuropathy. Skilled touch has helped many people through the pain of procedures, such as biopsies and catheterizations. Other treatment-related pain, such as shingles or bone metastases, will remain unchanged by bodywork.

CHAPTER 5
FIRST DO NO HARM:
ADJUSTING FOR COMMON
SIDE EFFECTS OF CANCER
TREATMENT
111

You don't try to change other people. Only their difficulties and their pain will transform them. Nothing that you specifically do or say will change them – except perhaps that by living your life and being an example or beacon or torch, you can help light their way.

— BERNIE SIEGEL, MD,
*HOW TO LIVE
BETWEEN OFFICE VISITS*

Therapists Ask

Q *What if clients request or even demand deep massage?*

A This can almost always be avoided by explaining to clients prior to the first massage that their body has a "new normal" and that there is no way for them or the practitioner to know what that "new normal" is. Together you must slowly and cautiously discover what the body and psyche can tolerate. Explain to the client that gradually increasing to deeper pressure is the best method of approach. Also tell them that within 48 hours of each session, a follow-up phone call will be made to see how they felt after the massage. If there was no deleterious outcome, we will inch forward the next time. When clients know that they eventually will be able to have pressure that is firmer, they are very agreeable to this systematic plan.

Practitioners must take a stronger leadership role in guiding the massage sessions. Clients, and even their health care providers, don't usually understand the effect of massage on the body. Rather than caving in to what the client wants in the moment, the bodyworker must educate the patient before the session begins and explain the principle of "inching forward."

The third category of pain, non-cancer related issues, can be influenced by massage, depending on the origin of the pain. Musculoskeletal conditions are most readily addressed by massage.

When pain is of unknown origin, the therapist is better off applying non-invasive techniques, such as craniosacral therapies or Healing Touch, until the source is determined by the oncologist. This is especially true for people with advanced cancer whose pain may be the result of bone metastases, nerve impingement, or tumor invasiveness, all of which can masquerade as muscular problems.

Specific massage adjustments are not given for the Pain section due to the complexity of the subject. The best advice has already been given: 1) seek the source of the pain and 2) realize that massage is not a "magic bullet" that can cure everything.

PERIPHERAL NEUROPATHY

Just as there are many different cancers, there are also many different chemotherapies, each of which has unique effects. Some chemotherapeutic agents consistently cause nausea, others affect the skin and hair, while a few leave the patient with tingling, numbness, or the sensation of "pins and needles" in the hands or feet. This condition, known as peripheral neuropathy, is caused by demyelination of sensory nerves and/or degeneration of axons. Radiation can sometimes be the cause of peripheral neuropathy, but most commonly it is a response to three chemotherapies – vincristine, cisplatin and paclitaxel.[18]

While neuropathy may seem trivial when compared to some of the other side effects of chemotherapeutic agents – e.g., permanent hearing loss or heart damage – the discomfort of peripheral neuropathy greatly diminishes quality of life. People with this condition are more likely to have greater fatigue and emotional distress. For some, their sense of well-being and ability to perform activities of daily living are impaired.[18]

Over time, peripheral neuropathy can abate. For those cases in which improvement is possible, touch therapies can help the affected areas return to normal sensation more quickly or get a few days of relief from the discomfort.

Massage Adjustments

Pressure:
- In cases of extreme pain, the pressure must be no more than is needed to apply lotion.

- Deep massage is inadvisable; clients cannot give accurate feedback.

Site:
- Some clients will request the affected area to be avoided when there is severe pain.

Other: • For those with painful neuropathy, describing the touch therapy as "lotioning" is often more appealing than referring to it as "massage."

CHAPTER 5
FIRST DO NO HARM:
ADJUSTING FOR COMMON
SIDE EFFECTS OF CANCER
TREATMENT
113

SCARS AND ADHESIONS

By Jamie Elswick, LMT

People who have received radiation or surgery as part of their treatment for cancer may be left with scarring and/or adhesions. Releasing of scar tissue for these clients has many considerations for the touch therapist. The practitioner must determine how to work toward the health of these compromised areas and not take away from the energy needed for the whole organism to heal from the cancer treatments. It is not like working with an athlete who has just had surgery to repair a tissue tear or is recovering from a broken bone. Working with a scarred Achilles tendon is worlds away from massaging tissue damaged by radiation, in which the complex and delicate lymphatic system must be taken into account, as well as the effect of radiation on blood vessels, fascia, muscle, and even bone.

Two of the primary treatments for cancer, surgery and radiation, have a significant effect on the layers of skin, including the subcutaneous layer with its vascular, lymph and nerve components, fascia, and muscle tissues. Skin has a number of important functions. One of the most evident is protection from the external environment. This is the job of the epidermis, or outer layer, which is composed of several layers. The deepest of these is the germinal layer where new cells are constantly dividing to replace those sloughing off at the superficial layer. Underlying this is the highly vascular dermis complete with collagen and elastin in a ground matrix. Both surgery and radiation can bring about reduced flow of blood, lymph, and possibly nerve conduction in this layer of the dermis.

Surgery and the resulting repair process leaves scar tissue behind. The severity of the scar is dependent on size of incision, health of the tissue, and in some cases, as in keloid or raised scars, the body's immune response. The layers of tissue can arrange themselves in such a way that they match up fairly well, or they can line up like along a fault line, where superficial layers are adhered to deeper layers. This slows the flow of blood and lymph to various degrees.

Radiation, too, affects the skin and tissues in the pathway of the radiation. As skin is repairing from the radiation process, extra collagen is laid down in response to the additional stress. This causes a thickening of the tissues, which creates obstacles for the fluidic waterways within the body. The previously-mentioned germ layer of the skin is also at great risk as the demand for dividing cells to repair the injury is increased. The time for cells from the germ layer to move to the surface is 14 days; this coincides with the time that skin damage from a radiation treatment manifests.

Studies have been done on how radiation affects blood vessels, particularly the endothelial or innermost layer. Vascular re-

---

Phyllis

Phyllis started massage school after months of treatment for breast cancer. During school, she asked fellow students to stay away from the scar because it was sensitive. One day, an instructor overheard her saying this and said, "Oh, but you need your scar touched!" and proceeded, with only weak permission from Phyllis, to massage it. Phyllis had rarely cried throughout her cancer treatment, but she burst into tears as the scar was touched in class.

This story teaches us several things – take care not to impose your agenda on the client; be sure to have the person's permission before starting; and be mindful that cancer treatment can leave a person vulnerable. Demonstrating on a cancer client in a large group setting may feel violating.

— AUTHOR

sponsiveness is slowed or even stopped by the damage. Over time, radiated tissue can be affected by necrosis, fibrosis, and edema, all side effects of vascular injury.[19,20]

Radiation has a mutating effect not only on the cancer cells but also on newly dividing, healthy cells which, unfortunately, remain largely immature and unable to contribute fully to the healing process. The treated cells may continue to be vulnerable to the normal wear and tear of daily life, perhaps forever. This is an important piece of knowledge for a therapist, as one might assume that as soon as the redness of the superficial layer goes away, the tissue is healthy.

Massage therapists must exercise caution when working with clients treated for radiation. It is not possible to be certain what radiation-induced damage has occurred underneath the surface. It is helpful to ask a client what angles of treatment were used and look at an anatomy book to get a clear picture of what structures might have been in the pathway. This can provide valuable additional information for understanding other symptoms the client might be having post-treatment. For instance, a person treated for a head and neck tumor may suffer affects to the cervical lymph nodes, taste buds, salivary glands, esophagus, larnyx, and thyroid as a result of tissue radiated in the field of treatment.

RELEASING SCARS AND ADHESIONS

Applying massage to soft tissues affected by radiation and surgery can be beneficial in many ways. Physiologically it can restore circulatory balance which feeds and oxygenates cells and removes waste products. Structural benefits occur from restoring range of motion to fascia, muscle, tendon, and ligaments, which improves normal daily activities. Equally important, attention to scarred areas can create emotional wholeness through the power of touch.

Sandi

Thanks again for a great massage, I floated down the road!! This was so different than what I had experienced in the past. After my mastectomy, the hospital physio was as useful as a chocolate teapot. I just was given a sheet of exercises and left to get on with it. I then went to a private physio who had never worked on someone who had had a mastectomy, chemo and radiotherapy. She did a lot of work with people who had back injuries, like police officers. Her style was pretty intense. She did a lot of stretching and 'stripping' down my arms. It was extremely painful. I was almost crying with the pain. However, the motto 'no pain no gain' kept coming into my mind, so I just went with it. I stopped going after about a year as I felt I had reached a point where I wasn't getting any real benefit.

After the sessions with Louise and Jamie, I noticed a warmth and tickling under the skin. I had never had this with the other physio. I felt instant results that lasted for a few weeks. It felt like something was healing and as if muscles that were tight or fused began to relax. I never felt it was invasive or painful, as more traditional styles seem to be. I think there is not enough information given out by the hospitals as to the importance of massage as opposed to exercises, especially the 'hard must be good' style that is on offer these days.

— CLIENT FEEDBACK TO JAMIE ELSWICK, ANCHORAGE, ALASKA
AND LOUISE ROY, EDINBURGH, SCOTLAND

In some instances, scar work with cancer patients is fairly complex and well beyond what can be learned from a book. It is only appropriate in this text to focus on those principles that are easiest to apply. One thing that will simplify the learning process, is to begin by performing scar work on those not at risk for lymphedema. However, therapists will eventually need an understanding of the lymphatic system in order to safely perform scar work with the vast variety of cancer patients. Lymphatic massage incorporated into scar work can help manage fluids so the system does not become overloaded as circulation is re-introduced. Knowledge of anatomy is essential in order to understand the orientation of muscles and fascia. Hands-on dissection or video tapes can help a therapist a great deal towards attaining this goal.

Tissue that becomes fibrotic is usually shortened and has lost its elasticity. The main goal is to create space, whether the affected area is skin, fascia, muscles, or even joints. Techniques such as gentle skin rolling, lifting of the tissue, side-to-side shearing, and longitudinal shearing will work through the layers and restore the circulation.

CHAPTER 5
FIRST DO NO HARM:
ADJUSTING FOR COMMON
SIDE EFFECTS OF CANCER
TREATMENT

115

Massage Adjustments

Pressure:
- Be gentle. Scar work should not be painful, nor should it create heat or redness to the skin.

- Work superficially at the start. Therapists should work through one layer at a time, gently rolling and lifting the tissue. Side-to-side shearing, longitudinal shearing, and light myofascial release are good for the skin and superficial fascial layers. Figures 5.16–5.18 show examples of these techniques. The same rolling and lifting techniques can be used for muscles. For instance, with those treated for breast cancer, the pectoralis major attachment often becomes restricted at the attachment site on the humerus. Unrolling the attachment out and away from the axilla can free fibers that overlap each other. This same principle can be used for the latissimus dorsi insertion, rolling it out to open the axillary space posteriorly.

- Deeper types of scar tissue work are contraindicated if the area has been radiated. Radiated tissue can be brittle, fibrotic, and excessively shortened.

Site:
- When surgical removal of such tissues as skin, fascia, muscle, and adipose occur, the layers left behind are often quite thin. Work an area for a minute or less and then move to a different part of the scar so that an area doesn't get overworked. There is time to work with a scar over several sessions, so there is no need to rush and create discomfort and excessive inflammation.

- Err on the side of caution. Perform scar massage with mindfulness. Remember that radiated tissues can be left

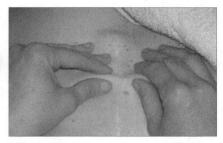

Figure 5.16 Skin rolling, gently working to separate the superficial layers first. Note: There is only a small amount of lift necessary.

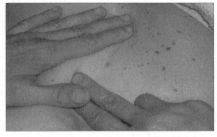

Figure 5.17 Cross shearing working perpendicular to the scar.

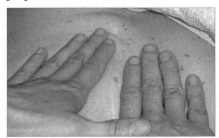

Figure 5.18 Longitudinal shearing along the length of the scar.

Photographs by Colleen Carroll

in a very delicate state and the total damage may not be apparent for years after treatment.

- Nerves are sometimes cut during surgery. The client will not be able to give appropriate feedback about pressure or discomfort in the treated area.

Positioning:
- Areas affected by scars or adhesions can have significantly less range of motion. Take this into consideration, particularly when positioning limbs to access adjacent muscles. For instance, a breast cancer client that has received radiation may not be able to have her arm placed overhead.

SKIN CONDITIONS

A variety of skin problems are created by radiation, chemotherapy, and other medications – dryness, rashes, burns, hive-like wheals, poor wound healing, disrupted integrity, hypersensitivity, itching, weeping lesions, and discoloration, to name just some. Attunement to the skin is the best assessment skill a therapist can cultivate. It can tell a therapist a great deal about a client's condition. Scars from surgery or medical devices, such as ports, are easily spotted. Tell-tale ink marks delineating the field of treatment of a radiation patient are subtle, but observable once the therapist knows what he is looking for. Darkened, tough skin also tells the therapist where radiation was given. Redness, puffiness, and warmth of the skin are the body talking to the therapist.

SKIN CARE DURING RADIATION

Most clients can tolerate gentle touch to the treated area for the first few weeks of treatment. After the skin becomes severely reddened, touch may need to be discontinued. Massage can usually be resumed to the treated area two to three weeks following the last treatment. Clients can guide the therapist about the use of touch or the amount of pressure during radiation.

Many types of lubricants are contraindicated during the time the person is receiving radiation, which can last up to eight weeks. Radiologists give their patients varying instructions on the use of topicals during treatment. Some may ask people to avoid all lotions, creams and gels and to use only the lubricant provided by the radiation oncology clinic. Other doctors may require that patients avoid specific skin products, such as powder or vitamin E oil. Check with the radiation oncology team before applying any substance.

One universal rule is – Never use oil or lotion on the field of treatment during the course of radiation treatment. These products can leave a coating on the skin that interferes with radiation and they can intensify the effect of the radiation to the skin. Many of the ingredients in lubricants also interfere with the skin's healing, e.g.,

INFO BOX

Lotions, Creams, and Oils

Therapists should be attentive to the lubricants they use on all clients, but particularly on those in treatment for cancer.

Products should be fresh and of food-grade quality. Consider lubricants as food for the body: instead of being administered orally, the food is being administered topically.

Use scent-free products. People in treatment for cancer may become nauseated around certain scents.

Choose the right type of lubricant. Heavy creams that require firm pressure to apply are inappropriate for many people in treatment. Those who bruise easily or have fragile skin should not receive the type of vigorous pressure needed to spread thick creams. Lotions that become sticky quickly should also be avoided. Choose a lotion or oil with good glide; friction is not needed in this setting.

Lubricant containers are important. Never use containers which you must dip into. If a favorite lubricant comes in this style of jar, transfer a single-use daub to a paper cup. Pump-top or squeeze bottles are better choices for this group of clients. In this way the cancer client is not coming into contact, via the lubricant, with the germs of other clients.

lotions containing alcohol and metals. Alcohol is drying, and metals, such as zinc oxide or aluminum stearate, can cause rashes to skin that is tender from radiation.

Pure aloe vera gel is usually safe for radiated skin. (Be sure the client checks with their radiation oncologist before using.) It decreases inflammation and rehydrates the skin. Take care, however, when purchasing aloe products. Some products on the market advertise themselves to be "100% aloe vera." However, if they are in a base of glycol they will sting when applied to already burned skin.

A final guideline – Do not use hot or cold packs on treated areas until the skin is recovered. Even though the skin may look healed, the subdermal tissue may take longer to rejuvenate. When first applying heat or cold, use the concept of "inching forward." Start with a warm cloth instead of a hydrocullator pad, or a cool cloth rather than an ice bag. Radiated skin can remain sensitive for a long period of time, sometimes forever.

CHAPTER 5
FIRST DO NO HARM:
ADJUSTING FOR COMMON
SIDE EFFECTS OF CANCER
TREATMENT
117

Susan

After finding a lump in my right breast, I was in the doctor's office at 8:00 the next morning. Within 10 days, we had determined it was cancer and the lump had been removed. A month later, the complete diagnosis had been made. I had a partial mastectomy with no lymph node removal and was scheduled for 33 days of radiation.

The doctors told me that the radiation would cause my breast tissue to shrink and to become harder. Since I was a practicing massage therapist, I requested permission from both my surgeon and the oncology radiologist to do self-massage to the right breast tissue. Both were supportive. Within a couple of days of surgery, I began gentle massage around the incision. When I saw the surgeon two weeks later, he commented on how well I had healed. I reminded him that I was doing massage to the tissue. He just laughed.

A week later, radiation treatments began. The radiation therapy was given five days a week for six and a half weeks. Every day I performed very gentle massage to the entire breast. I used no lotion, just a very gentle touch. I focused on the breast being a loved part of my body. After the initial gentle massage, I would seek out the areas of the breast that hurt. They were generally at the lower bra line and were sharp spots of pain. Gently I would set my fingers on the spots and just maintain contact. The spots would dissolve within a few seconds. I would spend a total of two to three minutes massaging my breast. Some days I massaged it several times a day.

Every Monday I saw my oncology radiologist. After about three weeks, he started commenting on the lack of redness in my breast tissue. I was five weeks into radiation therapy before the skin started to turn red. I talked to the doctor about the type of lotion that could be used for the dryness and began using it during the massage.

Two weeks after my radiation therapy was complete, I saw the surgeon again. He could not believe the condition of my breast tissue. He was expecting to see dry, inflamed, hard tissue. What he was saw and palpated was normal, soft breast tissue with just a light tan to the radiated area. This was the best tissue he had seen in twelve years of cancer surgery. I reminded him that I had performed breast massage throughout the process. He did not laugh this time and is interested in exploring how we can use massage in treatment. The oncology radiologist had similar comments and wanted to know exactly what I had done during my breast massage.

I also began Myofascial Release to the right pectoralis major about a month after radiation therapy to keep it from binding. I did it nearly every day for about two months. Seven months after radiation therapy, sore and dense tissue continues to appear in my right breast, but gentle massage keeps the tissue soft and pliable.

— SUSAN SHIELDS, LMT, BULL'S GAP, TENNESSEE

Massage Adjustments

Pressure:
- Be mindful of pressure on thin skin. The skin can thin as a result of long-term chemotherapy use. Lubricate it thoroughly in order to avoid tears.

Site:
- Avoid areas of skin that are not intact, contain vesicles, or are discharging body fluids.

- Areas of skin that have a rash that is not raised can often have gentle massage to the site.

- Skin with a raised, discolored lesion should be avoided until the doctor or nurse can be consulted.

- Avoid areas of the skin that have just been covered in topical steroidal cream. It can be absorbed into the therapist via the hands.

THROMBOCYTOPENIA

Low platelets, known as thrombocytopenia, can occur in cancer patients for a number of reasons – antitumor drugs, steroids, aspirin, anticoagulants, radiation, and specific cancers such as leukemia, multiple myeloma, or lymphoma. Platelets are the component of the blood responsible for clotting if the body is injured by trauma. Typically, a cubic millimeter of blood contains 150,000–400,000 platelets. These numbers are expressed as 150–400. (The normal range differs somewhat in different reference books and different laboratories. However, the differences are insignificant.) When the numbers of platelets are insufficient, people bruise and bleed more easily.

Thrombocytopenia is defined as a platelet count of less than 100. While this level is below the norm, it is not a highly dangerous level. Unless there are other influencing factors, clients can be given bodywork that is appropriate to their general health. However, when the count drops to 50, special attention must be paid to the amount of pressure used when giving bodywork. It should not exceed the superficial layer of musculature.

A platelet count of 20 or below is extremely serious! Health care providers or hospital staff often use this number as a cut-off point for massage because the person with a platelet count of 20 or lower is in serious danger of bleeding. Bleeding can occur either internally as would occur from a bruise, or externally, as from a cut or bleeding of the gums. The most serious bleeds are brain or retinal, which can occur spontaneously. Without sufficient platelets, any bleeding, no matter how minuscule, is difficult to stop.

The group of patients at the highest risk of severely low platelets are those receiving high-dose chemotherapy, those with acute leukemias, or those who are undergoing bone marrow transplants. These patients may have platelet counts below 10! This is a highly

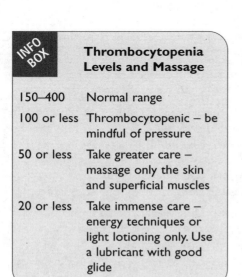

INFO BOX

Thrombocytopenia Levels and Massage

150–400	Normal range
100 or less	Thrombocytopenic – be mindful of pressure
50 or less	Take greater care – massage only the skin and superficial muscles
20 or less	Take immense care – energy techniques or light lotioning only. Use a lubricant with good glide

dangerous state. Systematic touch can be given with a very gentle effleurage stroke, similar to lotioning the skin. Techniques that do not employ pressure, such as cranialsacral therapies or Polarity Therapy, also are safe with these patients.

Patients with serious platelet disorders may be hesitant when a massage is offered, for fear the touch will be too heavy. And many health care providers are unfamiliar with the broad range of bodywork modalities that a therapist can turn to. The touch practitioner can help by using phrases such as "gentle massage" or "light touch." The term "lotioning" also works well and truly describes what will occur with these patients. Readers will remember from the review of the research in Chapter 3, that a number of studies have been safely done on bone marrow transplant patients. This affirms the feasibility of working with people who are thrombocytopenic.

CHAPTER 5
FIRST DO NO HARM:
ADJUSTING FOR COMMON
SIDE EFFECTS OF CANCER
TREATMENT
119

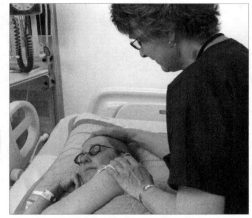

Figure 5.19 Hands that whisper to the body.

Photograph by David J. Lawton

Massage Adjustments

Pressure:
- Easy bruising or risk for bleeding is an indication for light pressure.
- When massaging severely thrombocytopenic patients, use a lotion with good glide to avoid friction to the tissues.

Site:
- Avoid areas with hematomas

THROMBOEMBOLIC DISORDERS

Thromboembolic disorders include superficial and deep vein thrombosis (DVT), and pulmonary embolism. Thrombosis, the creation of a blood clot that obstructs or partially obstructs a blood vessel, is a serious side effect of cancer and its treatments. Thromboembolic disorders affect 15% of cancer patients and they are the second leading cause of death in hospitalized cancer patients.[21] A thrombus can impede the flow of blood back to the heart, causing fluid and blood to pool distal to the clot. In the worst scenario, the clot can break off and travel to the lungs, resulting in death to the patient.

A variety of factors can contribute to the creation of a clot – surgery, immobility, venous access devices, hormonal and chemo therapies, and the disease process itself. Most practitioners are probably aware of the relationship between blood clots and surgery or venous stasis caused by immobility. However, the influence of certain IV catheters, medications, and the process of hypercoagulation caused by tumors may be new information.

Many of these factors cause injury to blood vessel walls, which draws platelet and inflammatory mediators to the area.[22] These substances stimulate platelets to adhere to one another and activate the clotting process.[21-23] Vessel walls can be damaged by surgery, radiation, chemotherapy, infection, tumor invasion, and in-dwelling

I massaged her as if she was a flower, or a piece of fine china. Those images helped me to stay soft.

— PAULA BENTLEY, LMT,
PORTLAND, OREGON

IV catheters. These devices increase the risk of thrombosis because their presence causes chronic injury to the endothelial lining of the blood vessel.[21] In addition, levels of fibrinopeptide A have been shown to increase during chemo infusion. This substance is associated with the rapid conversion of fibrinogen to fibrin, one of the prerequisites involved in clot formation. There is also a decrease in naturally-occurring plasma proteins with anticoagulant properties from the administration of many chemotherapies.[23]

Hypercoagulation is associated with a wide variety of cancers including ovarian, gastric, kidney, lung, prostate, and colon. Cancer doubles the chance of developing a clot following surgery as does hormone therapy, such as tamoxifen, and certain chemos – Cisplatin, etoposide, cyclophosphamide, methotrexate, flurouracil, doxorubicin, prednisone, thalidomide, and vincristine, for example.[21] Chemotherapy can damage endothelial cells lining the blood vessels. Damaged endothelium is unable to perform its anticoagulant and fibrinolytic functions. Substances that enhance clot formation may then be released.[23]

The incidence of thrombus increases in those with advanced cancer. Studies of large groups of patients show that men with lung and pancreatic cancer are most likely to develop thrombi, and women with colorectal, pancreatic, and gynecological cancers. Also at risk are patients with advanced brain tumors who are receiving chemo, recurrent rectal cancer patients receiving radiation therapy, and patients with advanced GI cancers.[21]

Normally, in people without cancer, thrombi lodge in the deep veins of the legs and tend to be solitary. A venous clot associated with cancer can be migratory and can be deep or superficial. They also affect unusual sites in the body, such as the arm and chest.[21]

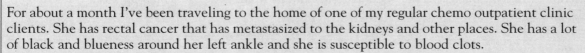

Ruth

For about a month I've been traveling to the home of one of my regular chemo outpatient clinic clients. She has rectal cancer that has metastasized to the kidneys and other places. She has a lot of black and blueness around her left ankle and she is susceptible to blood clots.

We've been doing 90-minute massages – side lying, due to her colostomy bag. I always felt my pressure was light enough, especially on her legs and feet. However, when I arrived today, she said her legs and feet were sore after the massage last week. She had bruises on her legs.

My insides turned over with guilt and regret. I apologized and told her I would avoid massaging her legs and feet but offered Reiki instead. I also suggested we only do one-hour sessions. She agreed.

The lesson here for me is to pay better attention, slow down and check in with my hands on pressure adjustment. I honestly thought I was going light enough. Obviously I was wrong. This was tough to face.

This was a huge wake-up call for me. I am thankful she didn't turn me away at the door. I spoke with one of the nurses today about what happened and she asked me if it would help if I saw the doctor's notes on her. Yes indeed! So now I have a much better idea of what's going on with her. She's in the advanced stage and basically it's all about pain management at this point. As far as I'm concerned, from here on out she's tissue paper in my hands.

— EILEEN HICKEY, LMT, PORTLAND, OREGON

Superficial blood clots are less worrisome. They present themselves differently than deep vein thrombosis (DVT). The surface of the skin may be red, warm, hard, tender, or contain a palpable cord along the vein.[24] The common signs of DVT include swelling, warmth, or reddish-blue discoloration on the side of the affected extremity. If the clot is in the leg, there may be pain when standing, fatigue in the affected side, or tenderness in the calf or thigh that intensifies over time,[21,22] unexplained abdominal or lumbar pain, or changes in neurologic status.[23] A DVT that has broken off and traveled to the lungs can result in chest pain with shortness of breath, a rapid heart beat, cough, or fever.

A client who presents with either group of symptoms should immediately see the doctor rather than having a massage that day. After physician care has been undertaken, a therapist's best course of action is to use low impact techniques.

The symptoms listed above are not unique to DVT and can be the result of other factors, such as lymphatic obstruction by a tumor, compression of a vein by a tumor, or an infection. Medical tests such as an ultrasound are needed to diagnose a blood clot. **The Homan's sign, commonly taught in massage school as a way to test for DVT of the leg, has a low reliability rate and should not be used.**[21] Readers should note, too, that many times patients with a thrombus show no symptoms. Half of all people who develop thrombosis have no symptoms.[22]

Massage Adjustments

Pressure:
- Remain mindful that many with advanced cancer are at increased risk of a thrombus due to the disease process.

- People in treatment are also at greater risk for clot formation for a variety of reasons. Do not go overboard with pressure.

- Decrease pressure for anyone on extended bedrest.

- Patients with a recent clot may be on anticoagulant medication. This is a bruising precaution.

Site:
- A limb with a known thrombus should not receive touch therapies that involve pressure or stroking. Static holds on the limb are permissible.

- Care should be taken when massaging the legs of post-op patients, especially when there is significant blood involvement. Wait until the doctor has approved before resuming circulatory massage to the legs.

- Central IV catheters (especially PICC lines) and inguinal catheters increase the risk of clot formation. Apply only energy techniques to an arm with a PICC line. Clots form easily in these veins because of their small size relative to the catheter. PICC-related clots are the most

CHAPTER 5
FIRST DO NO HARM:
ADJUSTING FOR COMMON
SIDE EFFECTS OF CANCER
TREATMENT

121

common ones. If the catheter is placed in the chest, apply massage gently to the adjacent arm up to the shoulder. If the catheter is in the inguinal space, massage can be given to the foot on that side, but no stroking movements or compression should be performed on the catheterized leg. The opposite leg can be massaged.[6]

FINAL THOUGHTS

People with cancer do not want those around them walking on proverbial egg shells or touching them as if they will break. They want to be touched fully with calm, confident, and loving hands. People want to be treated as normal. Their lives are filled with all of the same things as those without cancer – gardens, dogs, children, hobbies, and friends. They are living life. Bodyworkers should be at the forefront in embracing them and in teaching family and friends about the need for touch during this time.

REFERENCES

1. Tait N. *Anorexia-Cachexia Syndrome in Cancer Symptom Management*. Boston, MA: Jones and Barlett, 1999.

2. Schulmeister L. *Nutrition in Oncology Nursing*, 4th Ed. St. Louis, MO: Mosby, 2001.

3. Smukler A, Govindan R. Management of Bone Metastasis. *Contemporary Oncology*, 2002;1(13):1-10.

4. Preece J. Introducing Abdominal Massage in Palliative Care. *Complementary Therapies in Nursing and Midwifery*. 2002;8(2):101-105.

5. Walton T. Cancer and Massage. *Massage Therapy Journal*. Fall 2000, p. 68-80.

6. MacDonald G. *Massage for the Hospital Patient and Medically Frail Client*. Philadelpia,PA:Lippincott Williams and Wilkins, 2005.

7. Hand-Foot Syndrome. Available at: http://chemocare.com/managing/handfoot_syndrome.asp. Accessed Oct. 30, 2006.

8. Roche Pharmaceuticals. Cancer Chemotherapy and Hand Foot Syndrome. 2004.

9. Zuther J. *Lymphedema Management: The Comprehensive Guide for Practitioners*. New York, NY: Thieme Medical Publishers, 2005.

10. Zuther J. Traditional Massage Therapy in the Treatment and Management of Lymphedema. *Massage Today*, June 2002:1.

11. Burt J, White G. *Lymphedema: A Breast Cancer Patient's Guide to Prevention and Healing*. Alameda, CA: Hunter House Publishers, 1999.

12. Swirsky J, Nannery D.S. *Coping With Lymphedema*. Garden City Park, NY: Avery Publishing, 1998.

CHAPTER 5
FIRST DO NO HARM:
ADJUSTING FOR COMMON
SIDE EFFECTS OF CANCER
TREATMENT

123

13. Leonard K. *Massage for People with Cancer: A Teaching Manual*, 2nd Ed.(self-published). Fayetteville, NY, 2005.

14. Otto SE. *Protective Mechanisms in Oncology Nursing*, 4th Ed. St. Louis, MO: Mosby, 2001.

15. Wujcik D. *Infection in Cancer Symptom Management*. Boston, MA: Jones and Bartlett, 1999.

16. Paice JA. *Pain in Cancer Symptom Management*. Boston, MA: Jones and Bartlett, 1999.

17. Swenson CJ. *Pain Management in Oncology Nursing*, 4th Ed. St. Louis, MO: Mosby, 2001.

18. Wilkes GM. *Neurological Disturbances in Cancer Symptom Management*. Boston, MA: Jones and Bartlett, 1999.

19. Reide UN, Werner M. *Color Atlas of Pathology: Pathologic Principles, Associated Diseases, Seguela*. New York, NY: Thieme Medical Publishers, 2004.

20. Robbins KC. *Basic Pathology*, 6th Ed. Philadelphia, PA: WB Saunders, 1997.

21. Van Gerpen R. Thromboembolic Disorders in Cancer. *Clinical Journal of Oncology Nursing*. 2004;8(3):289-299.

22. Goldsmith C. Hidden Danger: Venous Thromboembolism. *Nurse Week*. May 23, 2005, p.19-21.

23. Dell D. Deep Vein Thrombosis in the Patient with Cancer. *Clinical Journal of Oncology Nursing*. 2002;6(1):43-46.

24. *Mayo Clinic Women's Health Source*. Learning More about Deep Vein Blood Clots (Thrombosis) – An Interview with Scott Litin, MD July 2005. p. 7-8.

COMMON PRESSURE, SITE AND POSITION ADJUSTMENTS FOR CANCER PATIENTS

Pressure Adjustments

Systemic restrictions are those in which the therapist must moderate the pressure used throughout the entire body. **Localized** restrictions are those requiring less pressure in a narrow, defined area.

Systemic Restrictions:	Localized Restrictions:
anticoagulant medications	central IV catheters
bone fragility	constipation
bruises easily	edema
cachexia	lymphedema
extended bedrest	lymph node removal in neck, axilla or groin
fatigue	peripheral neuropathy
fragile veins	a quadrant affected by radiation to neck, axilla, or groin
major organ complications	
neutropenia	
pain medications	skin (fragile or sensitive)
recent history of blood clot	
recent surgery	
skin sensitivity	
thrombocytopenia	

Site Restrictions

The left column presents scenarios in which the area should NOT be touched. The right column presents scenarios in which touch is allowed but with great mindfulness.

Do Not Touch:	Be Mindful When Touching:
severe bone mets	alopecia
incision (recent)	blood clots (recent history)
medical devices	intervention site (i.e., biopsy)
skin condition (open or communicable)	phlebitis
	skin condition (closed and healed)
	tumor (only "resting hands")

Positioning Adjustments

Positioning usually needs to be adjusted for the following conditions. Next to each condition is the typical adjustment.

ascites (supine only)	lymphedema (elevate affected limb)
breathing difficulty (no prone, elevate head)	medical devices (often no prone)
coughing (no prone, elevate head)	mucositis (often no prone)
edema (elevate affected limb)	nausea or cramps (minimal repositioning)
incision (usually no prone)	tender skin due to radiation (sometimes no prone)
lung mets (no prone, elevate head if needed)	tumor (case by case)

Chapter 6

Strengthening the Body

The Use of Touch Techniques to Support the Body During and After Treatment

By Isabel Adkins, BA, CMT

The bedrock of *Medicine Hands* lies in the use of comfort-oriented touch for people in treatment for or recovering from cancer. Intangible and surprising results often occur when the session is given with just that intention, the intention of comfort. Therapists and patients have reported that despite no attempt to create a specific outcome, such conditions as insomnia, fever, and anxiety have decreased and those such as a sense of being whole, calm, and loved have increased.

Comfort-oriented bodywork can always be safely given. However, bodywork can also be administered with the specific intent of remedying some of the side effects of cancer treatment, such as neutropenia, fear, or cachexia. This chapter focuses on the use of bodywork techniques to purposefully address specific side effects of cancer treatment. These treatment-oriented techniques might be interspersed into comfort-oriented sessions, used entirely on their own, or perhaps given on an as-needed basis, alternating between comfort-based sessions and treatment-oriented sessions. They should not, however, take the place of medications or other interventions

Softness triumphs over hardness, gentleness over strength.

— LAO TZU

All through my cancer diagnosis and treatment, the only time someone touched me and it didn't hurt was on the massage table. It was like an oasis in the desert.

— COMMENT BY A FRIEND OF
BRUCE HOPKINS, LMT,
PORTLAND, MAINE

that the person's oncologist has prescribed. They are meant to be used alongside of mainstream health care.

It bears emphasizing that when administering techniques to strengthen the body from the side effects of treatment, the approach must still be mindful and careful. Therapists should continue to implement the notion of being less demanding and inching forward. Nearly all types of bodywork can be given to cancer patients if the right adjustments are made. In this chapter, concepts from Chinese medicine will be applied to reflexology and acupressure in order to demonstrate how bodywork techniques can strengthen the vital organs, immune function, and psychological response. An entire book would not be enough to completely cover this topic. A chapter can only serve to plant seeds or function as an appetizer. Readers should approach this material as a simplified starting place.

VITAL ORGAN SUPPORT

Because the impact of chemotherapy and radiation causes permanent and detrimental changes in the cells, ongoing organ support is helpful in diminishing the symptoms caused by treatment. In Western anatomy and physiology, the organs are known only on the basis of their physical functions. The liver, for example, cleanses, produces cholesterol, stores glycogen, and has a hand in platelet functioning, to name a few functions. In Chinese medicine, the organs are more than just an anatomical body part. Besides their connection to bodily functions, they are viewed as having likes and dislikes, as having spirit, and as having specific emotions related to them. The Chinese concept of organ consists of a wide range of functions and processes that take place in many different aspects and sites of the bodymind.[1] For example, in Chinese cosmology, Liver* rules muscles and joints on a physical level and psychologically; it is the force that motivates people to move forward in a desired direction. In the same way, Kidney physically rules the reproductive organs and psychologically it is associated with the will to live, or interest in life. The Info Boxes "Nature of the Organs" and "Spirit of the Organs" contain details about other organs.

Acupressure points allow access to the organs through meridians, which are deep, interconnected pathways that distribute Chi, or vital force, through the body. Chi, like electricity, flows in a current. Although it cannot actually be seen, the effects and manifestations of Chi can be noticed and felt. It is like the flow of blood through the body.[2] Chi, according to Chinese medicine, represents actual life.

---

* ***Please note:*** *Each time an organ is mentioned in relation to Chinese medicine, or it is mentioned as a system that should be worked on through reflexology or acupressure, the organ name will be capitalized. When the organ being referred to is the anatomical organ, the organ name will begin with a lower case letter. For instance, to work on symptoms related to liver toxicity, it will be recommended to work the Liver points and zones.*

Without it, there is no life. So when practitioners are working with these channels, they are tapping into the body's own healing abilities, a healing that occurs by balancing from the inside-out rather than from the outside-in.

Bodywork that focuses on the organs occurs at a very deep level. For practitioners and clients that like so-called "deep tissue massage," it is important to realize that bodywork doesn't get any deeper than focusing on organs. Although acupressure and reflexology are subtle and less invasive ways to impact the body, they reach down to muscles and bones. For instance, perhaps a client's leg cannot be massaged for some reason. By working the reflex zones of Liver and Spleen, the client will leave the table feeling as if the leg had actually been massaged. From a Chinese Medicine point of view, this makes sense, not only because the Liver and Spleen meridians run through the legs, but also because Liver rules muscles and joints and Spleen rules the limbs.

CHAPTER 6
STRENGTHENING THE BODY:
THE USE OF TOUCH TECHNIQUES
TO SUPPORT THE BODY DURING
AND AFTER TREATMENT
127

Nature of the Organs

In Chinese medicine, the nature of each organ is broader than in Western medicine. For instance, in Western understanding, the kidney functions in such actions as purification of fluids and the maintenance of electrolyte levels. As can be seen in the list below, Chinese medicine attributes far more functions to Kidney. Understanding an organ's nature helps a therapist to better address a patient's symptoms.

Kidney: Called the House of Chi, relates to immunity, bone, bone marrow (consequently stem cell production), brain, skeletal structure, spinal cord, central nervous system, ears, and adrenals. It is also associated with reproductive organs, libido, and purification of fluids.

Lung: Associated with physical vitality through breath and oxygenation. Rules skin, strengthens protection from foreign invasion, playing a part in the body's ability to defend itself. In common terms, lung and skin are both about oxygenation and elimination, and, consequently, protection.

Liver: Called the General, it watches over the functioning of the entire system. The liver's well-being impacts all of the organs in the digestive system. It rules muscles and joints, eyes, nails, head hair, genitals, sexual performance and breast. The liver governs the diaphragm, impacting digestion and breathing.

Spleen-pancreas: Has a relationship to the lymphatic system and white blood cell production. The spleen is also responsible for the body's ability to absorb and process food into nourishment.

Stomach: Associated with appetite and digestive fire, the health of the stomach will determine whether the body has the fuel it needs to generate energy.

Intestines: The Small Intestine is associated with filtering physical nourishment, the Large Intestine with release and elimination of waste.

Heart: The heart is associated with mental functioning, circulation and spirit.

© Isabel Adkins

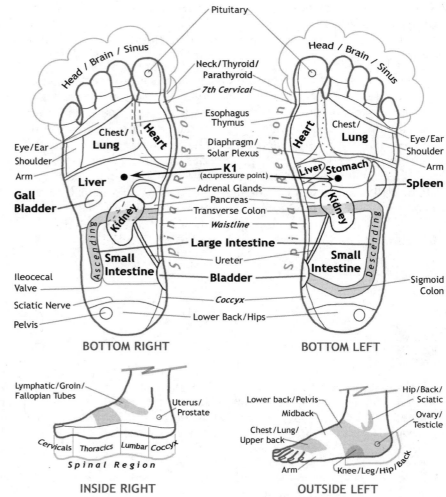

Figure 6.1 Foot reflexology map

Adapted by Nicki Hansen-Dix based on an image from Robin Varga,
Flocco Method Reflexology Instructor

The following symptoms and side effects are common among cancer patients. Listed next to the condition are possible ways to address them through foot reflexology, bladder meridian points, and other acupressure points. Foot reflexology zones are pictured in Figure 6.1, above. Bladder meridian points are in Figure 6.2, page 131, and other acupressure points can be found in Figure 6.3, page 139. Please take note of the guidelines listed on pages 137 and 138 for helping the therapist to decide which organs to focus on.

Addressing Common Symptoms and Side Effects

	Foot	Bladder points	Others
Anorexia	Spleen, Stomach, and Heart	20, 21, 22, 38, 47	Sp6, St36, P6, CV17
Bone Fragility	Kidney	11, 23, 47	K1, K3, K27
Breathing Difficulty	Lung, Diaphragm, and Liver	12, 13, 17, 18	P6, Lu1, K27, St16, CV17
Cachexia	Spleen, Stomach, and Kidney	20, 21, 23	St36, Sp6
"Chemo-brain" Concentration	Liver and Spleen	18, 20	Lv3, Sp6
Confusion	Liver and Heart	18, 15	Lv3, H7, CV17
Memory	Liver and Heart	18, 15	Lv3, H7, CV17
Constipation	Liver and Large Intestine	18, 22, 25	Lv3, CV4, CV6
Diarrhea	Liver, Spleen and Intestines	18, 20, 22, 25, 27	Lv3, Sp6
Fatigue	Liver, Kidney and Lung	13, 18, 23	Lv3, Sp6, St36, Lu1, K1, K3, K27
Impotence	Liver and Kidney	18, 22, 23, 42, 47	K1, K3, K27, Lv3, CV4, CV6
Insomnia	Heart and Liver	14, 15, 18, 38, 42	Lv3, H7, CV17
Libido	Kidney	22, 23, 47	K1, K3, K27, CV 4, CV6
Mucositis	Small Intestine and Heart	14, 15, 27,	H7, CV17
Nausea	Liver, Stomach and Spleen	18, 20, 21	P6, St36, Lv3
Neuropathy	Kidney	23	massage affected area with Mahanarayan oil.
Skin Problems	Lung and Liver	12, 13, 18	Lv3, Lu1, St16

CHAPTER 6
STRENGTHENING THE BODY:
THE USE OF TOUCH TECHNIQUES
TO SUPPORT THE BODY DURING
AND AFTER TREATMENT
129

Composing a Symphony

I have never been able to draw, sing or play an instrument. Poetry and dancing come only with great effort. But I have found a powerful creative impulse deep inside. I have touch equivalents for color and texture, harmony and discord, silence and thunder, overture, melody and reprise. I have a powerful need to express myself, to communicate through touch. For me doing massage is like composing a symphony to be heard only one time by just one person and then lost forever.

— BRUCE HOPKINS, LMT, PORTLAND, MAINE

Additional Resources

- Levine P, Fredrick A. *Waking the Tiger: Healing Trauma.* North Atlantic Books, 1997.

- Sohn T, Sohn R. *Amma Therapy: A Complete Textbook of Oriental Bodywork and Medical Principles.* Healing Arts Press. 1996.

- Dougans I. *Complete Illustrated Guide to Reflexology, Therapeutic Foot Massage for Health and Well-Being.* HarperCollins, 2001.

SUPPORTING THE IMMUNE SYSTEM

When preparing to give bodywork to a person with cancer, it is not the cancer that should necessarily be the prime focus. Most of the health care providers and family members are already giving plenty of attention to the cancer itself. One of the main areas the touch therapist should focus on is the immune system and how to build it. The immune system knows best how to respond to the cancer.

There are at least three ways in which the immune system and cancer are in relationship. First, it is this system that best knows how to deal with abnormal cells traveling throughout the body. One of the differences between a person who has cancer and a person who doesn't is the immune system's ability to identify cancer cells and the strength of it to eliminate those cells. Second, the immune system may be impacted by the disease. Leukemia, a disease that overproduces white blood cells, is a good example. Unfortunately, leukemic white blood cells are immature and poorly functioning, which suppresses the immune system. A third way that cancer and immunity can interrelate is the result of treatment side effects. Chemotherapy and radiation can both compromise the immune system because of their destruction of white blood cells, an important aspect of the immune system.

From the point of view of Chinese medicine, every vital organ in the body has a relationship to immunity. For instance, Large Intestine assists with immunity by eliminating toxicity. However, the three organs most associated with immunity are Kidney, Spleen, and Lung. Kidney, known as the House of Chi, is closely associated because of its relationship to bone, bone marrow, and, consequently, stem cell production. In Chinese medicine, Spleen is connected to the production of white blood cells and the lymphatic system. Lung's relationship with immunity is through its role in oxygenating and detoxifying the body via lung and skin. Also, Lung rules something called Wei Chi, a circulating layer of energy that resides below the skin. This layer protects the body from pathogenic invasion.

When choosing the ideal acupressure points or foot reflex zones with which to address a certain symptom, a bodyworker should look for those points or zones that can both assist with relief of the symptom and provide support for the immune system. For example, St36 is a classic point that supports digestive symptoms and immune function. The following symptoms relate to suppressed immunity. Listed next to the conditions are ways to address them through reflexology zones and acupressure points.

CHAPTER 6
STRENGTHENING THE BODY:
THE USE OF TOUCH TECHNIQUES
TO SUPPORT THE BODY DURING
AND AFTER TREATMENT
131

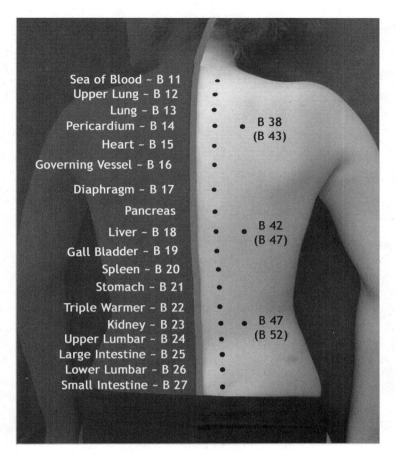

Sea of Blood ~ B 11
Upper Lung ~ B 12
Lung ~ B 13
Pericardium ~ B 14
Heart ~ B 15
Governing Vessel ~ B 16
Diaphragm ~ B 17
Pancreas
Liver ~ B 18
Gall Bladder ~ B 19
Spleen ~ B 20
Stomach ~ B 21
Triple Warmer ~ B 22
Kidney ~ B 23
Upper Lumbar ~ B 24
Large Intestine ~ B 25
Lower Lumbar ~ B 26
Small Intestine ~ B 27

B 38
(B 43)

B 42
(B 47)

B 47
(B 52)

Figure 6.2 Bladder Meridian Shu Points.

Photograph by Nicki Hansen-Dix

* *Note to the reader:* On the model's right side are points that have been parenthesized. They are part of a new acupressure numbering system. Some teachers still teach the old points, which are not in parentheses.

Symptoms that Relate to Suppressed Immunity

	Foot	Bladder points	Others
Anemia	Kidney, Lung and Liver	11, 12, 13, 17, 18, 23	K1, K3, K7, Lu1, St16, Sp6
Engraftment rate	Kidney and Spleen	11, 17, 20, 23, 47	Sp6, K1, K3, K27, CV4, CV6, CV17
Fatigue	Kidney, Lung and Spleen	12, 13, 17, 23, 47	K1, K3, K7, St36, Lu1, CV4, CV6, Sp6
Flu-like symptoms	Kidney, Diaphragm and Lung	12, 13, 17, 23, 47	K1, K3, K7, Lu1, St16, CV4, CV6, CV17
Herpes or Shingles	Kidney and Lung	12, 13, 23, 47	K1, K3, K27, Lu1, CV17
Lymphedema	Spleen, Lung and Kidney	12, 13, 20, 22, 23	Sp6, K3, K27, Lu1

Neutropenia	Kidney and Spleen	11, 17, 20, 23, 47	K1, K3, K27, CV4, CV6, CV17, Lu1, Sp6
Thrombo-cytopenia	Kidney	11, 17, 23, 47	K1, K3, K27

PSYCHOLOGICAL SUPPORT

For a few people, the hospital experience, both inpatient and outpatient, translates to feeling cared for, attended to, and, in a way, saved. For others, the experience generates feelings of being powerless and in danger. They may also suffer a degrading shift in which they are transformed from a "person" to a "patient." This shift, in which the person no longer exists but becomes a tumor that needs to be removed or abnormal cells that need to be destroyed, fosters a sense of disrespect, disregard, and humiliation. These feelings are lived in silence and their suffering tends to be downplayed and unattended, being considered minor in comparison to the cancer and its physical consequences.

Receiving a diagnosis of cancer impacts the core of a person's being on a very profound psychological level. It may trigger emotions of guilt (if I had only …), betrayal, loss (losing life, losing life as it is, losing your healthy identity, losing body parts, losing friends and even losing family members), despair, and fear. Where there is the possibility of loss, especially the loss of life, there comes a sense of threat.

Threat is typically perceived by the reptilian part of the brain which is responsible for survival. It knows only three possible responses: fight, flight or freeze. Many things can feel threatening, receiving a cancer diagnosis, for instance. This experience is filled with fear which can trigger the need not just to fight but also to run and, for some patients, freeze. Often, the language used in relation to cancer is borrowed from military verbage, such as "battling cancer," "winning the fight," or imagining cells to be "soldiers." That alone could awaken the person's reptilian brain, altering the ability to both think and feel. Patients may then relate to their diagnosis and make decisions about their treatment in a state of panic.

The reptilian part of the brain does not differentiate between a medical procedure, such as surgery, and any other type of attack. Both register as threat. Any experience that leads to a sense of threat will trigger a response in the central nervous system and the adrenal glands which produce stress hormones. If the body receiving these messages is not able to fully release all the biochemical responses triggered into it, individuals may develop trauma, with the most severe level being Post Traumatic Stress Disorder (PTSD).

Patients who undergo numerous surgeries in a short period of time combined with long hospital stays, can develop some symptoms of trauma. The signs of trauma can be a sudden onset of irritability, feeling disconnected from others, the need to recoil, and difficulty expressing feelings. Just the idea of going to the cancer clinic for a blood draw can trigger a certain panic. Insomnia may occur if the person has a fear of not waking up or simply feeling that it is not safe to relax, to surrender. Breathing may also become erratic, and at moments, even difficult. This is not to say that undergoing surgery or hospital stays will automatically trigger trauma or cause PTSD. In her book, *Invisible Heroes: Survivors of Trauma and How They Heal*, Belleruth Naparstek writes that many different conditions within a person's life story and within their system will determine their predisposition to developing PTSD as a result of trauma.[3]

Without a doubt, a cancer diagnosis and treatment cause an emotional reaction. A clear relationship has been established between the mind, emotions, and the health of the immune system. Scientific research, such as that done by Candace Pert, former chief of the section on Brain Biochemistry, Clinical Neuroscience Branch of the NHI, shows the presence of limbic brain cells, referred to by her as "molecules of emotion" throughout the body, including the immune system.[4] Research done at the University of California San Francisco, led by assistant professor Elissa Epel, shows the relationship between stress levels and premature aging of immune cells, possibly creating a predisposition to developing cancer at an earlier age.

Massage therapists need to take into consideration a cancer patient's mental and emotional state when planning the massage session. Touch therapies consistently affect emotional states known to directly impact immunity. Anxiety is an excellent example of this. It is one variable in which the evidence is incontrovertible. Across the board, among a variety of sample groups, both healthy and sick, anxiety decreases immediately after massage.

Tiffany Field, from the Touch Research Institute (TRI) at the University of Florida, has done a number of studies with a wide variety of subjects, that indicate massage lowers cortisol levels.[5] Cortisol is a stress hormone released by the adrenal glands. Too much of it is has deleterious effects on the body. Although the sample sizes in the TRI studies are small and not yet totally embraced by mainstream researchers, evidence is mounting that touch techniques can be effective in supporting people on a psychological level, which in turn benefits the body.

The following symptoms can occur when patients are emotionally distressed or affected by trauma, including PTSD. Touch therapies can be used to address these side effects:

CHAPTER 6
STRENGTHENING THE BODY:
THE USE OF TOUCH TECHNIQUES
TO SUPPORT THE BODY DURING
AND AFTER TREATMENT
133

Areas that Address Psychological Support

	Foot	Bladder points	Others
Anger	Liver and Heart	15, 18, 38, 42	Lv3, H7, CV17
Anxiety	Heart	14, 15, 17	H7, CV17
Confusion	Heart and Small Intestine	15, 20, 27, 38	H7, CV17
Depression	Liver and Diaphragm	17, 18, 19, 42, 47	Lv3, Lu1, CV17, K27
Disrespect	Lung and Diaphragm	12, 13, 17	Lu1, CV17, St16
Fatigue (stress-related)	Kidney, Adrenals and Heart	14, 15, 23, 47	P6, H7, K27, CV17
Fear	Kidneys and Adrenals	23, 38, 47	K1, K3, K27, P6, CV4, CV6, CV17
Feeling Confined	Liver and Diaphragm	17, 18, 42	Lv3, P6, CV17
Guilt/Shame	Large Intestine	13, 25	P6, CV17, Lu1
Hopelessness/ Disappointment	Kidney and Stomach	13, 21, 23, 47	K1, K3, K7 K27, St36, St16, CV17

To Whom Are We Relating?

R. came to me very ill, undergoing chemotherapy after having surgery for breast cancer. Her physical appearance had been altered by her illness and subsequent treatment as well as by the sudden death of her husband during her own chemo process. Mr. R had a heart attack on the day of her surgery and died 40 days later without leaving the hospital. I was aware of a sick, bald, grieving widow with a lot of will to live. That is the impression that I related to. In the back of my mind somewhere there was the knowledge that this person must not have always looked like this, but I was relating to the facade. One day R. told me that prior to her illness she had been a biker along with her husband. She explained how she had started out with a smaller, less potent bike but then wanted more power, and got a Gold Wing 1000. I had been seeing R. probably twice a week throughout her treatment, yet this story revealed to me a whole different side of R. I was struck by the fact that she was something quite different from what I had imagined. I asked for a picture of her on one of her bike trips. She brought in a picture which was about a year old. It revealed a long-haired, beautiful woman astride a motorcycle. I realized that this was who R. truly was and I started relating to THAT woman. I did not negate what was happening in the present moment, but I did start relating to her differently. Even though I didn't ever think that she was only the consequences of her cancer, until that picture, I mostly related to that aspect of her. Since then, every time I work with a patient who comes to me altered by this disease process and treatment, I always find an appropriate situation where I may ask, "Oh really? I would love to see a picture of that." Seeing a small picture that is brought in always gives me a more holistic sense of the big picture of this person's being.

— ISABEL ADKINS, PRACTITIONER OF ORIENTAL BODYWORK, NEVADA CITY, CALIFORNIA

Inability to interact with others	Heart and Spleen	14, 15, 20, 38	H7, P6, Sp6, CV17
Insomnia	Heart and Liver	14, 15, 18, 38, 42	Lv3, P6, H7, CV17
Irritability	Liver	17, 18, 42	Lv3, P6, CV17
Unsettled/ "feeling lost"	Heart and Spleen	14, 15, 20, 38	H7, P6, CV4, CV6, CV17

CHAPTER 6
STRENGTHENING THE BODY:
THE USE OF TOUCH TECHNIQUES
TO SUPPORT THE BODY DURING
AND AFTER TREATMENT
135

2/3 of help is to give courage.
—IRISH PROVERB

Spirit of the Organs

An organ's spirit is related to emotional and psychological aspects of health, to its likes and dislikes. Because the cancer experience triggers such an emotional reaction, it is an important component to attend to. Chinese medicine gives bodyworkers the tools to address feeling states.

Kidney: Associated with the will to live, consequently it is about both interest in life and survival. It is mostly associated with the emotion of fear. This makes good sense because fear arises in the same place where there is a concern for survival. Kidney is nourished by beauty and awe and is very aware of danger signals.

Lung: Called the Father, the Lung is about boundaries, both emotional and physical. It is nourished by respect and impacted by experiences of vulnerability and lack of consideration. It is mostly associated with the emotion of grief, which is natural given the connection between loss and the disruption of comfortable boundaries.

Liver: The Liver is the force that motivates us to move forward, to move in the desired direction; nourished by freedom to flow, to be, it responds negatively to experiences of confinement, lack of liberty, and inability to choose. The emotions most closely associated with liver are anger and frustration. For an organ to which free will is so important, anything imposed upon it will naturally trigger irritability or rage.

Spleen – Pancreas: Called the Mother, this organ is about nourishing others and self. It is also associated with thoughts and feelings of concern. One's ability to be comfortable with the body is directly related to spleen energy. The spleen is mostly nourished by touch and a sense of home. This is the organ that suffers with instability, unattended suffering, worry and mental clutter.

Stomach: Associated with the emotion of sympathy, the stomach reacts strongly to outside physical and emotional influences. In stressful circumstances, depending on the individual, the stomach will create the desire or lack thereof for food. It will also impact the ability or inability to digest. The phrase, "I don't have the stomach for this right now," says it all.

Intestines: The Small Intestine filters and sorts life experiences while the Large Intestine provides the process of managed elimination of the sorted matter, generating change through letting go.

Heart: In Chinese medicine, the heart, mind and spirit are considered as one. The heart is nourished through relationships with others and with the divine. It likes meditation and its natural state is considered to be joy. Nourishment of the heart assists with openness, and the avoidance of isolation. The heart is associated with excited emotions, such as joy or anxiety. It is troubled by too much chatter (both mental and verbal) and lack of opportunity for clarity.

Therapists Ask

Q *How can I integrate acupressure points into a regular massage session?*

A Supporting the organs will not only have an impact on how the body receives and deals with the toxicity from chemotherapy, other drugs, and the on-going degenerative effects of radiation, but will also be, in itself, de-toxifying. If you plan to integrate reflexology/acupressure in to your regular massage, whatever modality that might be, it is important to work in a way that you are not giving the body too much to process all at once. For instance, when I integrate reflexology and acupressure in to my work, I do not add it to a full body relaxation massage. I will usually start by giving twenty minutes to the feet working on specific organs, then fifteen minutes of acupressure, followed by 25 minutes of oil massage on any part of the body that could use some relaxation or is in pain. If we remember that the organs are networking, by the time you have completed the reflexology and acupressure treatment alone, it is already as if you have given a full body massage.

DETOXIFICATION

All bodywork that promotes circulation and lymphatic movement causes detoxification. Modalities such as Swedish Massage do this, as well as Ayurvedic massage, Acupressure, and Trigger Point Therapy, to name just a few. Detoxification has a place in oncology massage, but there are three very important matters that must be considered. The first consideration is "when" to start detoxifying work. Most assuredly, it should not begin during treatment or immediately after it has ended. Clients require time to recover from treatment before beginning detoxification. Second, the therapist and client must determine at "what pace" to promote this detoxifying. All at once is not the answer. Detoxing should be done at a speed that does not cause severe discomfort to the client. The third matter to be aware of is the "degree of toxicity" that the client has. This can be gauged by such factors as the length of time clients have been in treatment and the number and type of treatments received, their nutritional status, age, and energy level.

Chemotherapy, and the many other medications that patients take, accumulate in the body. Detoxification can be as demanding and exhausting as is the buildup and storage of toxicity. Therapists must be aware that each client has a different constitution, making their detoxification process very individual. In some cases, detoxification generates more troubling side effects than the actual chemotherapy does. For instance, one chemotherapy patient who went for a colonic had such a severe reaction that she had to be treated in the emergency room. When the time is right to begin focusing on detoxification, touch therapists must be sure that the clients feel that they have recovered at least 60–70% of their energy. This indicates a Kidney Chi that will probably be strong enough to process waste.

The three organs that are most affected by the toxic by-products of cancer treatment are Liver, Kidney and Spleen (due to its relationship to the lymphatic system – the body's sewer system.) It will also be these three organs that are the focus of detoxification, as well as any other organ that seems to have suffered the most during treatment. For instance, some patients were most distressed by constipation. When this is the case, the massage plan should include attention to the Intestines. For other chemo patients, skin rashes were the most severe side effect. For this, the bodywork plan would include Lung. Some patients had diarrhea as an ongoing symptom. The therapist would then work with Kidney, Liver, Intestines and integrate Spleen into the session because this is the organ that is out of balance when moisture presents where it should not be.

When detoxification work is started, the therapist needs to return to the same state of mindfulness and gentleness that was used when the client was in treatment. Bodyworkers need to check in with clients after each session. Asking the following day how he or she responded to the session will help the therapist to determine whether she can inch her way forward or whether she needs to work in an even more conservative fashion. One symptom that cancer patients resent the most is the loss of their energy. Bodywork aimed at detoxification should not restimulate that exhaustion. It is possible to release toxicity from the body effectively and yet at a measured pace without tiring the person. For some people, it may take the body over a year to rid itself of the toxins.

CHAPTER 6
STRENGTHENING THE BODY:
THE USE OF TOUCH TECHNIQUES
TO SUPPORT THE BODY DURING
AND AFTER TREATMENT
137

DECIDING ON WHICH ORGANS TO FOCUS

There will always be reasons, either at a physical or psychological level, to work with all of the organs. Listed below are guidelines that will help practitioners better choose which organs to focus on. It is important to follow these guidelines when working with cancer patients, irrespective of how much experience a therapist may have in the use of acupressure and reflexology.

- **Prioritize what seem to be the most important symptoms to address.** These symptoms are usually those that are related to pain or other physical symptoms that compromise vital needs, such as nausea, shortness of breath, or neutropenia.

- **Look for the common thread among the many symptoms.** For instance, a client that is undergoing chemotherapy may be affected by nausea, leg pain, and constipation, all of which can be addressed through Liver. Fatigue, low blood counts, and lack of libido can be addressed through Kidney. Once practitioners notice that a certain organ is a common denominator, which is referred to as "organ networking," they can narrow down which organs to work with.

- **Be aware of what is causing the symptom.** This will affect which organ that is attended to. For instance, fatigue was listed in three different places in this chapter – under the areas of organ support, immune support, and also psychological support. Fatigue caused by chemotherapy toxicity is first met by working Liver. Fatigue that is caused by compromised immunity is best met by Kidney, Lung and Spleen points. And the fatigue caused by stress is best addressed through Kidney, Adrenals and Heart.

- **When working with acupressure points, if in doubt about being in the right place, ask your client, "Does this feel useful?"** For a few therapists this may seem strange. But most clients are aware if something feels right or not, even if they don't necessarily have the specific knowledge to determine that. Many times when the therapist is holding points that are fundamental to addressing the client's condition, the clients say "Wow, that feels great!" Others will ask, "What is that point?" Still others will discreetly nod their head in affirmation, mostly without being aware of it. Through time, as therapists hold these points, they will notice a pulsing sensation or vibrating quality. Even if a

Cancer is something to be embraced, not resisted; something to be heard and attended to. Bodywork sessions should be a place that allows cancer to be met as it is with no judgment.

— ISABEL ADKINS,
PRACTITIONER OF ORIENTAL
BODYWORK, NEVADA CITY,
CALIFORNIA

We leave traces of ourselves wherever we go, on whatever we touch.

— LEWIS THOMAS

bodyworker does not feel this from the start, it doesn't mean that it is not happening. Trust this. Doing acupressure with cancer patients is very different from working with a healthy client due to how weak their system is and how long it sometimes takes for their Chi to rise.

- **Be creative in integrating these points.** For instance, for lack of appetite caused by liver toxicity, the practitioner might want to hold Lv3 with one hand while holding St36 with the other. Or, they might want to hold both the right and left St36 at the same time for boosting energy levels.

- **Inch forward and be undemanding** in the same way that is needed when giving a comfort-oriented session. At first, integrate in a few key organs while doing foot massage or only one or two acupressure points.

- **Do a follow-up call the next day** to see how the client is doing: Did they sleep better or worse? Do they feel flu-ish or do they feel stronger? This will help the therapist to determine if the sessions need to be less demanding or if he can inch his way forward the next time.

- **Touch techniques must be applied conservatively, humbly, attentively, and always with much reverence.** These patients are often very ill and sometimes traumatized. Independent of how good they look or how positive their frame of mind is, they still need to be touched with great mindfulness. Hard pressure does not need to be applied to the zones or points in order to be effective. Sometimes it is enough to just lightly hold or touch the point.

ACUPRESSURE POINT LOCATIONS

All acupressure points are bilateral except Conception Vessel and Governing Vessel points.

The Bladder (B) meridian acupressure points that run closest to the spine correspond to the vital organs in the body. These are called Back Shu Points. For example, B13 corresponds to the lungs and B15 to the heart. Please refer to the Bladder Meridian Shu Point Illustration, Figure 6.3, for location of other points. All of the points are two finger widths lateral from the spine.

- B11 through B17 start at T1 and end at T7.
- B18 through B21 start at T9 and end at T12.
- B22 through B27 start at L1 and end at the first sacral foramen.

Continued on page 142

CHAPTER 6
STRENGTHENING THE BODY:
THE USE OF TOUCH TECHNIQUES
TO SUPPORT THE BODY DURING
AND AFTER TREATMENT
139

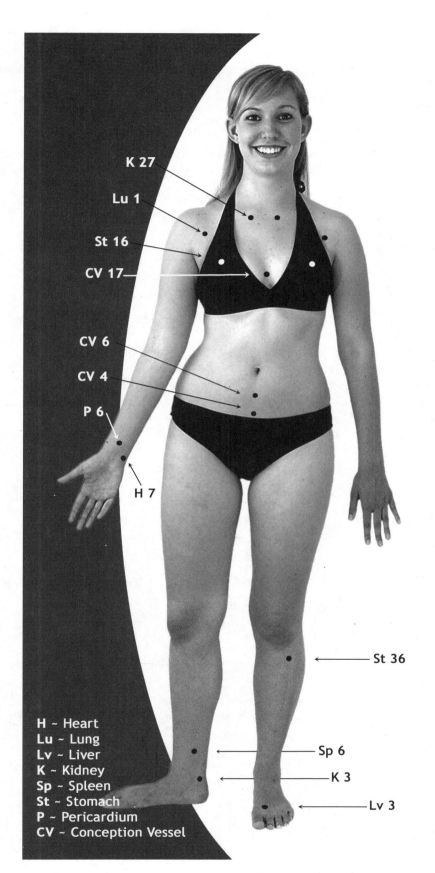

K 27

Lu 1

St 16

CV 17

CV 6

CV 4

P 6

H 7

St 36

Sp 6

K 3

Lv 3

H ~ Heart
Lu ~ Lung
Lv ~ Liver
K ~ Kidney
Sp ~ Spleen
St ~ Stomach
P ~ Pericardium
CV ~ Conception Vessel

Figure 6.3 Selected Acupressure Points.

Photograph by Nicki Hansen-Dix

CASE

Oncology Massage Intake & Session

Patient Name:	"S"	*Age:*	40-yr-old	☒ Male	☐ Female

Date: 4/28/06   *Name of Practitioners:* Paige & Jeannette

Patient's History: Rectal bleeding in 2002 – misdiagnosed – treated for hemorrhoids

Problems off and on for 3 years

Performed sigmoidoscopy in October 2005

Diagnosed with colorectal cancer in November 2005

> Underwent low anterior rectal resection with ileostomy on 12/27/05 with abdominal lymph node biopsy
> Prior to surgery, received 6 weeks of combination therapy with 5-FU IV once a week and 5 days a week radiation therapy to rectum
> Eight weeks following surgery started on Folfax (combination of chemotherapy agents 5-FU and Oxiliplatin) IV, every 2 weeks for 3 days to a total of 8 treatments
> Scheduled to have the ileostomy reanastomosed on June 20, 2006
> He has a right upper chest Portacath

Current Blood Counts: High WBC

Current Treatment:: Two days ago finished a 3-day chemo cycle. Has only 2 more cycles.

"S" began oncology massage therapy, focusing on organ and immune support, after 2 chemo cycles and received massage every week for 14 weeks.

Current Medications: Emend for nausea, Decadron, Compazine, Protonix

S (Subjective)   *What patient is reporting today:*

Current Major Complaints:	slight nausea, tiredness, pain in hips, cold feet with neuropathy and tingling in hands with acute sensitivity to cold.
Sleep:	intermittent, wakes up every night for a couple of hours
Appetite:	low for about 5 days after chemo, can't swallow cold for first 3 days after Oxiliplatin.
Physical pain:	stiff hips
Urination:	normal
Bowel movement:	normal
Moods:	emotional, feels it is probably due to lack of sleep
Overall energy:	on treatment week, low; off-week, better "out and about", works in the yard

CHAPTER 6
STRENGTHENING THE BODY:
THE USE OF TOUCH TECHNIQUES
TO SUPPORT THE BODY DURING
AND AFTER TREATMENT
141

STUDY

Symptoms marked on the intake form related to Chemotherapy/Radiation/Surgery

☒ Diarrhea	☒ Nausea	☒ Emotional Upset	☒ Thirst
☒ Decreased Taste	☒ Irritability	☒ Neuropathy	☒ Loss of Appetite
☒ Fatigue	☒ Muscle Aches, region: hips		

○ **(Objective)**   *Visual/palpable observations by Therapist; Treatment Plan*

"When we first saw him, we were both surprised — he didn't look sick. When you first described "S" we were both afraid. Not only did he have cancer but he had surgery, radiation, an ileostomy bag and a port. We were quite nervous. Yet, he is muscular, good color, very easy to talk with. The intake went well — all three of us were talking with each other. I soon realized that the cancer and treatments happened to him — it was not about him."

Treatment Plan   Foot: Heart (feet and hands, "intermittent sleep")
Kidney (immunity, hip pain, fatigue, bone support — Decadron leaches calcium from bones)
Liver (chemo toxicity, intermittent sleep, nausea, thirst, irritability, decreased taste, loss of appetite, muscle aches, fatigue — chemo related)
Intestines (colorectal cancer, resection with ileostomy)
Stomach (lack of appetite, nausea)

Acupressure: Along the spine: Bl 23, Bl 47, Bl 18, Bl 42, Bl 15, Bl 38

Other: Lv3, Sp6, St36, H7, P6, CV17, K27

Quadrant Protocol: No risk for lymphedema in any of the quadrants

Effleurage: Hands, with Mahanarayan oil. Neck, shoulders and back with organic sesame seed oil at a 2-3 pressure.

Session's Flow: Start with 20 minutes on the feet focusing on the specific organs, then integrate the acupressure points on the legs and feet for about 10 minutes.
Massage hands and hold H7 with P6.
Perform light effleurage on neck and shoulders integrating it with CV17 and K 27 for about 15 minutes all together.
Work on the Bl points and massage the back for about 10 minutes.
End with Reiki on the hips.

A **(Assessment)** – *Post treatment assessment*

Client felt relaxed, the hip pain subsided. "S" wanted to know if he could come back for the next student supervised clinic that will be in 4 weeks.

P **(Plan)** – *Follow up*

Next time "S" comes to the student clinic he will have finished chemotherapy and will be doing surgery to reverse the ileostomy in two weeks. At that time, besides current symptoms, the focus of the session will be immunity to strengthen the body for surgery, especially since he will not have had a lot of time to recover from the chemotherapy.

Instead of approaching a client with a Zen mind, a beginner's mind, imagine that this is the last time you will ever massage them. Without a doubt, this brings us into the here and now.

— Patsy Carlow,
Massage Therapist,
Edinburgh, Scotland

The following are good introductory points. They were chosen for their effectiveness, encompassing qualities, and direct relationship to immunity. All of these points together are a good immunity boost. Notice their names. They are very significant and give a sense of what they are about. See Figure 6.3 for locations.

Introductory Acupressure Points

K 27 *Elegant Mansion:* in the space between the protruding edge of the clavicle and first rib.

Lu 1 *Letting Go:* three finger widths down from the clavicle on the outer part of the chest.

St16 *Breast Window:* along the nipple line (running vertically) in the dip between third and fourth ribs.

CV17 *Sea of Tranquility* (Conception Vessel): at the center of the sternum. From the base of the bone it is three thumb widths up.

CV4 *Gate Origin:* in the lower abdomen, four finger widths down from the navel.

CV6 *Sea of Energy:* in the lower abdomen, three finger widths down from the navel.

P6 *Inner Gate:* between the radius and the ulna, two and one-half finger widths from the wrist.

Lv3 *Bigger Rushing:* in the groove between the big toe and second toe, on the top of the foot.

K3 *Bigger Stream:* midway between the medial malleolus and the Achilles tendon.

K1 *Bubbling Springs:* on the sole of the foot at the center of the reflex zone for the diaphragm.

St36 *Three Mile Point:* starting at the patella, four finger widths down and one finger width outside of the tibia.

Sp6 *Three Yin Crossing:* acupressure point where Liver, Spleen, and Kidney meridians cross. From the medial malleolus, four finger widths up.

H7 *Spirit Gate:* at the crease of the wrist on the little finger side.

B47 *Sea of Vitality:* four finger widths lateral to the second lumbar vertebra (L2).

B38 *Vital Diaphragm:* four finger widths lateral to the fourth thoracic vertebra (T4).

B42 *Soul Door:* four finger widths lateral to the ninth thoracic vertebra (T9).[6]

FINAL THOUGHTS

Through reflexology and acupressure, specific physical and emotional symptoms can be targeted. This type of treatment-oriented approach is preferable to some clients and therapists rather than the more random results brought on by comfort-oriented massage. Both approaches are valuable.

Blending East with West, integrating acupressure and Chinese thought with traditional massage strokes, brings a meditative quality to the work. The stillness that happens when acupressure is being given allows the client a moment to integrate what is happening in the session. This meditative quality, which is very pleasing for Heart Chi, allows the client time in which they can "stop for their life" instead of "run for their life." For a moment the fighting ceases and the soldier finally rests.

Blending these concepts into the massage session allows for organs to be strengthened instead of weakened or stressed. It provides a space where the focus is on that which is healthy and vital in the body in spite of any disease. Complementary medicine works with the premise that the body-mind can heal on many levels. Each cell in the body, with its dividing ability, contains the promise for more life, new life. Hope is a part of our physical make up. Being aware of this as they work, therapists are not only touching life but touching promise for life, touching hope.

REFERENCES

1. Leggett D. *Recipes for Self Healing*. Devon, England: Meridian Press, 1999.

2. Connelly D. *Traditional Acupuncture, The Laws of the Five Elements*. 2nd Ed. Maryland: Tai Sophia Institute, 1994.

3. Naparsek B. *Invisible Heroes: Survivors of Trauma and How They Heal*. New York, NY: Bantam, 2004.

4. Pert C. *Molecules of Emotion: The Science Behind Mind-Body Medicine*. New York, NY: Touchstone, 1999.

5. Field T. *Touch Therapy*. Edinburgh, Scotland: Livingstone Churchill, 2000.

6. *Basic Acupressure: The Extraordinary Channels and Points*. Berkeley, CA: Acupressure Institute, 1995.

CHAPTER 6
STRENGTHENING THE BODY:
THE USE OF TOUCH TECHNIQUES
TO SUPPORT THE BODY DURING
AND AFTER TREATMENT
143

Pat

A year after treatment, Pat returned to massage. By then, the meaning of the sessions had changed. Before cancer, the massages had been an extension of her fast-paced life. When the session ended, she immediately stepped back into the high stress, all relaxation quickly forgotten. Now, time spent receiving massage is sacred and meditative. Pat is in the here and now; she tunes into her body; and touch is an experience that deepens her awareness. These days, Pat enjoys the good feelings massage brings to her body and holds onto those sensations as long as possible. Bodywork helps her let go of the tension, anxiety, and fear that accumulated over the months of treatment.

— AUTHOR

Chapter 7

Massage for Children Living with Cancer

Special Knowledge for Special Patients

By Shay Beider, MPH, LMT

It is very difficult to imagine that a child could contract cancer and even more difficult to imagine that some children will die of it. Fortunately, it is a rare occurrence. The National Cancer Institute reports that each year in the United States approximately 9,500 children and adolescents under the age of 15 will be diagnosed with cancer. Of those diagnosed with cancer, nearly 1,600 will die from the disease each year. This makes cancer the leading cause of death by disease of children under the age of 15 living in the United States. Thankfully there have been significant improvements in cancer survival rates for children. The five-year relative survival rate among children with cancer improved from 56% for patients diagnosed between 1974 and 1976 to 79% for those diagnosed from 1995 to 2001, the most recent years that data is available.[1] As a group, children tend to respond much better to cancer treatment than do adults. According to the Children's Oncology Group, the cure rate for all childhood cancers is approximately 78%.[2]

CHAPTER 7
MASSAGE FOR CHILDREN
LIVING WITH CANCER:
SPECIAL KNOWLEDGE FOR
SPECIAL PATIENTS

145

Just as Complementary and Alternative Medicine (CAM) use has increased among adults, it is also increasing among pediatric populations because parents are instrumental in determining their children's health care choices.[3] A study of the use of alternative therapies for children with cancer found that 65% of patients in the cancer group were using some form of alternative therapy.[4] A survey of parents of children with cancer in British Columbia revealed that 66% of pediatric oncology patients were reported by their parents to have used massage therapy during their cancer treatment.[5] In this particular study, the reason most frequently cited by parents for the use of CAM therapies was to do everything possible for their child. Parents who did not use CAM therapies stated the foremost reason as being that they did not know about them. Parents indicated that they feel CAM helps to take their child's mind off pain and other side effects of treatment, which in turn helps them to sleep better. Because the treatment that children receive for cancer is generally more aggressive than for adult cancers, parents may be more likely to seek out alternative options such as CAM to help children cope with the side effects of treatment.[6]

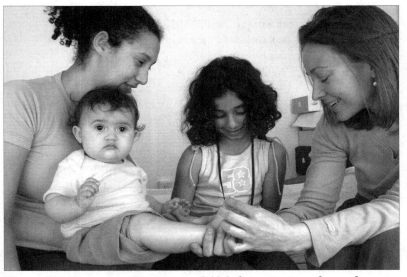

Figure 7.1 Parents are turning to CAM therapies in order to do everything possible for their child.   *Photograph by Andy Aryapour*

As CAM therapies have grown in popularity, research studies documenting their effects have increased in number. In the case of massage therapy, there is a growing body of evidence that massage therapy psychologically, physically, and behaviorally benefits children who are ill. Both single-dose (short term) and multiple-dose (long term) effects of massage are evident. A recent review of the pediatric massage literature found significant improvements in anxiety levels for children receiving massage.[7] These effects are strong and consistent with the effects found in adult populations.[8] Massage effects on pain and muscle tone also appear to be strong, but further study is needed in these areas. Other pediatric effects that are promising include massage therapy's effects on depression, negative mood, and certain types of behavior.

Of the randomized, controlled trials of pediatric massage conducted to date, only two have been published[9,10] and one has been submitted for publication.[11] Field et al. studied massage for children with leukemia.[9] The sessions were given daily for a month by their parents. At the end of the time, mood had improved and anxiety

It's time to embrace the invaluable effects of compassionate touch and massage and realize the biological and psychological benefit. Undergoing traditional western medical treatment can feel isolating and disconnected from the entire healing process. Massage can facilitate a person's complete body healing by reconnecting the medical profession and the patient with the entire mind-body process. Promoting sensory integration can minimize the debilitating effects of the common sensory deprivation in the traditional medical setting.

— JEFFREY GOLD, PHD,
CLINICAL PSYCHOLOGIST AT
CHILDRENS HOSPITAL LOS
ANGELES

decreased. The childrens' parents also reported psychological benefits from providing the massage.

Phipps et al. studied massage for children undergoing stem cell transplantation.[10] The patients were randomized to three groups: standard care, massage performed by a professional, and massage performed by parents. None of the primary measures (i.e., anxiety, discomfort, and mood) improved significantly. Nor did the secondary measures (i.e., use of nausea and pain medication, days spent in the hospital, and days to engraftment.) There was a positive trend, however. One of the trends, days spent in the hospital and days to engraftment, was a hopeful one. Not only would it mean being discharged sooner from the hospital but it would potentially save money. One significant finding was that the children massaged by their parents reached engraftment sooner. This means the child's immune system is working at a higher level.

Post-White and her colleagues measured the effects of full-body massage in children undergoing chemotherapy and the effects of a 15-minute seated massage on their parents. Pain, nausea, anxiety, fatigue, cortisol levels, and vital signs were examined in the children. There was no significant change in blood pressure, cortisol levels, pain, nausea, or fatigue. Heart and respiratory rate dropped, as did anxiety. Not surprisingly, all of the parents reported liking the massage and had less anxiety because of it.[11]

A study that did not use randomization, but instead used a longitudinal descriptive approach, documented the pain experience of children with acute lymphocytic leukemia (ALL), the most common form of childhood cancer. This study showed that leg pain was the most frequently cited pain, followed by abdominal pain, head/neck pain, and back pain.[12] Children with leg pain often reported that the leg pain occurred two days after chemotherapy treatment. Children also stated that their pain peaked at the beginning of the day and decreased gradually throughout the rest of the day. This is important information for massage therapists who are working with children who have ALL. Children may benefit from scheduling massage sessions in the morning when their pain experience is likely to be heightened. It may also be helpful to focus more time on the legs, abdomen, head, neck and back, since these areas are known to be the predominant sites of pain.

TYPES OF CANCER

Children tend to be diagnosed with different types of cancers than adults. Children's cancer is often not localized to specific organs but is more often systemic. Children are more likely to contract cancers of developing organ systems such as the blood, nervous system, and bones. Various forms of leukemia account for approximately one-third of all new cancer cases in children. Brain and other central nervous system tumors account for another 15–20% of childhood cancers. The most predominant types of cancer that affect children are leukemia, lymphoma, brain and neural tumors, sarcomas, Wilms' tumor, and retinoblastoma.

The causes of most types of childhood cancers are unknown. Several factors may contribute, including genetics, immunity, diet, hormones, viruses, socioeconomic status, lifestyle and other individual characteristics. Cancer therapies themselves are known to cause secondary malignancies. Certain types of chemotherapy, for instance, have been linked with an increased risk of developing leukemia.

Some suspect environmental factors as being related to cancer prevalence; however, there is not yet definitive evidence correlating this relationship, probably in part because different types of childhood cancers develop differently with multifactorial etiologies. This makes it difficult to establish a direct relationship between the environment and many cancers. Children with AIDS experience a higher risk of developing certain cancers, including non-Hodgkin's lymphoma, Kaposi's sarcoma, and leiomyosarcoma, a type of muscle cancer. Although parents sometimes experience feelings of guilt, cancer in children is generally not the result of any parental oversight or the result of any particular behavior the child may have engaged in.

TREATING CHILDREN FOR CANCER

Since the 1970's, both the incidence rates and the survival rates for some forms of childhood cancer have increased. For children younger than 15, the five-year relative survival rate has increased over the past three decades.[1] This is largely attributed to substantial advances in cancer treatment. The types of treatment that are used for childhood cancers parallel those used in adult populations, although they may be used with different frequency and intensity.

Much of the progress made in treating childhood cancers in recent years is due to advances made through clinical research. Family members of children undergoing cancer treatment may choose to enroll their children in clinical trials to test the effectiveness of new cancer treatments. Approximately 60% of pediatric cancer patients participate in clinical trials or research studies of cancer treatment. This is a much higher rate than with adult groups. The National Cancer Institute sponsors most pediatric studies. There are three primary groups that conduct these trials, including the Children's Oncology Group (COG), the Pediatric Brain Tumor Consortium (PBTC), and New Approaches to Neuroblastoma Therapy Consortium (NANT). It is important for everyone who is involved as part of the healthcare team for a child with cancer to be made aware of any research studies that the child is participating in. Research studies have strict clinical protocols with specific inclusion and exclusion criteria. Certain therapies, such as massage therapy, may not be allowed during the study period. Furthermore, it is of the utmost importance that every member of the child's team respect the study protocol so that the child's health is not jeopardized. For massage

CHAPTER 7
MASSAGE FOR CHILDREN
LIVING WITH CANCER:
SPECIAL KNOWLEDGE FOR
SPECIAL PATIENTS
147

Truth is fierce and unrelenting. We cannot change it, but we can change the way we live with it. Making mistakes, not being loved, and dying are inescapable experiences of being human; so is our fear of them. By facing those fears, we have a chance to step beyond them. When we are willing to do the best we can with what we know, to be honest with ourselves and others about who we are and what really matters to us, only then are the lives we live and the love we receive truly our own.

— MARIA HOUSDEN,
AUTHOR OF *HANNAH'S GIFT* AND
MOTHER OF A CHILD WITH CANCER

therapists, it is important to ask family members if their child is enrolled in any clinical trials. Once this information is obtained, the massage therapist can consult with the physician to determine if massage would be appropriate while they are enrolled in the research study.

Most children undergoing cancer treatment will attend school but they often find that they fall behind in their academic life because of extended absences or fatigue. Visible side effects of the illness or treatment can be a major source of discomfort for children undergoing cancer treatment. Children with cancer may show visible signs of hair loss, weight gain, or surgical disfigurement, which need to be explained to their teachers and peers so that their experience can be better understood. It is important for educators to work with students in the classroom setting to be able to explain what cancer is and how to most appropriately interact with their peers who may have cancer. It can be helpful to develop partnerships between the school, the hospital and the family to ensure as smooth a transition as possible. This is especially important because studies have shown that the best childhood predictor of adult adaptation is how well the child gets along with other children.[13]

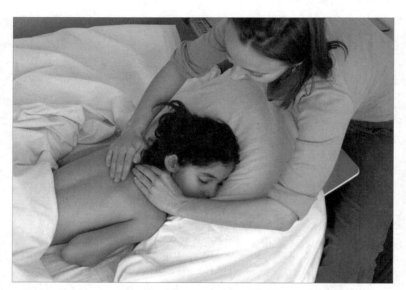

Figure 7.2 Through loving touch, massage therapists have the opportunity to show children that they are lovable and beautiful.

Photograph by Andy Aryapour

Because of the intimate nature of massage therapy, it is very likely that massage therapists will play a role in the child's process of coping with the physical changes they are experiencing. Children may discuss their uncertainty or discomfort with their physical appearance. For example, when surgery or chemotherapy have caused dramatic changes in their appearance, children will often express their concern and sorrow. One of the most valuable things massage therapists can provide in those moments is a willingness to listen – to really listen deeply. Through loving touch, massage therapists have the opportunity to show children in a very real way that they are lovable and beautiful. Massage therapy can help children to feel better about their changing bodies and can renew their self-confidence and self-esteem.

Another tool that is very effective in helping children cope with their cancer diagnosis and the effects of treatment are the camps that are made available to children with cancer. The Association of Hole in the Wall Camps is the world's largest family of camps for children with serious illnesses and life-threatening conditions.[14] Paul Newman, who started the first camp in 1988, founded this association. Children with cancer can attend the camps free of charge. They offer both summer and year-round programs that provide fun camp activities as well as medical supervision and psychosocial services. Retreats are organized for the children's parents, and siblings also have the opportunity to participate in some of the camps. For the massage therapist working with a child with cancer, it is very likely that the camp experience will play into their process of healing. In some instances, massage therapists may be able to join children on their camp outings. This is one of the experiences that is unique to working with children and that is noticeably different from working with adult patients. (See Massage is Like Mr. Freeze! on page 161.)

There are other notable differences in massaging pediatric and adult patients with cancer. Lymphedema, which is an important concern for adult patients with cancer, is extremely rare for children. Children do not tend to have lymph node resections, which explains some of the difference. Edema is also very rare for children with cancer but may occur in more advanced cases.

With adult patients, deep vein thrombosis (DVTs) can be an important concern, especially following surgical procedures. Among pediatric cancer patients, DVTs are not common. Massage therapists must show caution in treating patients who are at increased risk for DVTs, but it is less common for children with cancer to develop this complication than for adults.

Another difference between children and adults is that children aren't prone to having bone metastasis. This is because bone metastases are usually related to the primary cancer site and in children it is infrequent to see a primary disease that metastasizes to the bone.

The normal platelet range for children is similar to adults, about 150,000 to 400,000 (expressed as 150–400). The range for children with cancer is usually much lower and the medical staff is often satisfied if their platelets stay above 50 on their own. For children undergoing chemotherapy, the platelet range typically is between 20 and 100. A general guideline for massage therapists is that platelet counts of 10 to 15 are generally considered to be safe for massage. However, children with lower platelet counts may be massaged if great care is taken. In that case, it is essential to ask the medical or nursing staff about bruising and to maintain a close dialogue with the child to determine their ongoing comfort level.

Another difference between adults and very young children is that radiation therapy is infrequently used with children under three years of age because of concerns about the long term consequences. Sometimes young children with brain or solid tumors and leukemia and lymphoma patients with disease in the spinal fluid may receive radiation therapy. External beam radiation is mostly used with children. Internal radiation is not used and implants are very rare.

Children's white blood cell counts (WBCs) are comparable to adults, a normal range being between 4.5–10. Children undergoing chemotherapy may have WBCs in the range of 1.0–5.0 during treatment. If WBCs are in the range of 1.0–2.0 then another dose of chemotherapy can generally be administered. When treating children

CHAPTER 7
MASSAGE FOR CHILDREN
LIVING WITH CANCER:
SPECIAL KNOWLEDGE FOR
SPECIAL PATIENTS

149

I have a friend, a chemotherapy nurse in a children's cancer ward, whose job it is to pry for any available vein in an often emaciated arm to give infusions of chemicals that sometimes last as long as twelve hours and which are often quite discomforting to the child. He is probably the greatest pain-giver the children meet in their stay in the hospital. Because he has worked so much with his own pain, his heart is very open. He works with his responsibilities in the hospital as a "laying on of hands with love and acceptance." There is little in him that causes him to withdraw, that reinforces the painfulness of the experience for the children. He is a warm, open space which encourages them to trust whatever they feel. And it is he whom the children most often ask for at the time they are dying. Although he is the main pain-giver, he is also the main love-giver.

FROM *HOW CAN I HELP?*
BY RAM DASS AND PAUL GORMAN

*Don't turn your head. Keep looking
at the bandaged place. That's where
the light enters you.
And don't believe for a moment
that you're healing yourself.*

JELALUDDIN RUMI
FROM *THE ESSENTIAL RUMI,*
TRANSLATED BY COLEMAN BARKS

with cancer, low blood count scores during the first 30 days from the start of treatment are often tolerated and chemotherapy is delivered to try to get the patient into remission. This choice is made because studies have shown that children who are treated in the earlier stages of the disease have a much better chance of obtaining positive outcomes.

A course of chemotherapy for children is generally administered every four to five weeks for children between four months and three years of age, depending upon the type of cancer and the stage of the disease. Children with leukemia typically receive longer periods of chemotherapy (i.e., two to three years), whereas children with tumors are likely to receive shorter doses.

HOW CHILDREN DIFFER PHYSIOLOGICALLY FROM ADULTS

Children's bodies are quite different from adults'. First, there are significant musculoskeletal differences. As infants, the cranial bones are separated by soft spots called fontanels that enable babies to make their journey through the birth canal. Over the first two years of life, the fontanels gradually close and sutures form that allow expansion and development of the brain and skull. As adolescence is entered, these sutures become much more solid but never completely rigid. Because of the softness of the skull in early life, in some cultures infant's skulls are intentionally compressed for aesthetic purposes.[15] At a very early age, it is still possible to reshape the infant's skull using applied pressure. In the West Indies, for instance, some mothers have practiced a form of massage that literally molds the baby's head, nose, small of the back, and buttocks.[17] This example illustrates to bodyworkers the importance of taking great care in working with infant's skulls, with the full recognition and understanding that only light pressure should be applied.

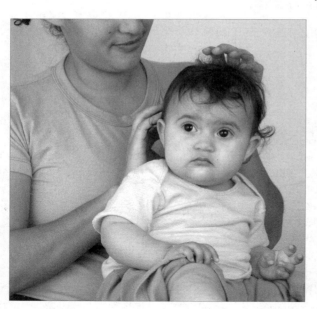

Figure 7.3 At early ages, only light pressure should be applied to the skull.

Photograph by Andy Aryapour

Children's bones are not as solid as adult's bones and are more vulnerable to fractures. This is because children's bones are not completely ossified. Ossification occurs gradually over time. Fortunately, children tend to heal fractures more quickly than adults because of increased bone blood supply and a thicker and stronger periosteum (the dense membrane that closely wraps around bones). Children with cancer can experience greater vulnerability in their bones because of medications, such as chemotherapeutic agents, which can deplete calcium and other important bone components. This may cause bones to become especially fragile.

At the ends of long bones are cartilaginous growth plates that can be damaged by excessive weight-bearing pressure or twisting. For this reason, it is very important to support the joints when working with children. A child's joints should never be forcibly manipulated and minimal torsional pressure should be applied. For all children with cancer, it is necessary to be clear whether they have developed any bone metastasis, even though this is very rare. Bone metastasis will make bones extremely vulnerable to damage, even with very light touch.

CHAPTER 7
MASSAGE FOR CHILDREN
LIVING WITH CANCER:
SPECIAL KNOWLEDGE FOR
SPECIAL PATIENTS
151

In general, children's muscles, tendons, ligaments, and joints are much more flexible than those found in adults. It is important not to overstretch children's bodies and to instead pay careful attention to their physical limitations. Since children's muscle tissue is not as developed as that of adults, they do not require the same depth of pressure. This is especially true for children with cancer who may only tolerate a light to light/medium touch. As with all cancer patients, firm pressure is never recommended. Because children's musculature is not fully developed, their posture differs from that of adults. Young toddlers tend to have lordosis (an inward curve of the lumbar spine), whereby their abdomens protrude slightly. This diminishes over time as muscular strength develops. Older teens tend to have reached maximal body strength unless a program of weight training is added later in life.

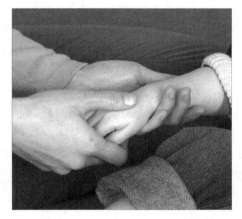

*Figure 7.4 **It is important to support the joints when working with children.***

Photograph by Andy Aryapour

Children's skin is more porous and more fragile than adults'. Also, it has more sensory receptors. Because children's bodies are smaller, the total skin surface area is smaller. An adult's hand can cover a very large portion of a small child's body. Therefore, careful attention must be paid to the impact of touch on body temperature. It is advisable to modify strokes to cover a smaller surface by using only portions of the hand, such as the fingers or palm. It is not necessary to use the full hand or hands at all times when working with children. If full hand contact is made, it is recommended that the therapist periodically remove their hands to give the child an opportunity to regulate their body temperature.

Children have more touch receptors per square centimeter than adults and can be over-stimulated by touch if it is not delivered with a careful hand. Because children's sensory receptors are still developing and their nervous system is not fully formed, they may not be as readily able to perceive temperature and pressure changes. When working with children with cancer, therapists need to be especially careful that the pressure errs on the lighter side and that the temperature in the room is sufficient.

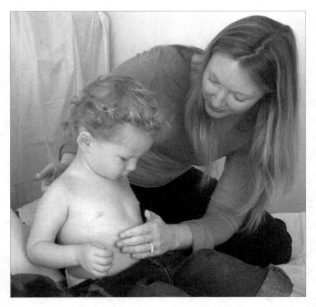

*Figure 7.5 **Modify strokes to cover a smaller surface by using only a portion of the hand.***

Photograph by Andy Aryapour

Practitioners should check in with the child frequently to see how they are feeling and if they are over-stimulated in any way. Children with cancer who experience fatigue may not always admit when touch is overly stimulating. It is the massage therapist's responsibility to check in with the child to see if they would like to take a break or if the child would like any changes to be made in the way they are being touched. Massage therapists must also make

Massage has been shown to be beneficial to children with chronic pain and especially those in palliative care. We have incorporated massage therapy as part of the UCLA Pediatric Pain Program since 1991 when the program was initiated. It has been one of the most valued parts of the program. Even children who have sensitivity in one part of their body can benefit from massage therapy in another part. I highly recommend massage therapy for newborns, sick children, those with chronic disease, and those at end of life.

LONNIE ZELTZER, MD,
DIRECTOR OF THE PEDIATRIC
PAIN PROGRAM AT UCLA

independent assessments of the child's well being based on color changes, body temperature, breathing patterns, and evidence of muscular relaxation or contraction.

Because children weigh less, they require smaller doses of medications and absorbed substances such as massage oils or lotions. For children with cancer, because chemotherapeutic agents can significantly weaken the immune system, practitioners may be informed by the medical staff that only certain types of lotions or oils that have been approved by the pharmacist are appropriate for massage. It is important to strictly adhere to their advice. Oils or lotions that are frequently used with healthy patients may introduce infectious agents that can be life-threatening for a child with cancer.

CHILDREN'S PSYCHOLOGICAL AND EMOTIONAL DEVELOPMENT

Children's psychological and emotional development changes significantly as they move through the different life stages. Those with serious illness, such as cancer, may experience periods of psychological and emotional regression in order to cope with the severity of their circumstances. It is helpful for massage therapists to have an understanding of what is considered to be generally consistent psychological and emotional development through the periods of infancy, early childhood, and adolescence.

INFANTS (UP TO 1 YEAR)

Infants who undergo cancer treatment have a deep need for maintaining a trusting and consistent relationship with their primary caregivers. Inconsistency in the parent-child relationship or separation from the primary caregivers can evoke a very primal fear. Infants are incredibly sensitive to their parents' emotional reality.[18] Babies look carefully at their parents' facial expressions to see what emotions are being communicated. Babies and parents frequently synchronize their emotional states. This emotional sharing gives them a way to communicate long before speech is developed. From this space of emotional attunement, secure attachment develops when a parent consistently senses their baby's desires and acts on them.

Young babies are not able to direct all of their own functions so they depend upon the information and stimuli from those around them to determine their

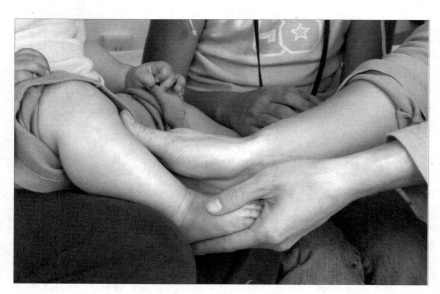

Figure 7.6 Infant massage is typically taught to parents who directly administer it to their babies.

Photograph by Andy Aryapour

experience. Infants' cardiovascular function, sleep rhythms, and immune function are all strongly influenced by their parents. Parents provide a form of physiologic governance until, over time, babies gradually internalize more of their regulatory functions. Because of these needs, infant massage is typically taught to parents who directly administer massage to their babies. Courses for massage therapists to learn infant massage instruction are widely taught and are necessary prerequisites to working with babies in this earliest life stage.

CHAPTER 7
MASSAGE FOR CHILDREN
LIVING WITH CANCER:
SPECIAL KNOWLEDGE FOR
SPECIAL PATIENTS
153

TODDLERS (1–3 YEARS)

Toddlers are beginning to differentiate themselves from their parents and are more able to regulate their physiological functioning. However, they still depend on their parents to provide positive reinforcement and a sense of secure attachment. Toddlers clearly recognize the difference between their parents and strangers and will want to have their parents very nearby when meeting someone new for the first time.

Because toddlers don't have a well-defined body image, they are very concerned about any procedures that are being done to their body. This can be particularly difficult for pediatric cancer patients who need to regularly receive physical interventions. Generally, toddlers' attention span is focused around the present moment, so it is important to communicate with them about things that are going to happen right before doing them. Toddlers' understanding of language is very concrete and they are unable to understand nuanced language. For this reason, a direct and simple communication style is the most effective.

Toddlers' understanding of cause-and-effect relationships is similarly limited and they may make inaccurate assumptions. For example, toddlers may think, "My parent left the room and my arm started to hurt. If my parent leaves the room my arm will hurt." This means that careful attention must be paid to the associations that toddlers link to a particular experience such as massage.

Toddlers' emotional expressions can be strong and immediate, as they are not yet adept at regulating their emotions. This makes dealing with stress particularly challenging for toddlers and sometimes they will feel the need to regress to younger behaviors to adapt to stressful situations. This indicates that they need to be soothed and comforted. Toddlers are often excited about exploring their environment and may enjoy a massage that is more active and engaging. For children with cancer, this will depend upon how they are feeling in the given moment. Games and stories can be useful adjuncts to providing massage therapy with toddlers.

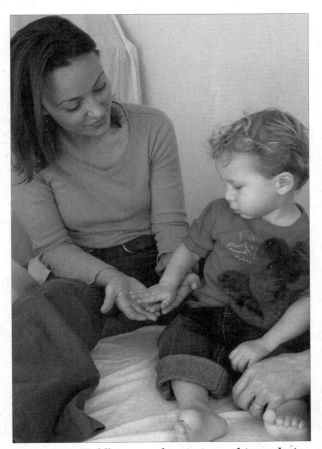

Figure 7.7 Toddlers are often interested in exploring their environment and enjoy massage that is active and engaging.   *Photograph by Andy Aryapour*

PRESCHOOLERS (3–5 YEARS)

Preschoolers are still very dependent on their parents for emotional support and security. They are beginning to learn basic concepts and enjoy asking questions. Typically, their vocabulary is limited to 900–1500 words and they tend to make sentences that are three to five words in length. Children at this age like to play make-believe, have imaginary friends, and engage in magical thinking. Because of their heightened capacity for magical thinking, they sometimes believe that their parents, or others, can make the illness go away.

At this age, children may become extremely anxious at the prospect of painful procedures. They are just beginning to have a concept of time and can have clear memories of their past medical treatments. Sometimes, preschoolers regress emotionally and behaviorally during treatment to help them cope with the situation. With preschool-age children it is important to maintain routines and family rituals and to provide opportunities for play and engagement. They can begin to learn self-comforting techniques, such as breathing awareness, and may enjoy having a favorite toy nearby during massage. Parent participation is especially helpful when working with preschool-age children and will help to alleviate some of their fears.

SCHOOL-AGED CHILDREN (6–12 YEARS)

For school-aged children with cancer, the most formidable issue often revolves around returning to school. A resumption of their school activities is essential for a positive transition. Involvement with their peers and teachers is crucial because children in this age group are increasingly concerned with their peers' opinions. Body image can be a real issue after cancer treatment. Not all children are compassionate when it comes to physical differences that are a result of cancer treatment, such as hair loss or amputation. Children who undergo cancer treatment often experience teasing about their physical appearance and may feel insecure. Through massage, a child's body image can be enhanced by reinforcing a sense of wholeness. Children can learn to accept their physical body and its limitations.

Children in this age group tend to be more fearful of bodily harm or injury. The experience of undergoing medical procedures can be particularly difficult. They may believe that they have done something wrong to cause their illness or that they are being punished for bad behavior.

School-aged children have a greater need for physical privacy and it is important to respect this during massage. Draping can be helpful in

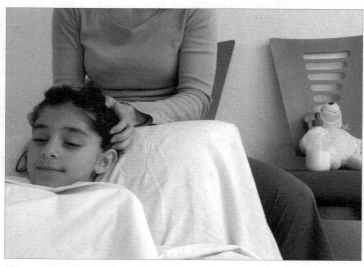

Figure 7.8 It is important to respect school-aged children's need for greater physical privacy.   Photograph by Andy Aryapour

establishing a safe boundary. For some children, wearing clothing may be comforting. In this age group, children begin to use cognitive operations to reach a logical conclusion. They have an increased attention span and begin to be able to see things from another point of view. Some children will experience cognitive delays as a result of cancer treatment, which can have implications for their future learning. This regression in cognitive skill can be troubling to the child and their family members and there may be some displaced anger as a result. Teachers need to learn to navigate this new hurdle with the family and discuss cognitive changes that they feel are significant.

ADOLESCENTS (13–18 YEARS)

With the onset of puberty, adolescence is a time of tremendous change. There is pressure to conform to one's peer group and to fit in. Some adolescents may have a negative body image and the difficulty of managing the physical changes that result from cancer treatment can seem devastating. Because adolescents have a heightened capacity to understand their illness, they are able to ask questions about the disease process and should be included in conversations and decisions around medical treatment and interventions. Fear of loss of control and identity as well as physical pain, disfigurement, or death can be deeply troubling concerns for adolescents with cancer. Teenagers may withdraw, become uncooperative or hostile, or engage in risky behavior. It is important to promote self-care and to nurture a safe environment that is honoring of their need for privacy, autonomy, and confidentiality. Visits and calls from their peers can be especially helpful, and encouraging verbalization of their feelings can help to keep things in perspective. Often, adolescents with cancer have many questions about their future and how this diagnosis will affect them for years to come. Massage can be a way to reconnect with the body and to release some of the pent-up anxiety that has developed.

PREPARING CHILDREN FOR MASSAGE

Massage for children with cancer requires heightened sensitivity and responsiveness to the needs of the child, their family members, and their caregivers. The treatment plan for any patient with cancer requires a delicate balance of listening, learning, and giving. Children with cancer bring an added dimension of complexity for massage therapists and other healthcare providers because childhood cancers are rare and because families are never fully prepared to receive such a diagnosis for their child.

One of the most important things for the massage therapist to establish with children and adolescents is that they are safe. This can be achieved in a variety of different ways, including carefully explaining what is going to be done before beginning the massage and establishing a comfortable relationship with the child's parents. This might involve having the parent approach the bedside with the

CHAPTER 7
MASSAGE FOR CHILDREN
LIVING WITH CANCER:
SPECIAL KNOWLEDGE FOR
SPECIAL PATIENTS
155

Live and love it up!

MICHAELA, 10-YEAR-OLD GIRL
LIVING WITH A BRAIN TUMOR

Start walking… your legs will get heavy and tired… Then comes the moment, of feeling the wings you've grown, lifting…

JELALUDDIN RUMI
FROM *THE ESSENTIAL RUMI*,
TRANSLATED BY COLEMAN BARKS

Do all you can with what you have, in the time you have, in the place you are.

NKOSI JOHNSON,
AIDS ACTIVIST WHO DIED
FROM AIDS AT THE AGE OF 12

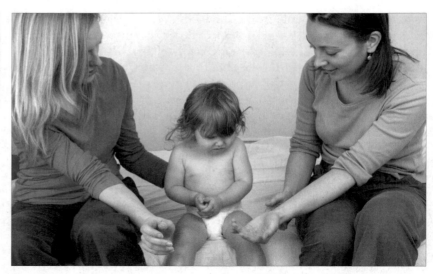

Figure 7.9 The massage therapist must etablish with children that they are safe.   Photograph by Andy Aryapour

massage therapist or asking the parent if they would like to learn some simple massage techniques.

Children pay careful attention to the way that people interact with their parents and they look to their parents for signals that someone is safe. It is always advisable that massage therapists introduce themselves to the parent and the child while maintaining eye contact. The therapist can touch the parent by shaking hands with them, which indicates to the child that their touch is safe. The massage therapist can also ask the parent if it would be all right to demonstrate massage on their hand or arm so that the child can begin to see what massage looks like.

When speaking with the child, massage therapists need to bend down so that their eyes are at the same level as the child's. This helps to establish a sense of equanimity and security. It is recommended for a first session that after the therapist introduces himself or herself they leave the room for a brief period. They can explain that they need to go get the lotion or oil for massage. This behavior tends to communicate to children that the massage therapist came by and nothing bad happened. This is especially important when working with toddlers or very young children who might not understand why the massage therapist is there initially. When the therapist returns, they will be remembered as someone the child has seen before who was safe. The massage therapist may also want to have a trusted nurse join them when they go in to meet the child and the parents for the first time. This can help to more quickly establish a relationship.

A massage therapist's appearance can also play an important role in the experience for children. Children will often look for objects such as necklaces or items of clothing that attract their attention. It is helpful to wear colorful clothing, pins, or necklaces that have animals or other fun symbols that children may enjoy. As the massage therapist becomes more familiar with the child's interests, they can choose to wear objects or clothing that the child is drawn to and finds comforting. A balance between professionalism in dress and wearing items that are attractive to children can easily be achieved.

It is best for massage therapists to begin the massage session by explaining or demonstrating massage on herself or himself or the parent. Massage can be explained as "good touch" to very young children. Let them know that it should always feel good to them. If they don't like the way it feels, the therapist can change what is being done or stop the massage. The child gets to choose. For children with cancer, the fact that they get to make choices around the way they are touched can, in and of itself, be very healing. Sometimes, being able to say "No" to massage is the most healing experience for a child in that moment because they are able to assert their control.

A massage therapist who worked with children with cancer for many years tells a story of a particular child she regularly visited in the hospital. This child would always say that he did not want a massage and the therapist would joke with him about it and talk with his mother about how things were going. After a few years of this, the massage therapist arrived one day and jokingly asked if the child would like a massage. The child said "Yes" for the first time. That was the massage therapist's only session with the child because he passed away very shortly thereafter. In some ways, the child was bringing the relationship to a close and honoring the importance of being able to make his own choices. For many of the treatments children will have for their cancer, they will not be able to say No and they will not be able to control the quality of the experience. Massage provides a special opportunity for children to use their voice and to be heard.

When explaining massage to parents, keep in mind that children are listening attentively to everything that is said. Always assume when communicating with the parent that the child is listening, even if they seem distracted or appear to be sleeping. It is also best for the therapist to adjust their language in an age-appropriate way when speaking with children so that they can fully understand what is being said. An adolescent might be very familiar with the benefits of massage, whereas a younger child may need to hear that "massage helps the body to feel good with gentle touch that is calming. It helps you to relax. It may also help some of the places that have pain to feel better."

Massage therapists need to be clear and direct with their body language so that the child can see they are not leaving and that they are paying attention to them. It is best to avoid turning one's body toward the door or lingering near the entrance of the room, unless it is time to leave. To physically demonstrate that the massage therapist is there to support the child, she can maintain close contact, position herself in a way that the child can readily make eye contact without having to turn his or her head in an uncomfortable position, and move gently with a slow steady rhythm that is supportive of the nature of the work. In a very real way, the physical movement of the body is an extension of the touch that is to come and children may interpret

Massage is a direct and benevolent way to benefit the person whose life we touch. Massage lets us "speak" deeply – though our hands and our hearts with purposeful presence. It is through this "conversation" in touch, our first language, that we may directly convey caring companionship and comfort. Massage allows us the opportunity to move beyond the diversity of languages, beliefs or cultural differences often present in health and hospice care. Massage may deeply affect one's experience in the journey with cancer, and serve as an important antidote to the by-products of this journey. These by-products may be the cycling through of various mental and emotional states that lead to anxiety, stress and prolonged suffering; as well as the physiological symptoms of the disease and the possible invasive, uncomfortable or painful procedures that are endured in treatment. Massage provides avenues for directly conveying compassion, acceptance, nurturing and loving-kindness. It is through experiencing these innate qualities that we are comforted in our journey, both as the receiver and as the giver. This positively impacts the experience of living and healing with illness including when the healing is to be into the journey of death and dying. Massage is a benevolent opportunity to console, serve and honor life.

KALENA BABESHOFF,
FOUNDER AND DIRECTOR OF
EDUCATION, A FOUNDATION FOR
HEALTHY FAMILY LIVING

the quality of the massage therapist's movements as an indication of how they will be touched.

Children tend to want to know about how the massage and the oil will affect all of their sensations. Adults never ask to taste the massage oil, but children frequently do. An example of this is a child who first asks what the massage oil smells like. After they are satisfied with that, they ask if they could taste it and if it would taste good. Because an organic, cold pressed, vegetable-based oil that is edible is typically used when working with children – especially very young children – it is safe for them to taste the oil. They may want to know if they will feel greasy. Some oil can be applied to the massage therapist's arm to demonstrate how the oil feels to the touch once on the skin. Children will want to know what else they might feel, hear, taste, touch and smell when they are receiving massage. They may ask how their muscles will feel and if they will feel any pain. They may not like the smell of the massage lotion or oil and may want it to be changed. Like most patients who are experiencing cancer treatment, children can become more sensitive to their body and their environment and may have strong reactions to particular smells. Massage therapists may need to discontinue using a particular lotion or oil if the child does not like it or is feeling nauseous as a result.

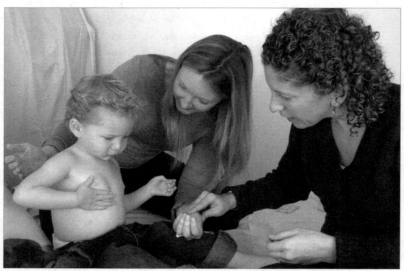

Figure 7.10 Explaining or demonstrating massage on herself or the parent is a good way for the massage therapist to begin the session.

Photograph by Andy Aryapour

Let the child know how they can participate during the massage session. The therapist can suggest that the child concentrate on their breathing while holding a favorite toy or a doll. Children always have permission to stop the massage and to tell the therapist that they do or do not want to be touched in a particular area. Check in frequently with the child throughout the session.

During the massage session, some parents will enjoy sitting quietly in the room and resting or observing the session. Other parents will want to remain at the beside, learning basic massage strokes from the massage therapist. One parent even liked to read a story to her daughter during the massage. The massage therapist performed strokes that interacted with some of the elements of the story. For instance, when the prince climbed up into the castle, the massage strokes included gentle "climbing" up the back.

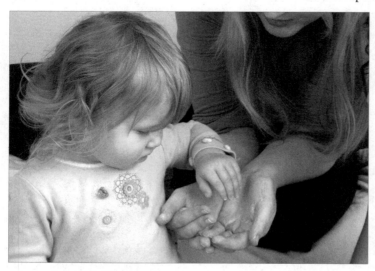

Figure 7.11 Children may want to know what the oil feels like.

Photograph by Andy Aryapour

Sometimes parents will ask if they can take a break and go do something else while their child is receiving massage. This is often a sign of trust and respect that they feel safe to leave their child alone with the massage therapist. There is no particular way the sessions must look. Each one may be quite different from the next. Be sensitive to the needs of the child and the parent in that moment and allow them to participate as they feel comfortable.

CHAPTER 7
MASSAGE FOR CHILDREN
LIVING WITH CANCER:
SPECIAL KNOWLEDGE FOR
SPECIAL PATIENTS
159

THE MASSAGE SESSION

One of the most important lessons when working in a hospital or hospice setting is for massage therapists to work collaboratively as part of the health care team. As with adults, standard precautions must be followed, which includes careful washing of the hands before and after every interaction and paying careful attention to infection control guidelines. It is important to follow all posted guidelines for precautions, which are typically found on the door to the child's hospital room. Children are more likely than adults to catch infectious diseases. Children with cancer who have compromised immune systems are particularly vulnerable. They must be carefully protected and massage visits should not occur when the therapist is feeling even the slightest bit ill.

Prior to beginning the massage, it is important to orient oneself to the child's medical equipment and to know what lines are inserted and where they are inserted. Find the precise location of the central venous line or PICC line. Maintenance of intravenous access and other medical equipment is critical and lines should never be disconnected by the massage practitioner. As appropriate, the nurse or another member of the health care team can make adjustments to the medical equipment. It is generally considered inappropriate for the massage therapist to do so. If a line accidentally comes out, a member of the health care team needs to be immediately alerted.

Before beginning massage, children must be safely positioned and feel that they are comfortable. In order to accomplish this, great care in handling and moving children is needed. It is always recommended to have the support of another member of the health care team prior to making any physical adjustments.

Setting the tone for a positive massage experience is very important. When entering the room, the practitioner's energetic presence should be calm and loving. Music that is soothing to the child can be used during the massage and the lights can be dimmed when appropriate. Practitioners want to reassure children that there will be no surprises during the massage session and that they will be in charge. It is important to recognize that different cultures have very different ideas around touch and how and when it is appropriate to be touched. A review of the child's touch history as well as the family's cultural touch practices can be helpful in clarifying the type of touch that will be seen as appropriate and most helpful.

Cancer awakens the need to honour our spirit. The resiliency of the human spirit helps patients and families find strength and hope and move forward on their journey. As oncology [practitioners], we empower families by connecting with and sharing our own spirit, honouring and being present to their journey, and guiding them forward as they anticipate challenges ahead. Caring isn't about doing for, but being there and being the wind behind the sails. When we connect with our spirit, we stay open to the unfolding mystery of life. Allow mystery and discovery in your life to drive your spirit of caring and to remind you to look for the rainbows.[16]

— JANICE POST-WHITE, PhD, RN,
UNIVERSITY OF MINNESOTA
SCHOOL OF NURSING

Continued on page 162

Massage is like Mr. Freeze!

When I met Jonathan, he was a brave twelve-year-old boy whose leg had been amputated because of osteosarcoma. Soon after, he returned home where he received physiotherapy and for almost a year he lived peacefully in remission. In the spring of the following year, he returned to the hospital. The tests revealed aggressive secondary cancers in the lungs and in his other leg. A few days passed, I bumped into him in the hall and he told me "This is my last summer, I'm going home and we'll make the most of it!" Stunned, I asked him, "Will you be attending the summer camp?" "Sure," he replied.

So, in August, escorted by his brother and his parents, Jonathan participated as much as he could in the camp activities in his wheelchair. With the help of the camp monitors and the nurses, he managed to participate in excursions – even canoeing! When the activities were out of reach, he would come and see us, which happened quite often. We would offer a massage, a facial or even a footbath – anything that appealed to him that day. Together, we laughed a lot; we even nicknamed him our V.I.P.!

At the end of October, the pain became severe; the doctors installed pumps to regulate stronger painkillers. During that week, I massaged him every day. Jonathan was expected to go back home on the weekend, and we knew we would not get to see him again. On Friday, I went to say goodbye and told him how fortunate I was to have met him.

Monday morning came around. I went to the hospital early and as soon as the nurse saw me she said, "Lyse, somebody is asking for you!" Surprised, I asked: "Who?" "Jonathan!"

The pumps had not relieved his pain. When it became unbearable, his parents had to bring him back to the hospital. He could not even tolerate a sheet over his skin! I was afraid I would not be able to help him at this stage, but the nurse insisted he was waiting for me.

I gathered my things for the day and walked straight to his room. "Good morning Lyse, I want my usual massage," said Jonathan. "I'm afraid it might not help you right now, you are in so much pain. Maybe we should wait for the medication to lower the level of the pain and then decide about the massage later?" "No, I want my usual massage now!" "Fine. Jonathan, I'll wash my hands and you choose the oil; but as soon as you tell me it hurts, I'll stop. Deal!"

Deep down, I was convinced I would not be able to touch even his little toe. But, I reached within myself, visualizing the Tree of Life, moving closer to his bed. His mother looked at me and I could read the despair in her eyes. I started with his leg; my hands ran like feathers. I very delicately patted his skin. Right away, he dozed off. With the gentlest touch, I went up to his hip, down his leg, softly, softly.

All of a sudden, he came out of his sleep and said, "Remember Lyse, how much fun we had this summer at the camp. I used to fall asleep on your massage table!" "Yes, these are wonderful memories, my sweet V.I.P.," I replied.

All was going well with the massage, so I decided to slowly move my hands to his stomach, although it was very swollen. He closed his eyes for a while. Then all of a sudden he said, "It was frightening this weekend, Lyse." I turned to his mother and she signaled her approval. "You want to tell me about it?" I asked. "The medication wasn't helping me at all. Mom and Dad got very concerned, and I was in constant pain. All of us were so scared."

"I'm happy you came back to the hospital," I told Jonathan.

CHAPTER 7
MASSAGE FOR CHILDREN
LIVING WITH CANCER:
SPECIAL KNOWLEDGE FOR
SPECIAL PATIENTS

161

"At least I got to say goodbye to my room, and to my house," he added.

I listened carefully, moved by his courage. I knew now I could move my hands to his torso and his arms. As I finished patting the arm, Jonathan said, "You know Lyse, your massage is just like a Mister Freeze [flavored, frozen water drink]!"

"You mean my warm hands feel like a frozen Mister Freeze?"

He looked me straight in the eyes, and said, "It's been three weeks now that the only thing I can eat is a Mister Freeze. It freezes my inside and it is soothing. The massage feels the same way on the outside. Do you understand now?"

He made me understand in his own words that my gentle patting was easing the pain. What a flattering remark! "Thank you, Jonathan." I moved to his neck, then his head, as he dozed off again. He woke up all of a sudden and said, "It's not fair you know, I never hurt anybody in my life and real criminals don't even have a cold! He better have some answers for me."

"Who?"

"Jesus."

I smiled and told him to carefully prepare his list of questions. He earned the right to be answered.

Jonathan was more and more relaxed. He insisted that I massage his back. He needed every inch of his body to be touched one more time, to be honored.

From then on, only his parents were allowed in his room. Jonathan left peacefully, but not before teaching me much about massage and life. The massage therapy provided a form of relief for Jonathan, but over and above alleviating his pain, it enabled his body to remember and re-enact some beautiful memories. Jonathan exercised his power of visualization. Touching his legs (motion center) brought him back to the camp activities. When I reached his stomach (emotional center) he remembered the distress of the weekend. On his torso and his arms (social center) he thought of his father and brother who supplied him with Mister Freezes.

When I finally got to the neck and the head, it was time to talk about life itself and all the questions he still had.

In so many ways, Jonathan reminded me of the true power of therapeutic touch, something I had introduced him to years earlier. He made me understand that the body is not only a physical entity, but a guide to a spiritual memory. Jonathan had mastered and applied all my knowledge of massage therapy.

That day, I received a gift that will be with me forever: to recognize the human body as a living temple, that its flesh is to be honored and respected in life and death. I am grateful to you, Jonathan.

Lyse Lussier,
Director of Programs, Services, and Research at Leucan*;
Massage Therapist member of the
Fédération des Massothérapeutes du Québec (FQM)

* Leucan is a non-profit organization whose mission is to enhance the well-being and healing of children suffering from cancer in Quebec and to ensure support to their families.

When moving from one area of the body to another during the massage, let children know what is being done and always ask their permission. "Is it all right if I massage your leg now?" They will enjoy being given the opportunity to say Yes or No. Sometimes children will not verbalize their discomfort, but subtle changes in their body will be evident. Their breathing may become shallow or they may appear to withdraw. If the practitioner senses that the child may be uncomfortable, they can start a dialogue with them so that their feelings become clear. The practitioner can also explain how the massage might feel. "My hand may feel warm and you may begin to feel more relaxed. Your body may get a little cooler as we do the massage so we'll have a blanket nearby in case you need it." The practitioner can also reinforce what the child seems to enjoy. "You seem to like it when I massage your feet."

Summary List of Guidelines for Massaging Children with Cancer

1. Obtain consent in writing from the physician and parent of the child who will receive massage.

2. Do some research before working with a child with cancer. Read about the type of cancer they are living with and have a good understanding of the disease process. Pay special attention to how their cancer impacts them physically, the stage of their illness, and the various treatments they may have experienced.

3. Ask the physician and nursing staff questions about the child including the child's response to their cancer treatment and what might be important considerations when providing massage to this child. Ask specific questions about safe positioning and any limitations, injuries, or fears this child may have.

4. Assess the child's touch history (positive and negative) in addition to their medical history.

5. Obtain verbal assent from the child whenever possible. When verbal assent is not possible, work carefully, repeatedly checking for engagement and disengagement cues.

6. When first meeting the child and their family member(s), make an introduction being mindful of the verbal and non-verbal communication that is being conveyed to the child and parent(s).

7. Ask questions about how touch is incorporated in their household and what the family's cultural beliefs are around appropriate or inappropriate touch.

8. Ask if the child has ever had a massage before and if they are familiar with the word "massage." Massage can be explained as "good touch" to very young children.

9. Explain massage to the child and parent(s) and demonstrate on the massage therapist's arm or a parent's arm.

10. Let the child know the areas of the body that can be massaged (i.e., arms, hands, legs, feet, head, face, neck, back). Ask where they would like to be touched and if there is anywhere they don't want to be touched.

11. Always ask permission to touch each area of the body where massage is to be provided.

12. Tell the child that they are in control and can stop the massage at any time.

13. Use appropriate draping guidelines and never partially undress a child who does not specifically give their consent beforehand.

14. Ask permission before touching each and every area of the body that the child said it is okay to massage (i.e., "Now that I have massaged your right leg, is it all right if I massage your left leg?").

15. Ensure that the child is safely positioned.

16. Report any concerns to the medical staff and the parent(s).

17. Remember to empower and respect the parent(s) at all times and to make them the expert on their child's health and well-being.

Always check in with the parent and child after the session to make sure that everything is all right. Be sure that the child is left in a safe position where they cannot accidentally roll out of bed. It is actually quite easy for a child who is ill to fall out of bed, so side rails must be returned to their original position and therapists must ensure that children are safely positioned. You can give parents and children feedback around what you experienced during the massage session and ask for suggestions for the next time you see them.

WORKING WITH FAMILY MEMBERS

Children are integral members of an entire family unit. The family must be respected and their feelings and wishes must be taken into consideration when providing massage therapy. Parents, guardians, siblings, and other relatives serve a vital role in supporting and sustaining children during their cancer treatment and it is essential that massage therapists include the entire family in the experience of the massage. This may involve the teaching of very simple, gentle massage strokes to family members. It may also mean demonstrating massage with the parent before working with the child. It is helpful to assess the family's comfort level with touch and to ask, "Do you do massage or any type of special loving touch with your child already?" Often parents will indicate places where they are already rubbing or massaging their child. This conversation can then be used to form a bridge into the beginning of the massage session: "Wonderful. Since you already massage your child's back and you know that feels good, we can begin with the back." Parents may also have ideas around touch that they find distasteful or areas of the body that they do not want massaged. Remember, it is important to have an understanding of their family and cultural beliefs around touch before beginning the massage session.

In some cases, parents will enjoy sitting quietly in the room during the massage because of the peaceful, calm atmosphere that is created. This can be very healing for them and it is important to give them the opportunity to be present in this way. In other cases, parents may want to take a break to go to the cafeteria or have some time for themselves. Especially after they feel comfortable with the massage therapist, parents are likely to make a request from time to time to leave for a short period.

Whenever possible, it is important for parents to be able to receive some massage therapy themselves. This can allow them to be more supportive in meeting the needs of their child with cancer and can help them to receive self-care at a time when it is easily forgotten. It can be wonderful to save time after the child's massage to provide a 10–15 minute massage for the parent or sibling. In viewing the family holistically, the importance of this extension of care is evident.

One of the greatest difficulties for siblings of children with cancer is that they often feel neglected. Despite the best intentions, family members' attention is frequently so highly focused on the child who is

CHAPTER 7
MASSAGE FOR CHILDREN
LIVING WITH CANCER:
SPECIAL KNOWLEDGE FOR
SPECIAL PATIENTS
163

ill that other children in the family do not receive the level of attention they are accustomed to. This can create a difficult emotional dynamic for siblings of children with cancer who may feel both a deep sorrow for their brother or sister's illness, and a personal loss in their relationships with the rest of the family. One way that massage therapists can address this is to include siblings in the massage experience.

Parents can be shown simple massage strokes that they can do with the patient's sibling while the massage therapist works with the child with cancer. Siblings may also want to receive massage from the massage therapist. A good way to incorporate this is to spend some special time at the end of the massage session telling the sibling a story while providing nurturing massage. There are several good massage stories for growing children that can be used with siblings.[19] Massage stories can help siblings to feel that their needs are important, too, and can help to ameliorate feelings of sorrow and jealousy that may be present during this difficult time. A wonderful example of a massage story is *Planting the Garden*, by Kalena Babeshoff.[20] In this story, a garden is planted on the child's back and they choose what seeds they would like to plant in their garden. They may want seeds of "love" or "ice cream," or sometimes "bicycles." Storytelling enables children to engage their imagination in the massage process and to interact with the therapist.

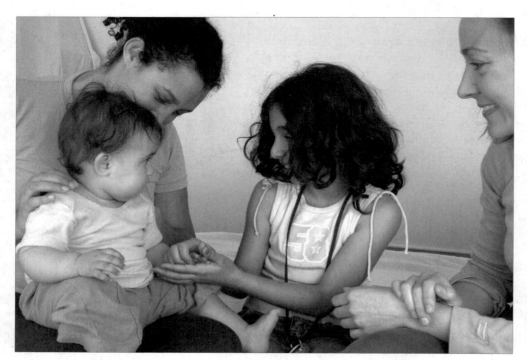

Figure 7.12 Including the entire family in the experience of massage is important.

Photograph by Andy Aryapour

If, as we believe, hospice care is about living, there is no greater way to honor a life than by compassionate touch – one to another – a soul to soul connection that knows no bounds.

— PENELOPE PECK THOMASON, RN,
DIRECTOR OF VOLUNTEER SERVICES
FOR TRINITYCARE HOSPICE AND
TRINITYKIDS CARE,
SOUTHERN CALIFORNIA

END-OF-LIFE ISSUES

In the U.S., federal eligibility guidelines for the Medicare hospice benefit, designed for adults, are often improperly applied to children. Under these rules, patients must have a terminal illness defined by a life expectancy of six months or less. Children at end of life often underutilize hospice because their parents do not want to discontinue curative treatment and this is currently a requirement for entering hospice. New approaches are being taken to help resolve this dilemma, such as introducing palliative or comfort care early in the disease process and integrating palliative therapies across the continuum of care. Palliative care is an extension of the hospice philosophy, and is now being introduced in a growing number of oncology centers that can serve as integrative models for programs around the country.[21]

Some of the challenges of pediatric palliative medicine include the fact that death is rare in this population (only about 2% of deaths occur in childhood) and that a child's death is seen as unnatural. In addition, there is often uncertainty of diagnosis and death can be unexpected. Medical insurance restrictions may create dynamics in which parents are given the choice to pursue curative treatment for their child or for their child to receive palliative care services. The choice for parents becomes one of "fighting for life," which is associated with curative care, or "giving up," which is associated with the palliative care alternative. Given this choice, parents rarely choose hospice or palliative medicine. This is unfortunate, because no parent wants to see a child suffer and hospice can be a way to reduce suffering for everyone. Parents are also not always aware that children can be discharged from hospice at any time should the child suddenly make unexpected improvements. Parents may also need to be supported in recognizing that rather than "fighting for life," fighting for the best quality of life may be the right decision.

In providing massage to children at end of life, there are several physical and emotional considerations that must be thoughtfully navigated. Fatigue is a common concern at end of life. Mornings tends to be a time when children experience more energy, whereas adolescents may have more energy in the late evening. Providing massage when children's energy is lower enables them to spend higher energy moments with family and friends.

Dyspnea, or shortness of breath, can be a cause of discomfort for children at end of life. Elevating the torso during the massage will make the child more at ease. And increasing airflow to the face by adding a fan also can help to minimize feelings of breathlessness.

Constipation or diarrhea can also occur at this stage of illness. In this case, belly massage can be quite helpful. There are specific stomach massage routines that were initially developed for treating colic in infants that can help to reduce constipation.[22] Nausea and vomiting may sometimes be lessened with gentle massage. Essential oils such as peppermint can be used along with a carrier oil. However, therapists must use care with providing scents and always ask the child to smell it before applying any to the skin. Rocking movements, which are sometimes incorporated in massage, should not be used for any patients with nausea or vomiting concerns. Bleeding and seizures are common at end of life and it is recommended to use darkly colored sheets and towels to lessen the possibility of children becoming frightened by the sight of their own blood. Massage therapists, like all healthcare providers, need to follow standard precautions that prohibit direct contact with blood and bodily fluids. In some cases, gloves may need to be used when providing massage at end of life.

CHAPTER 7
MASSAGE FOR CHILDREN
LIVING WITH CANCER:
SPECIAL KNOWLEDGE FOR
SPECIAL PATIENTS
165

It requires a leap of faith to accept that part of what you're there for is not just to fix what's broken, but to be with people through the brokenness that can't necessarily be fixed but can sometimes be healed.

— STEPHEN LIBEN, MD,
PEDIATRIC PALLIATIVE CARE,
MONTREAL, QUEBEC, CANADA

One of the most revered spiritual teachers of this century once asked a small group of listeners what they would say to a close friend who is about to die. Their answers dealt with assurances, words about beginnings and endings, and various gestures of compassion.
Krishnamurti stopped them short. There is only one thing you can say to give the deepest comfort, he said. Tell him that in his death a part of you dies and goes with him. Wherever he goes, you go also. He will not be alone.

LARRY DOSSEY,
HEALING WORDS

When working with children at end of life, it is important for massage therapists to allow themselves to attend the funeral whenever possible. It can be shocking to experience the sight of a tiny casket for the first time, but it enables an opportunity for grief to be expressed and for the family to recognize the love, commitment, and support that is available to them. The massage therapist may also be encouraged to maintain telephone contact with the family after the death. The bereavement period in pediatric hospice typically extends for the first 13 months following the loss of a child. If the massage therapist is able to make periodic contact during this period, it is most helpful. The first six weeks after the death are particularly important, as are special occasions such as the child's birthday. These phone calls become a natural extension of the care that has been provided.

Siblings of children who die from cancer may experience somatization, a transformation of the pain of the loss into physical pain. Massage can be very beneficial for minimizing these painful symptoms. Working with siblings and providing massage therapy during the bereavement period can help the sibling to work through their grief and pain. Maintaining close contact with the family and continuing to provide massage therapy will encourage a sharing of grief that can be very beneficial and healing.

Continued Presence

Soon after birth, an infant was diagnosed with a rare form of cancer that was very difficult to treat. The baby received massage for the first fourteen months of his life until he passed away. The massage therapist attended the funeral and stayed in contact with the parents and the older sibling of the infant. Some months later, the mother became deeply depressed. She discovered that she was pregnant again and she feared that this infant, too, would have cancer. The massage therapist continued to visit periodically and to stay in touch with the family. One week before the due date, the mother discovered that the infant passed away in utero and he was stillborn. The family had experienced the loss of two children in less than two years. In a letter to the massage therapist, the mother wrote explaining how supportive and comforting the relationship she had with the massage therapist had been during these difficult times. The massage therapist's presence continued to help the family to heal, as she provided gentle massage to the mother and surviving sibling after the second infant's death.

SHAY BEIDER,
MASSAGE THERAPIST,
DIRECTOR OF INTEGRATIVE TOUCH FOR KIDS

FINAL THOUGHTS

CHAPTER 7
MASSAGE FOR CHILDREN
LIVING WITH CANCER:
SPECIAL KNOWLEDGE FOR
SPECIAL PATIENTS
167

Along with the recent advances in cancer treatment and research, there is a real need for children with cancer to receive gentle, nurturing touch. As cancer treatment becomes increasingly "high tech," it is important that it also becomes "high touch." Children who undergo cancer treatment experience long-term health consequences that affect their physical, mental, and spiritual beings. The holistic nature of massage helps to encourage healing on multiple levels and reintroduces positive touch in environments where painful touch is often necessary. Massage therapists have the opportunity to bridge the world of painful cancer treatment with the pleasurable world of loving touch. The role that massage therapists can play in the future of medicine is one that is essential, effective, and very healing.

Until recently, there have been few opportunities to provide massage to children in hospital and hospice settings and even fewer chances to train in this area. However, an increasing number of pediatric hospital and hospice-based programs are including massage therapy in their services. And courses are available for massage therapists who want to work with children in medical settings with specific health care needs. The importance of training to work with infants and children affected by cancer cannot be overemphasized.

REFERENCES

1. National Cancer Institute Research on Childhood Cancer. Available at:
    http://www.cancer.gov/cancertopics/factsheet/Sites-Types/childhood/.
    Accessed July 29, 2006.

2. A Model of Medical Excellence: COG Collaborative Research.
    Available at:
    http://www.curesearch.org/support_curesearch/eblast.aspx?id=3062.
    Accessed July 29, 2006.

3. Post-White J, Hawks R, O'Mara A, et al. Future Directions of CAM Research in Pediatric Oncology. *Journal of Pediatric Oncology Nursing.* 2006;23(5):245-48.

4. Friedman T, Slayton WB, Allen LS, Pollock BH, Dumont-Driscoll M, Mehta P, Graham-Pole J. Use of Alternative Therapies for Children with Cancer. Available at: http://www.Pediatrics.org/.
    Dec 1997;100(6).

5. Fernandez CV, Stutzer CA, MacWilliam L, Fryer C. Alternative and Complementary Therapy Use in Pediatric Oncology Patients in British Columbia: Prevalence and Reasons for Use and Nonuse. *Journal of Clinical Oncology.* 1988;16(4):1279-86.

6. Barakat LP, Kazak AE, Meadows AT, et al. Families surviving childhood cancer: A comparison of posttraumatic stress symptoms with families of healthy children. *Journal of Pediatric Psychology.* 1997;22:843-859.

Resources

- Gentle massage for children:
  www.massageforchildren.com

- Integrative touch for kids:
  www.integrativetouch.org

- Leucan:
  www.leucan.qc.ca/index_en.asp

- Make a Wish Foundation
  International: www.worldwish.org

- Outlook: Life Beyond Childhood
  Cancer: www.outlook-life.org

- Sinclair M. *Pediatric Massage Therapy,* 2nd ed. Philadelphia, PA: Lippincott, Williams and Wilkins, 2004.

7. Beider S, Moyer CA, Randomized Controlled Trials of Pediatric Massage: A Review (eCAM 2006, in review. http://ecam.oxfordjournals.org).

8. Moyer CA, Rounds J, Hannum JW. A meta-analysis of massage therapy research. *Psychological Bulletin.* 2004;130(1):3-18.

9. Field T, Cullen C, Diego M, Hernandez-Reif M, et al. Leukemia Immune Changes Following Massage Therapy. *Journal of Bodywork and Movement Therapies.* 2001;5(4)271-74.

10 Phipps S, Dunavant M, Gray E, et al. Massage Therapy in Children Undergoing Hematopoietic Stem Cell Transplantation: Results of a Pilot Trial. *Journal of Cancer Integrative Medicine.* 2005;3(2):62-70.

11. Post-White J, Fitzgerald M, Sencer S, et al. Massage Therapy in Childhood Cancer. (Submitted for publication.)

12. Van Cleve L, Bossert E, Beecroft P, Adlard K, et al. The Pain Experience of Children with Leukemia During their First Year After Diagnosis. *Nursing Research.* 2004;53(1):1-10.

13. Hartup, WW. Having friends, making friends, and keeping friends: Relationships as educational contexts. ERIC Digest. Champaign, IL: ERIC Clearinghouse on Elementary and Early Childhood Education, 1992.

14. Association of Hole in the Wall Camps. Available at: http://www.holeinthewallcamps.org/htwc/index?page=home. Accessed July 30, 2006.

15. Hopkins, B. Culturally Determined Patterns of Handling the Human Infant. *The Journal of Human Movement Studies* 1976;2:4.

16. Post-White J. The Spirit of Oncology Nursing Care. *Canadian Oncology Nursing Journal.* 2003 Spring;13(2):84-94.

17. Hopkins, B. Culturally Determined Patterns of Handling the Human Infant. *The Journal of Human Movement Studies* 1976;2:12.

18. Idea discussed throughout the book *A General Theory of Love* by Lewis T, Amini F, Lannon R. First Vintage Edition, January 2001.

19. *The Massage Fairy Tale* by Rolf and Irene Elmstrom of the Axelsons Institute in Sweden is a wonderful massage story for children.

20. Babeshoff K. Planting the Garden. A Foundation for Family Living http://www.healthyfamily.org/.

21. Beider S. An Ethical Argument for Integrated Palliative Care. Evidence Based *Complementary and Alternative Medicine.* 2005 Jun;2(2):227-231. Epub 2005 Apr 27.

22. Schneider McClure V. *Infant Massage – Revised Edition: A Handbook for Loving Parents.* New York, NY: Bantam Books, 2000.

Chapter 8

BE-ing Is Enough

Comforting Touch for the Dying

In the late 1960's and early '70's, many people re-embraced the idea and practice of giving birth at home. As result, most hospitals now provide a home-like atmosphere that fully incorporates the family into this holy event. At about the same time that home birthing was making a comeback, a similar, but quieter, renaissance was happening as the modern-day hospice movement began. It, once again, placed the care for the dying in the hands of family with help from a team of health care professionals.

Interestingly, these two parts of life, birth and death, have comparable stages. Even so, death is generally not accorded the same sacred status as birth. It is instead regarded as a failure by some, and at the very least as an unwelcome event by most. Many patients and caregivers, however, have found comfort in approaching the end of life just as they would the birth of a long-awaited child. And just as home births are attended by a midwife, so too is home death. These midwives are the caregivers, family, friends, and hospice staff who approach the death of their loved one or patient as a blessed, miraculous event, lovingly prepared for; they commit to be "present throughout [the] journey toward death"[1]; to courageously accompany them to the doorway of the next world.

What does it mean to travel with a person who is dying? It means being able to temporarily leave a world that is earthly, solid, and linear and enter into a state that is ephemeral, porous, and circular. The life of a person who is healthy has a forward-moving pattern to it. The weeks and months of this life can be plotted out more or less on a straight line. On Monday she does this, on Tuesday she does that, and on Wednesday she does something else. The days in the life of an ill or dying person are indistinguishable from one another. Time becomes circular. Sunday is no different from Wednesday. Each day circles into the next, spinning a hazy cocoon around those caught in its web. The dying person cannot come "out," the therapist must go "in" to them. Therapists must travel between two worlds, leaving daily life at the patient's front door – the world of doing, moving, and productivity – and enter a world of being, stillness, and reflection.

Relationships often revolve around what we do together, but when illness and death become part of life, there must be a transition from "doing" to "being." New ways to relate must be found. Massage can bridge the gap between doing and being and help one to enter into the world of the person who is at the end of life. Through massage they can simultaneously be "doing" while "being" with their friend, client, or family member.

TOUCH AT THE END OF LIFE

Just as touch is one of the first forms of communication a newborn receives, it may be one of the final ways we talk to the person who is dying. However, Jan Bernard and Miriam Schneider comment in *The True Work of Dying* that many caregivers are ill-at-ease about touching someone who is dying, uncertain about what will feel good or fearful of hurting them. However, "When an infant is not nurtured with touch and caring, he does not thrive. When a dying person is not cared for in the same way, she cannot achieve all the healing possible through the process of dying."[1] Through the act of compassionate touch, bodyworkers can be instrumental in showing families that, despite the decline in their loved one's body, it is not something to be afraid of. The body of someone who is in the last stage of life, even though frail and dependent, is worthy of the same tenderness, care, and unconditional love as is a new baby.

In his classic book, *Birth Without Violence*, French obstetrician Fredrich LeBoyer gives us clues about touching the newborn. But they could just as well be instructions for touching the one who is departing:

The baby is on the first step of a glorious adventure – and yet it is transfixed with fear. Do not move. Do not add to the baby's panic. Just be there. Without moving. Without getting impatient. Without asking anything. At this point, out of consideration for her child, out of real – not egocentric – love, a woman will simply place her hands on its body. And leave them there, immobile. Hands that are not animated, agitated, trembling with emotion, but are calm and light. Hands of peace. Through such hands flow the waves of love which will assuage her baby's anguish.[2]

During the last stages of life, there is a place for touch given by a professional massage practitioner and by family and friends. Like an infant, the dying person needs to be touched frequently, not just during the weekly, or even twice weekly, sessions a professional might give. Having a professional's help, however, provides relief and respite for caregivers. The easing of their family member's pain, anxiety, and suffering lifts an emotional, unspoken burden, at least momentarily.

The professional touch therapist also gives the patient someone to interact with who is not in the immediate social circle. Patients sometimes withhold information or feelings from their loved ones, believing they are protecting them from further emotional pain. Callanan and Kelley refer to this as a "compassionate conspiracy."[3] During the relaxed atmosphere of a massage session, the one who is dying may feel freer to admit things she has been withholding. The touch practitioner may become a witness to thoughts or feelings the patient still wants to share. Ron, who was dying of leukemia, felt everyone around him was walking on egg shells. No one showed their true feelings or talked to him about his. It was only during his Reiki sessions that he could let down.

Connie, a bone marrow transplant patient who was nearing the end of life in the hospital, also withheld information from her family. Before and after each massage, the massage students at OHSU ask the patients to rate their pain, fatigue, physical and emotional comfort. Connie's husband was in the room while the student collected this information. Initially, Connie rated her comfort as fairly high, but as soon as her husband left the room, she changed her ratings, admitting that she was very uncomfortable and in pain.

TEACHING FAMILY TO GIVE MASSAGE

One of the major contributions a bodyworker can make is to instruct family caregivers on basic massage strokes or touch techniques and to encourage them to follow their heart about ways to touch the dying person. When Jane's father was dying of throat cancer, she wished someone had suggested massage to her. Not only did the cancer leave him unable to speak, but he was also deaf, leaving Jane sitting at his bedside feeling helpless and disconnected. By the simple act of stroking his skin, Jane could have communicated with her father, conveying through her hands the love she felt.

Most people have an innate instinct about giving massage, and need only a little tutoring. Touch is the language spoken between mother and child, lover and beloved, comforter and sufferer. The massage therapist can build on this and teach family and friends other forms of touch and areas of the the body that may benefit from touch. One of the best ways to teach family and friends is for the practitioner to have the family member work side-by-side with him, each massaging a foot, hand, or leg. The family massage giver can then experience how gentle the touch must be, can emulate the slow, tranquil pace, and can get a better sense of timing.

Often, touching brings the greatest comfort and is ultimately the healing needed for the heart for both the care giver and care receiver.

JAN SELLIKEN, ND, RN,
AND MIRIAM SCHNEIDER, MSN,
THE TRUE WORK OF DYING

Health care workers at the VA Medical Center Hospice in Palo Alto have seen the family unit strengthened through massage. They believe it to be a method that assists patients and families to communicate more openly, and has "the effect of strengthening the family bonds in a time of crisis."[4] Helen Campbell, a massage therapist in the Palo Alto program, tells the story of a lung cancer patient who had been estranged for years from his 17-year-old son. The man wished to see his boy before dying. The son reluctantly agreed to come and sit in his father's room, but did not want to talk to his father. When the young man arrived, Helen was massaging his father's feet. The son "sat down noisily in a chair by the window, as far away as possible from his father. His body language was full of resentment." Eventually, however, Helen was able to coax the boy up to where she was and to work along side of her on his father's other foot. When this raging son put his hands on his father's foot, everything changed. Forgiveness happened "in the giving and receiving of gentle, caring touch."[5] Helen did not have to massage the man again, because the son came every evening after that and massaged him.

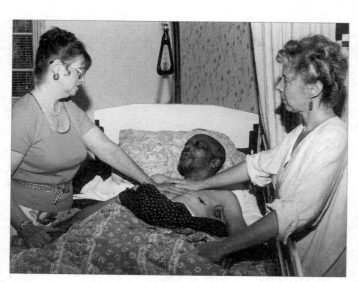

Figure 8.1 The massage therapist and patient's wife minister to him through touch.   *Photograph by Don Hamilton*

Skilled, supportive touch offers the same benefits for those who are at the end of life as it does for those who are in the middle of life. It helps dying persons know they are important and loved. Hospice nurse Alina Egerman believes that massage allows the person who is dying to escape reality for a moment. "We all need a vacation periodically," says Egerman. "When we can get away for awhile, life often looks different when we return." During massage, the recipient becomes quiet and is able to get in touch with what he is feeling. Gentle massage can help the patient surrender to the process and let go of the body. Ron felt clarity and peace of mind from the touch sessions he received from Sheila. His acceptance of the situation made it possible for Ron to help his mother let go of him.

Reiki Master Phil Morgan assembled a team of practitioners to provide Reiki for his wife when she was diagnosed with pancreatic cancer. The team hoped that the disease would be defeated, but eventually they were forced to let go and allow her process to unfold in its own unique way. Phil felt that because of the healing, supportive touch, his wife needed less pain medication, which allowed her to be less drugged and more present with her experience. The Reiki helped Phil's wife let go, moving her through to death more quickly and gracefully than anyone had anticipated.

ALLOWING FLEXIBLE BOUNDARIES

Being midwife to a dying friend or loved one is not "business as usual" for the professional bodyworker. Sessions no longer fit neatly into a limited block of time. Instead of an hour, the practitioner/friend may give touch over a period of hours. When Ron was dying in the hospital, Reiki Master Sheila King administered Reiki for four to five hours at a time. This relieved his discomfort and gave him the opportunity to rest.

The professional massage therapist will be accustomed to following a code of conduct concerning boundaries, both physical and emotional boundaries. However, when caring for a friend or family member who is dying, the boundaries may need to be more flexible to allow for giving care at the deepest level. When giving Reiki to Ron, Sheila would crawl into bed with him when giving touch to his head. Although a practitioner would not use such a position with a healthy person, lying in bed and holding the person who is at the end of life may be the touch that is needed in that moment.

The emotional boundaries become fuzzy when caring for a person with whom there is a strong attachment; removing the agenda becomes more difficult. The therapist/friend can become more impatient, wanting the person who is sick to get well, to be fixed. Although being midwife for someone special is a rewarding experience, it is much more difficult than caring for a person the therapist does not know well. There is no recipe for unfolding these relationships. As best as they can, the midwives must try to put aside their preconceived notions about how the experience should occur and allow the loved one to direct her own dying.

Some people are averse to receiving massage during this time. They are afraid that if they relax too deeply they will let go and die.

Massaging Grandma's Feet

I was called on by a well-intending granddaughter to provide massage for her elderly grandmother. She knew her grandmother was in pain and felt that she had no way to help her. I agreed with her but also shared that a new person being brought in at the end of Grandma's life might be intrusive and disruptive, especially since she had never experienced massage. I suggested to the granddaughter that gentle foot and hand massage provided by her would be just as beneficial, if not more so. She was willing to have me come to her grandmother's house to demonstrate and share the guidelines for giving gentle touch.

After getting permission from Grandma to proceed, I demonstrated pressure levels on the younger woman's arms and hands. We then sat side-by-side, chair-by-chair, at the foot of the bed and began massaging Grandma's feet. After just a few minutes of this tutoring , the granddaughter felt comfortable enough to continue on her own. Soon she was showing her mother how to do this. "It is so good to be touched by those I love," responded the grandmother.

Upon my departure, we were all in tears. They were grateful that I had come, and I was delighted that they were willing to allow a complete stranger to share this precious moment. I was so profoundly moved that I sobbed as I walked the mile back to my office. It was then that I experienced the value and significance in sharing my skill. It was then that I witnessed a reawakening of souls, allowing family to connect once again through the simple act of gentle touch.

— MEG ROBSAHM, LMP, EVERETT, WASHINGTON

Touch professionals must honor this position and not push patients to accept massage if they are clearly against it. One of the tenets of hospice care is to allow the patient to control his experience.

SHARING TIME TOGETHER

Anyone who is providing touch for someone at the end of life, whether it be for a client or one's own family member, will want to read some of the books available on this subject. One short chapter is not enough to convey what is known about such topics as communication, grief, or what death will be like. A few basic guidelines for sharing time together are given below:

- **Listening is enough.** Listening is an act complete in itself, but believing that it is enough is difficult. Rachael Naomi Remen speaks often of listening and healing, reminding us that the simple human interaction of listening is the most powerful tool of healing. Healing is accomplished not by doing something, but by receiving the person.[6] People change when they are received and listened to.

  Bodyworkers are natural listeners. They have learned to move into a quiet, still space, to listen with their hands, to hear the non-verbal messages of the body, to communicate without words. In just this same manner they must allow their ears to hear, their voices to respond, to receive the dying one just as they are.

- **Follow the conversational leads of the patient.** Never force the conversation onto topics that the patient does not want to discuss, but if they do initiate the subject of their illness, allow them to talk about it rather than diverting attention away. Many well-meaning visitors try to distract the dying person with talk about what is going on in the outside world, the weather, what's happening at work, or gossip about family and friends. Visitors wrongly suppose that letting the conversation drift toward intimate topics such as death, fear, or the afterlife will upset their dying friend. More often than not the patient will be grateful for the opportunity to share honest feelings. Despite the attention of many loving people, illness can be a lonely experience when there is no one who understands and accepts the perceptions of the ill person.

- **Smile and laugh.** Serious illness does not put a ban on laughter.

- **Allow silence.** Love needs no words and silence can be as supportive and welcome as conversation. As death approaches, the one who is dying will withdraw and words become less important. The giving and receiving of touch allows both people to spend quiet time together in a pleasurable, undemanding way that needs no words.

- **You don't have to have all the answers.** In the PBS documentary, When Doctors Get Cancer, Dr. Balfour Mount

Listening does not require a response. We put ourselves under a strain when we believe a response is necessary and the effort gets in the way of hearing. Listening is effortless. To listen is to be relaxed and quiet. It happens in a silent mind.

— DARLENE STEWART

says, "As caregivers we think we have to have the answers. [But] we don't have the answers. If we are there to share the questions, that's what the person wants [and] needs."[7] At times there are no complete solutions. Accept that you are limited and do what you are able to.

- **Don't offer untrue statements.** If a patient isn't doing well, don't make remarks such as: "You'll be good as new before you know it." Or, "You're probably feeling down because of the weather." Acknowledge their feelings and the situation as it actually is, with comments such as, "It sounds as if you're really uncomfortable," or, "You seem frustrated."

- **Respect the privacy, wishes, and beliefs of the patient.** Call before you visit. Never assume you know what is best for them. Don't force your ides about illness or death onto the patient. Allow him to have his experience as he would like.

- **Respect the patient's wish to be touched.** Any sign, verbal or non-verbal, that the patient does not want to be touched must be respected despite our personal desire to provide massage.

- **Be there to support the person's process.** Have no agenda or expectations. Massage professionals are sometimes at a loss when they make a visit expecting to give a massage, only to have the patient decline. It is best to have no expectations about how the time will be spent. The focus should be on spending time together, not on massage.

- **Offer to help, but only if you can follow through.** Don't make idle offers. In their book *Final Gifts*, Maggie Callanan and Patricia Kelley suggest offering to help with specific tasks.[3] Rather than making a general comment such as, "Let me know how I can help," ask the patient (or caregiver) if you could do the grocery shopping once a week, take the kids to soccer practice, mow the lawn, or massage her feet. People who are in the final stages of life usually do not have the energy or even the interest to compile "to-do" lists when friends casually ask if there is some way they can help.

- **Allow the person to do what she can for herself.** Most people want to be as independent as possible for as long as possible. Even if there is a bit of struggle in putting on their own slippers or turning over in bed, this bit of autonomy gives people a sense of control.

- **Give the one who is ill the opportunity to be not only a receiver of help but also a giver of help.** Everyone wants to feel useful. Caregivers need to permit themselves to be receivers whenever possible. Not only will the dying one feel they are making a contribution, but the primary caregiver will lessen the burnout that often accompanies this situation.

You matter until the last moment of
your life, and we will do all we can
not only to help you die peacefully but
also to live until you die.

— DAME CICELY SAUNDERS,
FOUNDER OF THE MODERN-DAY HOSPICE
MOVEMENT AND OF ST. CHRISTOPHER'S
HOSPICE IN ENGLAND

SUPPORTING LIFE UNTIL THE END

When the physician feels that the patient has six months or less to live, the person can choose to enroll in a hospice program. The goal of hospice care is no longer to search for a cure, but to manage symptoms palliatively, allowing the patient's remaining time to be as peaceful and comfortable as possible. The hospice staff of doctors, nurses, social workers, physical and occupational therapists, massage therapists, and chaplains works with the family to care for the patient at home or in a home-like setting. Although not all cancer patients choose to die at home or to be served by a hospice agency, the hospice philosophy can be implemented anywhere. Hospice is not a place, it is a "concept of care"[3] that emphasizes helping patients live fully until the end.

Peoples' dying processes are as unique as their births or their lives, for that matter. Some patients remain fairly active until the last month and then quickly slip away. Others slowly decline over several years. The person with cancer who is preparing to depart this world will follow a series of stages that are more or less the reverse of those in the birthing process. These stages are especially applicable to the cancer process which unfolds slowly, unlike the suddenness of death caused by a heart attack. Familiarity with the stages of dying may help the bodyworker understand the behavior she observes from her dying friend or family member and therefore be more present with the process. Because the experience of giving birth is well known to many, it will be used as a springboard to understanding the stages of dying. The timelines, however, may not always follow those given in the sections below.

QUICKENING – A FEW MONTHS PRIOR TO DEATH

Around the fifth month, the fetus usually makes its presence known by kicking, stretching, and shifting within the womb. These first movements, referred to as the "quickening," are a time of excitement for the expecting parents, friends, and family. Placing a hand on the mother's swelling abdomen to feel these signs of life is a moment full of awe, curiosity, and excitement.

Death, too, often makes its presence known by some defining movement. These movements are not as noticeable, dramatic, or welcomed as those delivered by the developing fetus, and they may only be evident in hindsight. Ralph threw a big party for his friends the Christmas before he died, but he may not have been conscious that death was becoming present when he did so. However, when his friends looked back, they could see that it was his way of saying good-bye. Six or seven months before his death, Charles and his ex-wife prepared an advanced medical directive to insure that no heroic measures would be taken to keep him alive. Perhaps it was preparedness that motivated Charles, or perhaps he was becoming aware of death's proximity. Elsie called a meeting of her five daughters a few months before her death. One evening they all gathered at the nursing home where their mother was being cared for, to select a piece of jewelry from Elsie's treasure box.

Whereas the fetus becomes noticeably active during the "quickening" stage, the person preparing to depart the world becomes less active. They may sleep and nap more, have less interest in the outside world, and eat fewer solid foods. The physical life is gradually left behind.[8] Massage, however, is one physical experience that still holds pleasure.

MASSAGE COMFORT MEASURES

- During the quickening stage, bodywork sessions will be similar to those for people in treatment or for hospitalized patients. By and large, light to moderate pressure is used, with the emphasis on relaxation. The patient may need more assistance, may have position restrictions due to tumors or medical devices, sessions may need to be shorter or may need to be conducted in the home. John was housebound for several months prior to his death, but he continued receiving massage at home until the end. He insisted on receiving the sessions on a portable massage table rather than in his bed because he wanted to feel normal for as long as possible. Another homebound client also wanted to receive her sessions on a massage table. The therapist was able to help the patient accomplish this by raising the hospital bed to the same height as the massage table and then helping the patient roll onto the table. Esther, on the other hand, was still able to drive herself to weekly Reiki sessions and climb 13 stairs to the treatment room during this stage.

- Give patients choices. The choices may be between lotion and oil, a hand or foot massage, massage in their chair, the bed, or massage table, or a warm blanket or no blanket. Choice allows people to regain a sense of dignity and control over an uncontrollable situation.

- People with cancer, especially in the end stage of life, may be on morphine to manage their pain. One of the side effects of narcotics is the slowing down of the bowel which creates constipation. Hospice clients or caregivers can be instructed how to do two minutes of clockwise abdominal massage in the morning and evening to assist the bowels.

- Administering massage to the joints and performing passive or active range of motion exercises can contribute to patients' overall comfort, allow them to do more for themselves, and make it easier for care partners to provide care. The more mobile the patient is, the easier it is to accomplish daily care activities such as dressing, going to the bathroom, or turning in bed.

Additional Resources

- Callanan M, Kelley P. *Final Gifts.* New York, NY: Bantam Books, 1992
- Finch MA. *Care Through Touch: Massage as the Art of Annointing.* Continuum, 1999
- *Graceful Passages: A Companion for Living and Dying* (Music CD with messages)
- Hospice Association of America www.nahc.org
- Levine S. *Healing into Life and Death.* New York, NY: Anchor Books/Doubleday, 1991
- National Hospice and Palliative Care Organization www.nhpco.org
- Nelson D. *From the Heart Through the Hands,* 2nd Ed. Findhorn Press, 2006
- Rose MK. *Comfort Touch: Massage for the Elderly and the Ill* (DVD)
- Share the Care: How to Organize a Group to Care for Someone Who is Seriously Ill www.sharethecare.org

LIGHTENING – A Few Days to a Few Weeks Prior to Death

A few days to a few weeks before delivery, the fetus begins to move into the delivery position, usually with the head turned down toward the birth canal. In obstetrics this stage is referred to as "lightening" or engagement. This is the beginning of moving from an internal reality to an external one. During this time the baby takes in a lot of nutrition and puts on weight.

Conversely, a few days to a few weeks before entering the active phase of dying, the person will prepare by withdrawing from the outside world and move inward. Eating and drinking decrease, weight is lost, and breathing patterns and rates may vary. The patient's breathing may speed up one moment, slow down in the next, or may stop altogether for a short period of time before returning to an even pace.[1] These changes in the breath are due to the decrease in circulation causing body wastes to build up.[9] Other changes may include:

Skin: Fragile; pressure sores; rashes; bruising; bleeding; skin color may fluctuate from flushed to bluish or a pale yellow (not to be confused with the yellow of jaundice); the hands, feet, and nailbeds may become paled and bluish as the circulation slows.

GI Tract: Nausea; vomiting; constipation or diarrhea; dry or sore mouth.

Musculoskeletal: Weakness; fatigue; loss of movement; brittle bones.

Emotional: Can range from calm and accepting to anxious and agitated; depression; anger; impatience; restless; picking at the bed covers and other agitated arm movements. Some hospice workers believe these random-appearing arm motions are actually an indication that the dying person is experiencing something and that the picking and agitated arm movements are an attempt to communicate with someone who can only be seen by them.[3]

General: Pain may be present for some and absent for others; fluctuations in body temperature; varied sleeping and waking patterns; sensitivity to sights, smells, sounds, and movement; incontinence.[1,3,8]

Massage Comfort Measures

- If the patient is able to communicate, ask them directly, rather than the family or caregivers, what they want from the massage session. Continue to give the patient opportunities for choice.

- When offering to give massage, especially to someone who has not had one since becoming ill, make the offer specific, such as, "Would you like your feet gently massaged?" Most people do not realize that massage can just be given to a part of the body or that the pressure can be adapted to meet the needs of someone who is dying. They often imagine it will be a vigorous

---

Then Can We Rest?

We need to give hospice patients permission to tell us what they most need and then we need to truly listen. I worked with one hospice client who, after telling me she really didn't want massage that day, asked me if it would be okay to "just be quiet." I said of course and went on to say that it would even be okay for her to rest if she would like. "Will you rest with me?" she asked. When I told her that I would, she sighed a sigh of relief and promptly fell asleep.

As her quickening progressed, this was our custom during my 2–3 hour visit. I would ask if she would like a massage. She would reply, "maybe my hands or feet, then can we rest?" Many days she just wanted to rest. And we would rest, she in her chair and me in mine six feet away. In those quiet moments, I could never bring myself to do anything except "BE" with her. I could not read, I could not get up and do something else for her. What I felt most important was that I was with her, heart to heart.

— Meg Robsahm, LMP, Everett, Washington

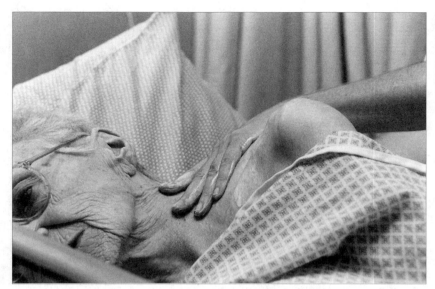

Figure 8.2 Light, gentle hands stroke the person who has entered the "lightening" stage.

Photograph by Don Hamilton

rub-down of the entire body rather than a soft, comforting experience.

- The range of bodywork given during this time is still fairly broad. Some people may want a light, full-body massage, others may want only parts of the body massaged, or just to have their hand held.

- Create privacy for the massage recipient if possible and appropriate. The dying one often will be surrounded by family and friends during this time. Ask the patient if he would prefer to have family remain in the room or would rather receive massage in private. Many people are more able to fully relax when they are left to themselves. In addition, the massage session is an opportune time for family and friends to refresh themselves with a walk, nap, or meal.

- Use increased gentleness when touching people at this stage. The skin and flesh may be tender or bones may be brittle.

- Skin care is vital for people confined to bed. If they can tolerate it, patients should be massaged daily with lotion. This may increase circulation and moisturize the skin, possibly decreasing the chance of pressure sores developing. Maintaining skin integrity becomes even more important as people lose weight. Pressure occurs where bones are close to the surface, causing the skin to break down and possibly allowing the bone to break through. Massage the skin covering joints to maintain its suppleness in these high risk areas.

- If a patient has a stage 1 pressure sore (reddened but intact skin), do not directly massage the spot, as further damage may be caused, especially in older cancer patients whose skin has

Continued on page 182

Hands that know the art of touch as "anointing" and treat the body as "sacrament" will never be without work. ...Massage as the art of anointing is a vocation, a call to loving work through our hands.... If our hands are prayers, then touching another person as in massage... is indeed an embodied way of praying our care for another person.

— MARY ANN FINCH, FOUNDER AND DIRECTOR OF THE CARE THROUGH TOUCH INSTITUTE, BERKELEY, CALIFORNIA

Animals Watch

Sometimes teachers appear when you ask for them. Sometimes they appear anyway. True teachers are often different from what we expect. Messier, strangely packaged or achingly familiar, insistent or just passing through, teachers nevertheless transmit whatever we need and are ready to learn. In my experience teachers run in packs.

The phone rang on a glorious autumn morning. A local woman wanted to schedule a massage for a friend of hers who was in the final days of metastatic cancer. Hospice had just been started and her friend was dying at home. I made arrangements with the client's husband to come over and provide a massage that day. A few hours later, I made my way to their house through one of those New England September afternoons. The drying leaves sharpened their orange edges on the brilliant blue space above me. I arrived at the house and moved into the soft, quiet interior.

A home where someone is actively dying is a different culture, with its own rhythm and code of behavior. The house has a palpable pulse: slower, deliberate, everything organized around the vigil. Conversations may be hushed or hollow, or may be especially warm or reflective. Pretense is often scrapped for the mean, authentic moment. Meals are skipped. Unopened mail lies in piles. Calls are screened and dishes pile up in the sink. Emotions tumble out in surprise attacks, or they are held close and dear until it's over. Necks grow stiff from sleeping in odd positions, then snapping to attention. Meaning stands out in sharp relief and can be found anywhere – in the patient's mumbled words, in the Luna moth hanging from the screen door, in the weather or the movement of the moon across a room. Voices are husky with unshed tears or strained from fatigue.

Whenever I enter this unusual world I am acutely conscious of being a stranger to it. I try to move unobtrusively and wait for the moment to weave myself in with the larger rhythm. It's a bit like calculating a jump from a fast-moving vehicle to a slower one. That first afternoon, I checked in with a few family members about the client's status, and went to warm my massage lotion in the microwave, removing a cold, forgotten dish of food from within. I washed my hands then climbed the stairs to the client's room, greeted her softly and began to set up the room for the session.

Suddenly two gatekeepers appeared. A huge gray cat flew in out of nowhere. It hurled itself across my client's bed and parked between us, an effective barricade. A half-grown silky-soft black dog skittered in and stood firmly in front of me, shadowing my knees as I tried to move about the room. I gently nudged the dog aside and peeled the cat away to insert a pillow under the client's knee. I draped and bolstered her thinning body and heard her quiet sigh of relief as she rested heavily on the pillows. As I began the massage, the dog put a paw on my leg, which stopped me. He looked into my eyes, barked once, growled quietly and stared at me for a full minute. His deliberate gaze said it all. Pay attention. Don't mess with her. For everyone's sake, be careful. Finally satisfied that I had heard him, he turned away to my ankles, carefully licking them while I stroked my client's back. He and the cat kept watch at each visit.

I was especially stirred by the dog's attentions. Only five months old, he had joined the family just a month before, the day her hospital called to release her from an experimental treatment and told her they could do nothing more. He landed in the family in the middle of this news. Once in their home, he sniffed the scene and immediately understood what was needed.

What was needed was help, real material help to get through what had to be gotten through… what could not be gotten around, but must be met, managed, and survived. He seemed to know they needed not only his love during this time, but also his strong sense of duty and his humble offer of distraction. Barely more than a puppy, he took his responsibilities seriously and rarely left my client's or her husband's side for long.

Upstairs with my client, I learned that her lower back gave her pain, that in addition to me and the animals, she saw other figures in the room, and that she was terribly parched but unable to drink without vomiting. Her body was drying to a thin film, to be borne away by the season. Her family, friends and animals kept watch and cared for each step of her passage.

Around the edges of her sessions I would sit on the porch and chat with her husband. I learned that it was his ten-day wedding anniversary. Partners for more than a decade, they were married in a small garden wedding at her mother's, when she was still able to stand.

My last session with her was on a Thursday night, a point when regular massage was too stimulating. She was barely responsive, and I simply held her head, her shoulder, stroked her arms. When someone is trying to leave their body, hold it quietly. Touch should not ask too much of the body, nor pull it too close. It should be cradled instead, letting it rest between efforts. I sat at her head. A friend of hers sat holding her feet, saying goodbye. Curtains fanned us from the open windows. When I left, my client slept in her darkening room, a luminous September moon sliding across her feet.

She died two mornings later.

I learned a great deal from these brief exchanges. There were teachers on every surface – the bed, the porch, the floor at my feet. The animals taught me that love and duty prevail in the toughest situations. My client and her husband taught me that beginnings and endings can be in the same sentence, such as, "They married two weeks before she died," or even, "the puppy joined the family to help as she was leaving." My client's husband showed me dignity and a bottomless connection to his wife, to everything that had ever happened and was about to happen to her.

At the center of this vigil, my client taught me that dying is hard work – that it's not for the faint of heart – and that a well-placed pillow matters in the scheme of things. Intent on her labors, she let everyone do their part. By her still, quiet example, she named herself beloved. She also taught me to name what you love and to let it surround you. She seemed to say, "Do this, even – especially – as you let it all go."

— TRACY WALTON,
LMT, CAMBRIDGE, MASSACHUSETTS

less elasticity and integrity. When massaging in the vicinity of a pressure sore, leave a one-inch buffer of healthy skin.

- Incorporate other activities into the massage time, such as music, aromatherapy, or relaxation imagery. Some people enjoy having guided meditations, prayers, or stories read to them. In his books *Healing into Life and Death* and *Guided Meditations, Explorations and Healings,* Stephen Levine has many wonderful meditations on pain, taking medications, letting go, and dying.

- Say good-bye each time when working with someone who has entered this phase of dying; leave nothing undone or unsaid with a person when you leave.

As the patient enters the final few weeks of life, eating and drinking decrease. Because food and drink are equated with nurturing, caregivers are often at a loss about how to provide sustenance.[11] Loving, gentle touch can be a form of nourishment, a spiritual nourishment that feeds caregivers and care receivers.

ACTIVE LABOR – A FEW HOURS TO A FEW DAYS PRIOR TO DEATH

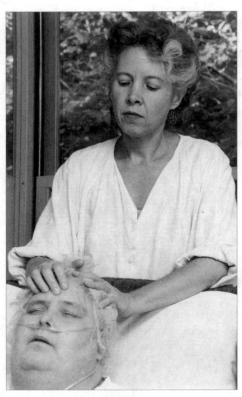

Figure 8.3 Some people request a gentle, full-body massage; others may want only parts of the body massaged.

Photograph by Don Hamilton

Active labor, or the onset of regular contractions, is the sign that the birthing process has begun. These contractions progressively create the opening in preparation for delivery of the baby. This process can begin hours or sometimes days before the actual birth. The one who is dying undergoes a comparable process a few hours to a few days before death. Active labor for the dying person is a series of physical processes that progressively shut down the body. The changes that occurred during the "lightening" phase generally become more intense. Additional changes that may occur include:

Skin: Extremities cool to the touch; mottling; lips and nails turn blue, hands and feet turn purplish; backside of the body becomes blotchy as well as the ankles, knees, and elbows.

GI Tract: Difficulty swallowing.

Breathing: Breathing pattern becomes very irregular; mucous gathers in mouth and congests in the throat or lungs causing the loud breathing sound known as the "death rattle"; there may be loud moans or sighs as the "letting go of life occurs."[1]

Muscoloskeletal: Weak and unable to do anything for self; unable to turn in bed; twitches; restless.

Mental Functions: Decreased awareness; inability to concentrate; can still hear even if other senses have faded.

Emotional: May be calm and accepting or fearful and anxious; may relax when family members are at the bedside.[1]

Spiritual: Out-of-body events; sense of connection to spiritual source;[1] may have a sudden surge of energy in which they are able to clearly speak to those around them or may wish to share a meal despite not wanting food for the preceding weeks.[3]

General: Sleep deepens, making the patient more difficult to rouse; deterioration of body, causing odors, incontinence, and secretions; urine output decreases and urine darkens.[1,3,8]

MASSAGE COMFORT MEASURES

- Continue touch to the end unless the person cannot tolerate or is distracted by it. It may be as simple as holding his hand or lying in bed and cradling her. Light, feather-weight stroking is often comforting at this time.

- Many hospice workers have commented that touching the body during the final days and hours seems to distract the dying person from letting go, bringing the attention back to the body. If this seems to be happening, hold and touch her energetically in your mind and heart as you sit with her. Even if you never put your hands on the one who is departing, it doesn't mean you haven't touched him. What is most needed at the end is presence, not doing.

- If the dying one cannot be touched directly, smooth the energy field above him with a long, effleurage type of stroke.

- Ascertaining tolerance for touch when the dying one is unresponsive can be difficult. Some practitioners prefer not to give touch to these patients in case it causes pain which the patient is unable to communicate. Subtle cues such as eye movements or breathing rate may indicate discomfort. However, if the massage giver is concerned about hurting the person who is dying, she can employ the suggestions given in the above sections rather than directly touching the patient.

- Hearing remains acute until death. Even if the person is in a coma, introduce yourself, explain who you are and why you are there. For instance, before touching her you might say, "In a minute I am going to put my hands on your feet." From time to time explain what you are doing. Sheila King talks to the dying person with her mind. As she worked with Ron during the last days of his life, he would mentally tell her where to put her hands.

- We touch the dying person not only with our hands, but with our eyes, our tone of voice, and even our thoughts.[9] People near death are sensitive to and perceptive of the thoughts and emotions around them.[1] Some hospice workers believe that the unconscious thoughts brought into the room by friends or caregivers can help the situation or can agitate the patient and slow down the dying process. Strive to face the fears or discomforts that arise from being part of someone's dying process. Being honest with yourself about how you feel will make your emotional energy field more calm and clear. If your distress makes it impossible to work in that moment, permit

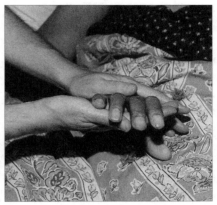

Figure 8.4 Near to the end of life, something as simple as holding a hand can bring comfort.

Photograph by Don Hamilton

Being with cancer patients is easy. With them, my best self comes out. I do this work because it makes me whole.

LIZ DAVIDSON, LMT,
PORTLAND, OREGON

Repeatedly, I am awed that the most wondrous of all the massage strokes is that of simply "resting" – resting my hands, resting my intentions, resting my heart as one would rest in contemplative prayer. Compassionate massage, then, also embodies contemplation. Silently, I am here, sheltering you through my hands with my own vulnerable and wounded loveliness. This is touch raised to the art of anointing, the art of prayer, and the sacrament of caring.

MARY ANN FINCH, FOUNDER AND DIRECTOR OF THE CARE THROUGH TOUCH INSTITUTE, BERKELEY, CALIFORNIA

yourself to leave the room. Massage givers must honor their process, too.

Therese Schroeder-Sheker, founder of the Chalice Repose Project, tends to the dying with music specially designed for their needs. She teaches her interns that they must "differentiate between music for the living and music for the dying. Music for the living is meant to be engaging, whereas music for the dying is meant to be freeing, to help them let go."[12]

Touch for the dying should also be freeing, allowing them to be unfettered rather than binding them to this plane. How could we touch someone in a way that does not hold them back, that allows freedom, and even encourages them to go deeper into the passageway? Our hands and heart must be open, not clutching; they must be light, still, and calm, asking nothing, offering thanks and release. We must create an emotional spaciousness within ourselves that allows the dying person the freedom to be on any plane necessary; and try not to pull the person out of the internal world she has entered and into our external one. The books, *Coma: Key to Awakening* by Arnold Mindell and *Final Gifts* by Maggie Callanan and Patricia Kelley, may teach the bodyworker to assist dying people in following the experience of dying.

THE MOMENT OF DEATH

Some births happen with just a few easy pushes while others are a long, drawn-out, Herculean task. The moment of death, too, is unique and can happen with gentle ease or struggle and effort. Each death is what it is. Like birth, death is a passage, not a success or failure. It deserves the same honor we reserve for the moment of birth whether it was a peaceful experience or a conflicted one.

At the moment of death, the following changes may occur:

- No pulse
- Skin color changes to gray
- Eyes lose focus and remain open at death
- Breathing gradually stops. It is sometimes difficult to decide if the breathing actually has stopped. The last few breaths may sound like a sigh.[3] Others have described the final breaths as "fish out of water" breathing.[8]
- Involuntary loss of stool or urine.[1]

MASSAGE COMFORT MEASURES

May the work of your hands be a sign of gratitude and reverence to the human condition.

— MAHATMA GANDHI

- Continue to move slowly and gently around the body, allowing a sacred space for the transition of spirit.[1] Many traditions believe that the soul leaves the body slowly.[11]
- Clean and prepare the body. (See *Judy's Last Massage*)

- Say good-bye through prayer, ritual, silent meditation. The good-bye is not only to the one who has died, but also to what has been lost because of the death. For the ones left behind, it often feels as if part of themselves has died. Reading special prayers or spiritual passages may also help the "newly released soul become free of suffering and find its way in the afterlife."[11]

Judy's Last Massage

For years I have received professional massage on a regular basis. When my sister Judy was being treated for a rare form of sarcoma, I thought massage would help her discomfort and tried to convince her to go for a session given by someone trained in the field. Judy, however, wanted me to do it. After being on the receiving end of so many wonderful massages, I needed no instruction, my hands instinctively knew what to do. Judy and I had been competitive swimmers as girls. The long, gliding strokes of massage reminded us of that time, a time that had been especially important to Judy.

I was born prematurely, weighing just under four pounds. When our parents brought me home from the hospital, Judy, who was three years old at the time, heaped love and attention on me. But as we grew up and our personalities evolved, the relationship became somewhat contentious. This continued on into adulthood and was not resolved until Judy's illness. The massage was one of the few ways Judy got relief from pain, but the sessions also played an important role in healing our relationship.

My mother and I were with Judy when she died. After she finally passed, I called the hospice nurse to have them come and take out the tubes, catheter, and remove the PCA pump. After the nurse had disposed of the impersonal, medical side of the experience, I took a new bar of Judy's favorite lavender soap, a wash cloth, and basin of water, and proceeded to clean, clear, rest, and settle her exhausted and spent body. In a rather horrified way, my mother asked what I was doing. I told her I was preparing Judy, not unlike she had done when she brought Judy into this world. My 79-year-old mother became very quiet and thoughtful, but without another word she got a wash cloth and towel and lovingly began to wash Judy's left side while I washed the right. After bathing her frail body, I gently massaged Judy with oil one last time, using the long, flowing strokes that she loved. When the massage ended, we smudged the room with sage and had a quiet time with Judy before calling the mortician. Then my mother and I dressed Judy in her favorite swim suit, a red and orange Hawaiian print that reminded her of swimming in the ocean. Now she was ready for the next big event.

— MARY BLAKE, SEASIDE, OREGON

Usually the bodyworker will not be with the patient when death occurs unless he is part of the immediate family. The moment of death, like the moment of birth or sex, is so private, that even though a massage therapist may have developed a close, intimate relationship over the months of massaging the patient, the dying person generally wants only a few special people with him at the end. Some people even prefer to have no one with them and will delay the moment of death until everyone has left the room.

During final labor, the patient sometimes feels free to die when she knows that her loved ones are being taken care of. This is something the touch therapist can do. By caring for family members he is indirectly giving help to the dying one.

Many of us have the privilege of being an angel to somebody in a moment of need. At such times, we are more than ourselves; we carry the forces of heaven with us.

JAN SELLIKEN, ND, RN,
AND MIRIAM SCHNEIDER, MSN,
THE TRUE WORK OF DYING

FINAL THOUGHTS

The act of giving touch to people at the end of life is simple. Professional bodyworkers may be skilled in a variety of massage modalities, but for people in the last months of life, touch techniques are less important than the quality of the practitioner's presence. Most of us, however, are not accustomed to interacting and being present with someone who is dying, and must seek out additional training and other sources of information. *Medicine Hands* should only be considered a beginning.

Walking the final steps with someone who is leaving this world is a privilege. The journey can be a meaningful process for the one who is dying and those around her, and is as important as any part of life. I have seen midwives to the dying shortly after being present at the death of their friend, patient, or family member. Their countenance is one of awe, light emanates from their face, and they temporarily seem to be on a higher plane. Those who attend a birth often reflect the same brilliance, mystery, and other-worldliness. Like birth, death is holy and worthy of embracing. Loving touch shifts us into that sacred place and reminds us that death is a blessed and miraculous event.

REFERENCES

1.   Bernard JS, Schneider M. *The True Work of Dying: A Practical and Compassionate Guide to Easing the Dying Process.* New York, NY: Avon Books,1996

2.   LeBoyer F. *Birth Without Violence.* New York, NY: Knopf, 1975.

3.   Callanan M, Kelley P. *Final Gifts.* New York, NY: Bantam Books, 1992.

4.   Ellis V, Hill J, Campbell H. Strengthening the Family Unit Through the Healing Power of Massage. *The American Journal of Hospice and Palliative Care.* 1995;12 (5):19-21.

5.   Campbell H. Why We Do What We Do: A True Story of Love and Forgiveness. Hospital Based Massage Newsletter. 1996; 2(3):8-9.

6.   Rachel Naomi Remen, interview by Bill Moyers, *Healing and The Mind* video (Wounded Healers segment). 1993.

7.   Balfour Mount, interview, *When Doctors Get Cancer,* PBS video: Station WHYY, Philadelphia. 1994.

8.   Karnes B. *Gone From My Sight: The Dying Experience.* Self-published. 1986.

9.   Nelson D. *From the Heart Through the Hands.* Findhorn, Scotland: Findhorn Press, 2000.

10. Huntington L. *Living with Hope, Dying with Dignity: Home Care for the Terminal Patient.* Master Books Publishers. 1988.

11. Peay P. A Good Death. *Common Boundary.* 1997;15(5):32-41.

12. Schroeder-Sheker T. Music for the Dying. *Noetic Sciences Review.* 1994. Autumn. P.32-36.

Acknowledgment: *The True Work of Dying* by Jan Selliken Bernard and Miriam Schneider provided significant inspiration for the framework of this chapter.

Chapter 9

Massage as Respite

Caring for the Caregivers

Caring for a seriously ill family member is emotionally and physically exhausting. Caregivers are required to perform tasks for patients that are physically demanding, such as bathing, assisting them to the bathroom, or making transfers from the bed to a wheelchair or commode. In addition to providing this extra day-to-day care, caregivers are left to manage the household chores on their own. As if all of this is not enough, they often have to rise many times during the night to attend to the patient, thereby diminishing their sleep. Not only does the body become over-extended from the increase in duties and lack of sleep, but it becomes tense and armored due to fear, grief, and even anger.

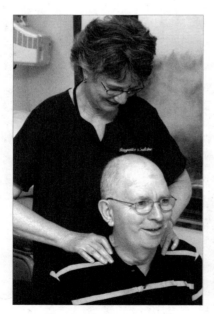

Figure 9.1 "Hey, what about me?" says the husband whose wife just received a massage during her chemo treatment.

Photograph by David J. Lawton

Robert

Robert was my first massage patient at OHSU. He had been in the hospital for weeks and more than anything was bored. For him the massage was a pleasant distraction and something new in an otherwise dull day. He enjoyed the session well enough. His wife Sharon was my second patient. Even though she was not the "designated" patient, Sharon needed care as much, if not more, than Robert. The couple lived on a small farm near the Oregon coast. When Robert became ill with leukemia, Sharon did the bulk of the farm and house chores as well

Continued on page 189

Scientific research supports the effects of caregiving on family and friends. Care partners suffer anxiety, depression, fatigue, sleep and eating disturbance.[1-5] Spouses report as much anxiety and stress as the person with cancer, which can have prolonged effects on the spouse's health and well-being. They may experience a higher incidence of hypertension, respiratory distress, and immunosuppression, all of which create a more stressful experience of caring for a person who is ill.[5]

Certain periods of time are more stressful than others.[5] These include:

- Before initial discharge from the hospital.

- Two months after being hospitalized. It is during this time that both the care partner and patient realize the impact of the disease on their lives.

- During outpatient treatment. At this time the patient needs more help with symptom management.

- The advancement of each stage.

THE HOSPITAL WAIT

After receiving the diagnosis, the first taste caregivers have of the cancer experience is often in the hospital when the patient begins treatment. Time in hospitals is characterized by endless amounts of waiting, waiting for loved ones to come out of surgery, "standing watch" for days or even weeks at the bedside, and enduring nights "sleeping" in a reclining chair. At the very least there are frequent day-long waits in the outpatient clinic while the patient receives chemotherapy or radiation. A short seated massage can give release to pent-up bodies and minds, provide a pleasant distraction, and allow those in the role of givers to receive, just for a moment.

Rexilius et al.[1] and Goodfellow[5] both have shown this to be true. Rexilius et al. examined massage and Healing Touch given to caregivers of patients undergoing stem cell transplantation. Participants received two 30-minute massages or Healing Touch treatments for a period of three weeks. The control group received standard care. Only the massage group showed statistically significant declines in three of the measured variables – anxiety, depression, and fatigue.

Goodfellow studied the effect of a single, 20-minute back massage on natural killer cell activity (NKCA), heart rate, blood pressure, mood, and perceived stress on spouses with cancer. Mood and perceived stress improved but no change occurred in NKCA, heart rate, or blood pressure. Even though there was no change in NKCA, a relationship was found between mood and NKCA. Those who had the highest negative mood scores had the lowest NKCA levels. The reader could extrapolate then that improving mood would be accompanied by increased NKCA levels. Weaknesses in the experimental design, however, kept the researcher from collecting the necessary NKCA data.[5]

Robert, continued
as maintain a part-time job. The physical and emotional burden was staggering. Driving 180 miles round trip to the hospital, feeding livestock, and parenting two sons plus her regular responsibilities had taken a toll on her body, especially her back and shoulders. For Sharon, the neck and shoulder massage was more than a diversion, it gave her time to rest for a moment, to stop and take a few breaths.

— AUTHOR

reading all the signs
for the umpteenth time
        — HANK DUNLOP,
    ABOUT THE OR WAITING ROOM

hospital vigil
the imperceptible shift
of clouds
        — FRANCINE PORAD

Hands of Clouds

She is much older than her 9 years, the girl who always accompanies her mom to chemo and radiation treatments. She acts as her translator, interpreting news and information that a young child should not be exposed to. One day, I was walking with the girl when we passed a patient who was very disfigured from a large tumor on the neck. Putting my arm around her, I quietly said, "You are too young to be exposed to so much illness." She looked at me and said, "It is okay, this is my normal."

Whenever I see her, I bring the girl into my massage room for a few minutes of pampered attention. I become her caregiver. She is a such a delight to talk to. You have "hands of clouds," she told me, the first time I massaged her back.

— TONI MUIRHEAD, LMT,
COOPER CITY, FLORIDA

My whole outlook changed.

— FAMILY MEMBER OF HOSPITAL
PATIENT AFTER A 15-MINUTE
SEATED MASSAGE

GUIDELINES FOR GIVING SEATED MASSAGE TO FAMILY CAREGIVERS IN THE HOSPITAL

- Observe intake protocols for giving seated massage, even if the session will only be ten minutes. Performance of a health intake before the massage is vital. Many cancer patients are in advanced years, which means that many family members are older and have a variety of medical problems. It is not uncommon to encounter such conditions as diabetes, prior cancer treatment, breathing disorders, fibromyalgia, or even mild congestive heart failure. The questions listed in the Info Box on page 207 will give the therapist enough information to safely administer a chair massage.

- Handwash before and after each session.

- Be adaptable and flexible with regard to time, location, and necessary props. Sometimes waiting family members only have five minutes to receive massage, or must leave suddenly part way through. Five minutes is better than nothing. Be willing to conduct the session wherever the caregiver is most comfortable. Sometimes people want to leave the room for a few minutes of rest and relaxation. At other times they want to remain in the patient's room. Learn to give a massage using only a regular chair. Often there is only a brief window of opportunity to give a session, and the moment can instantly evaporate if the therapist needs to leave to set up a seated massage chair or to get other props. If caregivers perceive that the bodyworker is going to a lot of trouble on their account, they will sometimes suddenly decline the opportunity.

- If the massage therapist and family member are both waiting for the patient to return from the lab, or to finish a session with the physical therapist, or to consult with physicians, suggest a neck and shoulder massage. In this situation, the caregivers feel as if they are not a bother, since the massage therapist is also waiting for the patient. Even if the wait is only going to be a few minutes long, offer to massage just the neck or just the shoulders. Any contact helps to develop rapport for the future. Many cancer patients are in and out of the hospital on a regular basis, so practitioners become familiar with them, their families, and friends. Ongoing relationships develop over time.

- Never pressure people to accept a massage. If the offer of bodywork is firmly turned down from the start, move on to the next potential recipient. Only offer again if caregivers are showing some ambivalence or confusion about what a seated massage entails. Perhaps they need a little encouragement to do something for themselves or need to get further information about the process of seated massage. Often caregivers may initially act excited at the prospect of receiving some TLC and then just as suddenly will back away with a comment such as, "I was just kidding," or, "Save your energy for the patients." Caregivers often feel guilty about accepting care for themselves when their loved one is sick.

- An unused overbed table positioned against the wall makes a good station from which to give a seated massage, especially if the caregiver wishes to remain in the loved one's room. Raise the table up to the most advantageous height and place several pillows on the top.

PROVIDING CARE AT HOME

Shorter hospital stays, increased treatment in outpatient settings, and longer survival rates have placed a greater responsibility on family members to provide care. While the hospital experience is distinguished by long periods of inactivity for care partners, caring for someone at home – whether recovering from chemotherapy or surgery, or in the last stage of life – is characterized by running from morning until night. Accepting support for themselves can be difficult for family care providers. They feel there isn't enough time, or if they relax they may never get back up. Some feel guilty receiving TLC for themselves when their loved one is sick or dying.

Marti, a massage therapist, was the primary caregiver (PCG) for her dying grandmother. She related that during the time she cared for her grandmother, she never had a massage for fear of falling apart. Marti was certain if she received a massage she would not be able to "hold it together" and would be unable to fulfill her responsibilities to her grandmother and her sons.

Caregivers may need to be encouraged and helped in learning to take time for themselves. They often don't understand that by taking care of themselves they can better take care of the patient. Bodyworkers, however, can only offer their skills as a way of helping family caregivers. If the caregiver's decision is "No," practitioners must accept it without exerting pressure. Other ways can be found to give support, such as staying with the patient while the PCG goes out or by doing the grocery shopping. The massage therapist can let her know that the offer is always there if she changes her mind. Very few families can afford to pay for extras such as massage during a serious illness. Even with good insurance coverage, the out-of-pocket expenses are financially depleting. Professional practitioners must bear this in mind when offering massage.

HOSPICE CAREGIVERS

Caring for a family member at home who is at the end stage of life is particularly demanding for primary caregivers. Some families provide all of the care themselves without the help of a hospice agency. But even with the assistance of a hospice program, the task for caregivers is overwhelming. Those unfamiliar with hospice care may erroneously think that the hospice agency provides the day-to-day nursing care, but it is usually a member of the patient's family who does this. The hospice team is there to make home visits, monitor medications, coordinate professional and volunteer caregivers, instruct family members in patient care, plus many other services. It is the primary

> ### Holding It Together
>
> Caregivers of the seriously ill often spend a good deal of their time trying to "hold things together," sometimes denying their own needs and feelings in order to be there for others. Such people may be afraid to relax even a little bit fearing that if they do, they will fall apart completely and not be able to carry on. They may sense that letting themselves be nurtured and cared for will make them feel vulnerable or bring up feelings that they are reluctant to face or accept. It is important to acknowledge and accept such fears or reluctance and not to challenge someone to move beyond what they feel they are capable of…. At the same time, one can offer support by encouraging a caregiver not to let their own needs go unmet for too long or to push themselves too hard without relief.
>
> — DAWN NELSON, FOUNDER OF COMPASSIONATE TOUCH ®

To take care of another is to take care of yourself. (I kanaaka no'oe ke malama é ke kanaka.)

— HAWAI'IAN PROVERB

caregiver, however, who performs the tasks of daily living, such as bathing, oral hygiene, special skin care, preparation of special meals, bowel care, assisting to the bathroom, or helping with exercise regimens. Caregivers often must learn special procedures to care for catheters or colostomies, to monitor IVs, or to keep track of the patient's fluid intake and output.

Successful hospice care is dependent on caregivers who are willing and able to attend to the needs of the dying loved one 24 hours a day, with infrequent help from the hospice agency. Generally hospice care is begun when the physician feels that the patient has six months or less to live. However, it is likely that the PCG has been attending to her loved one throughout the illness, so that by the time hospice care is begun, she will already be mentally, emotionally, and physically exhausted. Caregiver fatigue is one of the main deterrents to successful hospice intervention and is a fundamental reason patients must be institutionalized in the final phases of their illness.

The majority of hospice patients are over 65, so caregivers, too, are often in advanced years, with health problems of their own. One survey of a midwest hospice organization found that "the frail elderly individual is the most common problem regarding family caregivers."[6] Spousal caregivers, who comprise the bulk of hospice care partners, have been found to experience increased symptoms and a decreased sense of well-being before and after the death of the ill spouse.[7] Other stresses are isolation, lack of time for themselves,[8] the loss of physical affection from the dying loved one,[7] and the need to be more socially active.[9]

Supporting caregivers is highly beneficial during this arduous time. It is not uncommon for hospice patients to be admitted to the hospital or a care facility during some of their final days. This may happen because the family is unable to give the needed high tech care. Sometimes it is because the primary care giver is too exhausted to continue in their role. A patient with an exhausted caregiver is likely to spend more days in the hospital or is more likely to be permanently transferred to a care facility and is less likely to die at home. Therefore, directly caring for the PCG is beneficial not only to the patient, but to the providing agency, and in the long run also to society through reduced health care costs.

MASSAGE AS RESPITE

The hospice philosophy recognizes that cancer doesn't just happen to one person, it affects the entire family. The "unit of care" is not only the patient but the family too. Despite including the family in the unit of care, most of the direct care is still focused on patients. PCGs often express a desire for direct support "rather than being instructed about how to attain it through self-reliant means."[7]

Respite care is one way hospice programs provide for the needs of caregivers. Typically, when a respite volunteer comes in for a few hours, it allows the PCG a chance to complete errands, shop, or to keep an appointment. However, a pilot outreach program through the Oregon Hospice Association successfully used massage as a respite intervention. Massage therapists traveled with their tables to the recipients' home, which made it easier for the PCGs to participate in the program. Participants received a series of full-body massages, usually weekly or bi-weekly. On average, six massages were given in the series, although some received only three sessions, while a few received up to eight. The majority of recipients were women who were caring for male loved ones. Their ages ranged from 35 to 82, with nearly half being over 70. About half had never had a massage.

The project's primary objective was to reduce the fatigue and stress that compromise the PCG's ability to effectively care for the dying loved one at home. Feedback given at the end of the series of massages indicated that this objective was met for every caregiver but one. Data was collected prior to starting the series of massages and following the final session, on four items: emotional stress, physical stress, physical pain, and sleep difficulties. A decrease in emotional and physical stress was reported by 85% of the participants (n=13). Physical pain, which was defined as specific symptoms such as headaches, back pain, or pain from knotted or strained muscles, decreased in 77% of the group. Sleep difficulties were reduced for 54%.

Typical responses were, "The massages have been extraordinarily helpful. They were very successful in relieving built-up stress." A.M., a 71-year-old woman wrote, "I am sad the massages are almost over. I really looked forward to them each week and it's a good way to relieve physical and emotional stress. It is also very good therapy for the spirit." Before receiving any massages, R.B., a 74-year-old caring for her husband, reported, "…having some really bad days lately – no one left to share the burden." Following a series of eight massages, R.B. wrote, "I am more relaxed. I still have a lot of tension, but it seems easier to handle at times. I find I don't have to do everything right now, it'll still be there." S.K., a 35-year-old woman who cared for her mother in addition to her own family, reported, "I am surprised at how much the massages helped. I didn't think they would. They helped me realize where I carry my stress – the headaches are gone, and muscles are not tight."

Only one caregiver did not notice any long-term benefits from the three massages he received. Each massage felt great to him while it was happening and immediately following, but it was very difficult to return to the same stressful situation afterwards. Most of the relaxation was gone as soon as he left the room. This was one of the few PCGs to complete at least three massages who was also working full-time. The added stress of working and caring for his wife no doubt contributed to his incredibly high stress level. On the whole, a series of massages was not a successful intervention for caregivers who were also working full-time. Originally the idea sounded good to them, but their day was already so full that one more thing couldn't be squeezed in without its being an added stress. Most discontinued after one or two sessions. The greatest benefit was to those who were full-time caregivers.

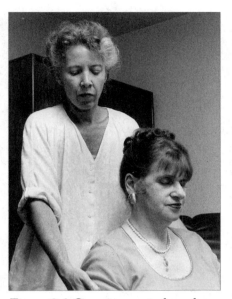

Figure 9.2 Caregiver rests for a few moments, gathering strength for her difficult job.

Photograph by Don Hamilton

SUPPORT DURING THE DYING PROCESS

As the patient enters the active stages of dying, the experience intensifies for the caregiver. During the final stages, they may react with physical symptoms such as headaches, fatigue, loss of appetite, insomnia, and muscular tension; and with such emotional symptoms as fear, guilt, anger, depression, sorrow, relief, withdrawal, or peace.[10] Care partners may need encouragement to take some care for themselves. A walk, nap, hot bath, or seated massage can help them preserve the energy and composure needed to sustain care for the dying loved one, as well as maintain a calm environment.

Vicky, whose 82-year-old father was dying in the hospital, was very distraught by her father's struggle to breathe. As the massage students were de-briefing, his nurse put her head in to the conference room and asked if someone would do an "emergency massage" for this man. Pam volunteered. When she entered the room the patient was having difficulty breathing. His daughter felt he should rest and was not in favor of her father being massaged. Pam gently asked if she could just hold the patient's feet, which Vicky consented to. At first he gave a couple of twitches and jerks. Pam thought he might die at that moment. But within five minutes his breathing calmed, along with the atmosphere in the room. Soon after, Pam gave the distressed daughter a seated massage in another room, enabling her to relax. The patient died the following day. The charge nurse reported that everyone was

---

Edgar

Edgar, 82 years old, is a sweet, soft, gentle man who is just about spent emotionally and physically. He has been caring for his wife Maureen, who is in the end stage of metastatic breast cancer to the lung, for several months. Taking care of her as well as maintaining the house and yard are overwhelming. He rated his emotional and physical stress at 4 and 4.5 respectively on a 1–5 scale, with 1 being low and 5 being high.

After the last time Maureen returned home from the hospital, stress fractures occurred at T10 – L4. Edgar feels they are a result of his emotional distress. The fractures cause him a lot of pain and make it difficult to lift and position Maureen, even though she only weighs 58 pounds. He rated his physical pain at a 5. Sleep too is difficult, which he rated at a 4. Every two to three hours he must rise to help Maureen. Usually Edgar sleeps until three A.M. and lies awake until it's time to get up. He just hired a caregiver because he is only able to manage now until two P.M.

WEEK 1. Because of the back pain, Edgar asked me to focus on that area as well as general relaxation. I used Swedish and Russian effleurage, petrissage, and friction, as well as gentle vibration and shaking to the shoulders, back, and gluteals. His pain didn't seen to be in the spine but in the left quadratus lumborum (QL). The new caregiver also had massaged the area, leaving it bruised and sore. Edgar reported that, "She really went after that spot!" I will show her how to work the area next week when I come.

WEEK 2. Edgar seems less stressed and his back is better. The hired caregiver and massage are helping a lot. I used Muscle Energy Technique to stretch and release the QL, as well as applying relaxation strokes.

WEEK 3. Maureen's son is visiting. He is here to make the final arrangements and yet talks as if his mother will recover. Edgar is sleeping better and his sense of humor is surfacing. Unless he lifts something, his back is all right. As I left, Maureen's parting comment was that she probably wouldn't be here next week.

WEEK 4. Maureen was asleep when I arrived. Edgar's daughter is visiting, which noticeably raised his spirits. She is a massage therapist in California, so I showed her what I've been doing with her father's back.

calmer that final day. It will never be known to what extent Pam's ministrations were helpful, but perhaps the massage played some part in making a painful situation more bearable.

Another family was momentarily transformed by the soothing effects of massage as they struggled to endure the discomfort of the dying man who was their brother, son, and husband. As the night wore on, different family members would leave the hospital room and wander the halls, the despair evident on their faces. In some miraculous way, each of those four people independently found their way to one of the massage students who had just started their first night of work on the oncology unit. When the student's evening ended, they all passed by the patient's room on their way back to the de-briefing room. The entire family, relaxed and smiling, came out to thank the students for their care. Allowing themselves to be massaged for just 15 minutes had palpably shifted the mood from anguish to tranquility.

EASING THE WAY DURING BEREAVEMENT

Often during the Massage Respite Project, the patient died before the caregiver had received all of the massages in the series. The sessions then became part of the bereavement process. One 56-year-old participant who received a series of three massages, all after her

I noticed my mood changed after each massage. I could face the world a little better. It was easier to go back and tackle things.

— K.C., 42-YEAR-OLD WOMAN WHO CARED FOR HER BROTHER

Edgar's back continues to improve, but he forgets to put on the back support when helping Maureen into and out of bed, which makes his back hurt.

WEEK 5. A couple of days ago Maureen fell during the night. Her cries for help eventually woke Edgar. He tried to help her up but couldn't, and hurt his back again. Together they crawled to the bed so Maureen could help pull herself up. He was especially glad to see me today, the back problem is really getting him down. I focused on the lower back from T10–L4. He soaked up the massage. Tomorrow Edgar leaves for a week to see his brother and is expecting flak from the family. He needs to get away from Maureen. Her anger and attitude is getting to him.

WEEK 6. Maureen is in great pain owing to muscle spasms from coughing. Edgar looks refreshed from his week away. The focus was on full-body relaxation.

WEEK 7. The house was quiet today. Maureen continues to be in pain from muscles spasms, but was asleep at the time. Edgar seemed in a good space today. I think he looks forward to the massage so much he automatically feels better on these days. His back is good. There were no situations this past week to stress or reinjure it. The massage session focused on the low back and shoulders. He always tells me, "I'll give you 24 hours to stop." We talked about how much better his back feels now and how grateful he is.

WEEK 8. Maureen is still having a lot of pain. She hurts too much to be touched and is on morphine now. Edgar is stressed again this week. The hospice nurse had been there just before my visit, to teach him how to administer morphine injections. Since this was his last massage as part of the Massage Respite Project, he asked for "one more good back massage." Since starting, his back is much better overall. Unless he does something to stress it, he is pain free. Before starting the series of eight massages, his physical pain was a 5. By the end of the series it had dropped to a 2. Edgar's emotional stress also dropped from a 4 to a 2, physical stress from 4.5 to a 2, and sleep difficulties went from a 4 to a 2. Thanks to the massages he was better able to care for his wife.

— COURTESY OF THE MASSAGE RESPITE PROJECT

Grief is ruthless. It has no boundaries and shows no grace. We cannot control it or organize it. The only thing we can do is bring consciousness to it and honor ourselves as we pass through it.

— IRENE SMITH,
*EVERFLOWING TOUCH TECHNIQUES
IN HOSPICE CARE*

husband's death, wrote, "It gave me something to look forward to and helped relieve the stress during this hard time. It was so nice to be taken care of after so many months of taking care of others." One of the most touching stories was that of a 68-year-old woman who anxiously asked the nurse, almost immediately after her husband died, if she would still be given the remainder of her massages. The caregiver was afraid that after her husband died she would no longer be eligible to participate in the Project.

Not only is caregiving deleterious to the PCG's health; so is the grieving process. The stress of bereavement has been shown to have a negative effect on components of the immune system. Calabrese et al.[11] in their review of literature in "Alterations in Immunocompetence During Stress, Bereavement, and Depression," cited studies of spouses with seriously-ill partners in which the T lymphocyte responses were adversely effected. Six weeks after the partners' deaths the lymphocyte responses were even lower than at the first sampling, leading researchers to suggest a "cumulative, time-dependent effect." Another study found reduced lymphocyte response in bereaved subjects who had scored high on a depression rating scale. A study of subjects that scored high on a loneliness scale exhibited decreased immunocompetence, a relevant finding related to grieving caregivers, as loneliness is one of the stresses reported by PCGs.[11] Schleifer et al.[12] also found lymphocytes to be depressed in the spouses of 15 women who had died of breast cancer. Bereaved women in another study showed reduced NKCA and increased cortisol levels.[13]

Although no significant research has yet been done to assess the immunological and psychological effect of massage on those in mourning, it is possible that receiving nurturing touch will be beneficial to caregivers as they grieve the death of their spouse, child, parent, or friend. A pilot study that examined the effect of Therapeutic Touch on four people who recently lost a loved one showed no consistent effects on immune function. The exception was lowered suppressor T cells, a type of lymphocyte that turns off the immune system, in all four subjects. By lowering the percentage of these cells, the immune system should function at a higher level.[14]

The dramatic results of the Therapeutic Touch study were on a psychological scale measuring positive qualities such as joy, vigor, contentment, and affection, and negative elements such as anxiety, guilt, hostility, and depression. The recipients showed significant increases in the positive characteristics and marked decreases in the negative ones.[14] However, the sample size of this study is too small to lead to any conclusions.

Evidence exists that those who care for a dying loved one at home over a long period of time find it more difficult to readjust during the early months following the death.[15] One of the primary needs during this time, if not the primary need, is for emotional support. According to Stetz and Hanson's study of caregiving demands during and after the experience, "...a primary intervention would be to assist the caregiver emotionally with his or her grieving".[7] Massage is such an intervention. Bodies that have become armored over the months and years are loosened and softened, allowing grief to move through with greater ease and speed.

People derive emotional support from a variety of avenues. For some, the deepest comfort comes from the patient's nurse, for others it is provided by the clergy or a social worker, while still others depend on family, friends, or even nature. Bodywork can be an equally viable source. During a massage the caregiver is not only able to rest and be physically cared for, but is simultaneously able to tell her story to a compassionate listener. Grief is not just an emotional process; a physical component is always involved. In order to truly assist the bereaved, hospice and home health care agencies should make a diverse and holistic group of support services available, including methods that integrate the body into the process.

RECOMMENDATIONS FOR GIVING BODYWORK TO CAREGIVERS IN THE HOME

- Being able to receive massage in the home is important. Many hospice caregivers are reluctant to leave, even for a while, in case something should happen to the patient.

- Put aside any preconceived notions about who would be open to receiving bodywork. Sometimes it is assumed that because of age, gender, weight, or religious conviction, a PCG would be opposed to such an opportunity. Predicting who would like to receive massage is impossible.

- Because many caregivers are in advanced years, with health problems of their own, it may be helpful to have them fill out a health history prior to the first session in case the person's physician needs to be contacted for approval or information.

- A seated massage can be an effective first session for some care partners. This allows those who have never received bodywork to ease into both the process and the relationship with the practitioner. Others are immediately ready for a full-body session. Sound out the caregiver on which would be more comfortable for her.

- Ascertain whether the patient can be left unattended for the hour it will take for the session. If constant care is required, encourage the PCG to arrange for another family member, friend, or neighbor to come to the house. This will make it possible for the caregiver to relax, knowing he will not have to get off of the table midway to help the patient.

- Call to confirm 24 hours before the session is scheduled and then call again the morning of the appointment to reconfirm. The situation can change drastically from one hour to the next when someone is seriously ill, and time can cease to exist.

FINAL THOUGHTS

The hospice model should be the universal standard of care in all situations of serious illness, not just for those families affected by a terminal disease. But even the hospice model needs expanding where caregivers are concerned. Hopefully the hospice and home health care team of the future will include a massage therapist. Bodywork practitioners bring unique skills and qualities to a health care staff. Not only do they have the training to work with sore muscles or stiff necks; touch professionals bring with them qualities such as restfulness, tranquility, deep compassion, and the ability to listen with their entire being. Through their hands these attributes are transmitted, momentarily easing the burden, nourishing the caregiver's body, mind, and heart.

Providing nurturing bodywork for care partners not only supports them but can also have an indirect benefit for patients. The caregiver who remains in good health will be able to care more easily for their loved one. Also, caregivers, family members, or friends who have been massaged are often then able to give compassionate, loving touch to the patient. Once they have personally experienced the sensations of increased physical and emotional well-being, and become familiar with the types of strokes, the depth of pressure, and pacing, some feel confident to carry this experience over to the patient.

Many, including some health care workers, see massage as an unaffordable luxury. But by offering services that support family caregivers directly, health care agencies and the families themselves may save money in the long run as caregiver demands on agency resources are reduced. A rested caregiver who is attending to some of her own needs will be able to provide more and better care for the patient.

REFERENCES

1. Rexilius SJ, Mundt CA, Megel ME, et al. Therapeutic Effects of Massage Therapy and Healing Touch on Caregivers of Patients Undergoing Autologous Hematopoietic Stem Cell Transplant. *Oncology Nursing Forum*. 2002;29(3):35-44.

2. Kurtz ME, Kurtz JC, Given CW, et al. Depression and physical health among family caregivers of Geriatric Patients with Cancer. *Medical Science Monitor*. 2004 Aug;10(8):CR447-56.

3. Glajchen M. The Emerging Role and Needs of Family Caregivers in Cancer Care. *Journal of Supportive Oncology*. 2004;2(2):145-55.

4. Sorocco KH, Belzer A, Teasdale T. Integrating Caregiver Health into Patient Care. *Journal of Oklahoma State Medical Association*. 2005;98(11):545-8.

5. Goodfellow LM. The Effects of Therapeutic Back Massage on Psychophysiologic Variables and Immune Function in Spouses of Patients with Cancer. *Nursing Research*. 2003;52(5):318-328.

6. Smith MA. Primary Caregiver Options in Hospice Care. *American Journal of Hospice and Palliative Care*. 1994;11(3):15-17.

7. Stetz K, Hanson W. Alterations in Perceptions of Caregiving Demands in Advanced Cancer During and After the Experience. *The Hospice Journal*. 1992;8(3):2-34.

8. Hull M. Sources of Stress for Hospice Caregiving Families. *The Hospice Journal*. 1990;6(2):29-54.

9. Martens N, Davis B. The Work of Patients and Spouses in Managing Advanced Cancer at Home. *The Hospice Journal*. 1990;6(2):55-73.

10. Bernard JS, Schneider M. *The True Work of Dying: A Practical and Compassionate Guide to Easing the Dying Process*. New York: Avon Books, 1996. P. 96-97.

11. Calabrese JR, Kling MA, Gold PW. Alterations in Immunocompetence During Stress, Bereavement, and Depression: Focus on Neuroendocrine Regulation. *The American Journal of Psychiatry*. 1987; 144(9):1123-1134.

12. Schleifer SJ, Keller SE, Camerino M, et al. Supression of Lymphocyte Stimulation Following Bereavement. *Journal of the American Medical Association*. 1983Jul15;250(3):374-7.

13. Irwin M, Daniels M, Risch SC, et al. Plasma Cortisol and Natural Killer Cell Activity During Bereavement. *Biological Psychiatry*. 1988 Jun;24(2):173-8.

14. Quinn JF, Strelkaukas AJ. Psychoimmunologic Effects of Therapeutic Touch on Practitioners and Recently Bereaved Recipients: A Pilot Study. *Advances in Nursing Science*. 1993;15(4):13-26.

15. Kirschling JM, Tilden VP, Butterfield PG. Social Support: The Experience of Hospice Family Caregivers. *The Hospice Journal*. 1990;6(2):75-93.

Acknowledgment: Parts of this chapter originally appeared in *Alternative Therapies in Clinical Practice*, May/June 1997, and were reprinted in *The American Journal of Hospice and Palliative Care*, January/February 1998.

Additional Resources

• Miller JE, Cutshall SC. *The Art of Being a Healing Presence – A Guide for Those in Caring Relationships*. Available at: www.willowgreen.com

• Cancer Care: On line Support Group: www.cancercare.org

• National Family Caregivers Association: www.nfcacares.org

Chapter 10
Gathering Information

An Essential Part of Safe Practice

C lients often walk in for their massage appointment seeming to simultaneously discard jewelry, kick off shoes, and pull sweaters over their head. Eager to get started, some are partway undressed before the therapist can leave the room. Being stopped for a health inventory is an annoyance to them. Therapists, too, sometimes feel that asking about a person's health status destroys their rhythm, unnecessarily takes up time better devoted to the hands-on aspect, or makes the experience seem too clinical.

Awareness of clients' health history is essential, but for the medically frail client, it is especially important. Reviewing treatment history, the side effects and length of time in treatment, and other health conditions will influence session goals, the type of massage modality used, the length of session, and the amount of pressure. Gathering health information about clients is part of being an ethical and safe practitioner. It is as much a part of the session as the hands-on component.

An entire chapter of stories that illustrate the need for performing intake could be written. These stories show what can happen when the intake is skipped or is insufficient. A couple of examples will suffice to make the point.

Adrienne, a nursing assistant in a bone marrow transplant unit, would stop at a moment's notice to get a ten-minute neck and shoulder rub from the massage students doing clinical rotation at the hospital. Suddenly and mysteriously, she no longer wanted the seated sessions. After nearly a year, Adrienne finally told the massage supervisor that after her last massage, many months ago, she developed swelling in her arm and was off work for two days feeling very unwell. Unbeknownst to the massage student, Adrienne had been treated a number of years previously for breast cancer. A lumpectomy, including nodal dissection, had been performed followed by radiation therapy. As the readers now know, this put the woman at risk for lymphedema. Without inquiring about her health history, the massage student could not have known about the need for caution. Adrienne was extremely muscular and healthy except for the breast cancer treatment. By looking at her, no one would have ever known about her prior condition without asking.

Gillian, a massage therapist, wanted to help her friend Lucy as she was going through cancer treatment by giving massage. Gillian wasn't accustomed to taking health history nor was she aware of the precautions needed when working with cancer patients. "What harm could come in giving my friend a 15-minute massage?" she thought. At the time that she was receiving the first massage, the pressure felt good to Lucy. Later in the day, however, she developed a headache and felt flu-ish. This went on for the next week, and she attributed it to the massage. That was the first and last time that she allowed Gillian to massage her.

The purpose of this chapter is to convey to readers the importance of performing a health intake. Methods of intake will be presented, along with sample forms and sections that address intake for full body and chair massage, as well as at special events. Documentation, however, is not covered in this text because information about it is available through other resources.

The spotlight of this chapter is on gathering information about a person's oncology history. Clients also may be affected by other health conditions unrelated to cancer, such as fibromyalgia, diabetes, or cardiovascular disease. It is not the goal of *Medicine Hands* to address those. It is assumed that the bodyworker is knowledgeable and experienced in performing a general intake. Also, the focus here is on performing intake with non-hospitalized patients. Instruction on working with people in the hospital is also available from other sources.

WHOSE RESPONSIBILITY?

Mona's client was receiving treatment at a pain clinic for a chronic condition. Due to an inadequate intake, this information did not surface and the therapist was unaware that her client was on pain medication. When the practitioner followed up the next day with the client, she was told that the massage, which had been fairly heavy, had

Interviewing is an information-gathering process.... There are two primary obstacles to gathering information – thinking that you already know the answer and being afraid to ask the question.

DIANA THOMPSON,
HANDS HEAL: COMMUNICATION,
DOCUMENTATION AND INSURANCE
BILLING FOR MANUAL THERAPISTS,
2ND ED.

**Examples of
Specific Questions for
Cancer Clients:**

- What kind of cancer were you treated for?

- What treatments were used? and where?

- When did you start the treatments?

- Did they remove or radiate any lymph nodes?

- How is your energy level?

- Are you bruising easily?

- Is your skin affected by the treatments?

- Are the treatments causing any nausea?

- Did any of your treatments cause peripheral neuropathy?

- Have you had a recent blood clot?

- Do you have any swelling or an area of excess warmth?

- How is your bone density?

- Do you have areas of pain?

- Do you have any medical devices?

triggered such severe pain that the client had to attend the pain clinic on an emergency basis. The touch practitioner was distraught that the client had not told her she was taking medication for pain.

The above story not only shows the need for collecting health information from clients but also provides a springboard into the question, Who is responsible for insuring that the massage therapist has all of the necessary medical information? Is it the client's responsibility? The doctor's? The massage therapist's? Or a combination of the above?

Ideally, patients are the quarterback of their health care team. After consulting with their practitioners, they should have the right and responsibility for choosing the interventions that best support their healing. However, many people feel more confident having their doctor's permission to integrate complementary therapies into their allopathic treatment regimen.

Many oncologists, surgeons, and nurses value massage, but don't yet understand its power. Believing massage to be mostly benign and incapable of causing harm, they often refer the patient without any precautions, trusting that all massage therapists are sufficiently trained to work with people treated for cancer. Clients, too, are not aware of what a bodyworker must know in order to create a safe massage plan. Therefore, the responsibility for collecting the necessary data about a client rests squarely on the shoulders of the bodyworker. Even if the doctor has written a script approving massage, it is still the touch practitioner's job to present the doctor or nurse with the specific questions that will elicit the needed information.

Massage therapists must realize that health care is so complex and specialized that doctors can't be expected to know more than the basics about other health care fields. While medical and nursing schools are more often incorporating information about integrative therapies into their curriculums, it is still not enough to enable health care providers to give detailed guidance to the touch therapist. Massage practitioners must work in tandem with the patient's care team, prompting them with the questions that will bring out the details of a person's health status. Bodyworkers must never assume that the client, nurse, or doctor will be able to list the precautions from the question, "Is there anything I need to know?" *Asking vague questions of the client or health care provider is insufficient.* Specific questions are needed.

While many people are referred by their physician, many others self-refer to massage, are referred through a friend, or are given gift certificates. Nearly half the time, the research shows, they do not inform their doctors that they are using CAM therapies in conjunction with the allopathic treatments.[1,2,3] What course does the therapist take in the case of a patient who is in treatment for cancer but has not yet conferred with their doctor about the use of massage? Rather than refusing to massage first-time clients until they have a doctor's note or have informed the doctor, practitioners can work with them in a conservative manner using non-invasive techniques. It is very disappointing for clients to be refused when they have been looking forward to a massage. Some will withhold information about their health status to avoid being turned away.

Patients should be strongly encouraged to make their physicians aware of the complementary modalities that they are using. Not only do physicians have responsibilities toward the patients; patients have an obligation to the doctor. The doctor-patient relationship works best when both parties uphold their end. When a health care provider agrees to treat and care for a patient, they are assuming great responsibility for that person. Having a complete picture of the patient's activities helps the physician or nurse practitioner give the best treatment and care.

One way that touch therapists can support their patients in informing the health care provider is to prepare a general letter briefly explaining their work with cancer patients. This can be taken to the next doctor's appointment. Informing the physician about the use of ancillary treatments does not mean that he or she is the final arbitrator of what patients can or can't do. It is acknowledging the need for full disclosure in order that the physician can give his or her input and help the patient make decisions that are in his best interest. The Info Box on page 204 illustrates one therapist's letter to a doctor.

Bodyworkers are often told in massage school to "Get a note from the doctor." In the ideal world, this would be possible. In reality, it isn't always easy or necessary. Physicians are limited in the amount of time they have for each patient. Filling out paperwork for a massage is near the bottom of the priority list.

Instead of the doctor, therapists should plan to be in contact with the nurse. In reality, the nurse is one of the best staff members to receive guidance from. She is often more up to date on the patient's complete health status, physical and emotional. And, because massage was at one time part of standard nursing in hospitals, nurses understand the benefits of it more readily.

When communicating with the health care staff, make it as simple as possible for them. Be brief, communicate initially in writing, create checklists, and use common language to describe the massage work. Instead of using the term "effleurage," use "stroking." Replace "petrissage" with "kneading."

Some offices prefer not to sign permission forms but will communicate via phone conversation. This is usually done with the nurse. The touch therapist should record in the client record what was said, who the conversation was with, the date, and time.

In some circumstances, orders from the doctor are absolutely necessary. One example is when a governing body, such as a state massage board, requires it. Another commonly required instance is for hospitalized patients. When bodyworkers are wanting to perform outcall massage for hospitalized clients, this can be easily accomplished by having the patient or a family member speak to the patient's nurse

> ### Alone and Dejected
> A man dropped his wife off for a massage during the period she was in treatment for lung cancer. An hour later he returned to pick her up, expecting to see his wife relaxed and rosy cheeked. When he arrived, she sat, alone and dejected, in the reception area, her coat still on. The massage therapist had not been willing to give the woman a session. Eight years later, the man's heart still hurts when he thinks of that day.
>
> — AUTHOR

Letter to the doctor

December 8, 2006

Dear Dr. Farrell,

I am writing at the request of your client Jane Smith and her family. A few weeks ago I sent you a standard permission request form for massage and manual lymph drainage for Mrs. Smith. Because of her history of blood clots you denied permission. Absolutely a history of blood clots is a contraindication for deep, general, "full body" massage.

However, Mrs. Smith is requesting gentle, palliative massage primarily for back discomfort and to be generally soothed. I believe Mrs. Smith can safely receive skilled and compassionate touch by taking **several precautionary measures.** These would be:

1. NO deep pressure work of any kind. She has many systemic, general precautions for the pressure of touch.
2. NO massage on the legs or abdomen due to history of blood clots.
3. NO positioning that requires moving from prone to supine, etc. Positioning precautions due to the chemotherapy port, the oxygen system and her age.
4. **Site precautions at the chemo port, lymphedema quadrant and lower extremities** (for blood clots). These areas would be avoided.
5. **NO lengthy sessions.** She has duration precautions due to her age and overall health, sessions are 15 to 40 minutes maximum.

The gentle, palliative sessions would include:

- Gentle & light foot, head & neck massage for relaxation.
- Gentle massage of the non-lymphedema arm and hand.
- Gentle back massage-which is Jane's primary concern.

With these considerations we are asking permission to give Mrs. **Smith some relief via skilled touch. We respect your expertise and will abide by your decision. Thank you for your consideration.**

If you have any further questions or comments, please contact me. I have many hours of specialized training and experience in working with oncology patients in all stages. I am also certified in manual lymphatic drainage and geriatric massage.

Sincerely,

Elle Lewellen
LMT NCTMB LLCC

ahead of time so that the order can be requested and recorded in the chart prior to the therapist's arrival. In this way, little time is wasted waiting for physician approval.

There is no black-and-white rule for when to require clients to provide a doctor's script. A reasonable guideline is to request that cancer patients who are within one year of finishing treatment provide a doctor's script. One year is the length of time that it commonly takes for people to recover after treatment ends. Other therapists may want medical approval for as long as the client is under the oncologist's monitoring, which is often up to five years but may be the remainder of the person's life. There is no absolute guideline. The bodyworker's comfort level may be the deciding factor in whether a doctor's note is required from the client or not.

Therapists Ask

Q *What about people not under the care of an oncologist or other doctor? Should I massage them?*

A Some bodyworkers prefer only to work with cancer clients who are under the care of a physician. Occasionally, a bodywork client, who is using neither mainstream nor alternative care, requests a massage. The decision to work with that client may be influenced by a variety of issues. The first is state or regional guidelines that require a physician's approval. If the massage therapist is not required by laws or guidelines, then the decision must be made based on his own belief system and comfort level. Some therapists may believe that a person's body is their own and they have the right to choose their own course of action. This might include no treatment or the use of only complementary treatments, such as prayer or visualization techniques. Other therapists may feel that the liability presented by the situation is professionally risky and they refuse to take on the client, choosing to refer them to another therapist who is more comfortable with the situation. Liability is a legitimate concern, especially if the person has a contentious attitude about mainstream health practices.

From a clinical perspective, the cancer patient who chooses not to receive treatment will have fewer massage precautions initially than the patient who is in treatment. Remember: for the most part, the adjustments to a massage session are the result of chemo, radiation, and surgery. If the disease eventually overtakes the person, the massage therapist will need to make significant adjustments to the touch sessions.

VERBAL OR WRITTEN INTAKE?

The gathering of client data can be accomplished in a variety of ways or combination of ways. If the person books the appointment in advance, the paperwork can be mailed ahead of time. The advantage to this is that the person can fill out the form at their leisure, which gives them time to give comprehensive answers. (See the Sample Intake Form on pages 214–215.) However, there is less verbal interaction with the therapist, and it is in the exchange between client and therapist that the stories surface.

Other therapists have the client arrive early for the first appointment, to fill out the health history form. This is a good method of gathering information, but people often are not thorough. Many clients just rush through the form, anxious to be on the table.

There are advantages and disadvantages to each style of doing intake. Written intake often occurs more quickly and can be done ahead of time. But it is more clinical and isn't as conducive to storytelling. Much is learned about the client that cannot be learned through a form. The chance to tell their story is often one of the highlights of the massage session.

Combining both the written and verbal methods is an excellent way to gather information. Clients can give their general health history on a written form, followed by an interview concerning the specifics of their cancer treatment. During this time, stories will rise unbidden. Healing often takes place when patients have the chance to be deeply heard.

SUGGESTIONS FOR PERFORMING VERBAL INTAKE

- Sit down face-to-face with the client. Do not stand above them.

- Be at ease and spacious. Imagine there is plenty of time.

- Sometimes clients withhold their cancer history for fear they will be turned away from massage. It is important at the very start to communicate to clients that everyone can be massaged, despite any medical conditions. But, it is important that they tell the therapist their history.

- Ask specific questions. A common intake question asked by therapists, "Is there anything I need to know today?" will not get the job done. Clients don't know what information bodyworkers need in order to create a safe massage plan. Frequently they surprise a therapist part-way into a massage. Many times it has happened that a client suddenly remembers their cancer history from a dozen years ago, conveniently putting it into the background until the treated part of the body is touched. Asking specific questions decreases the chances of these surprises.

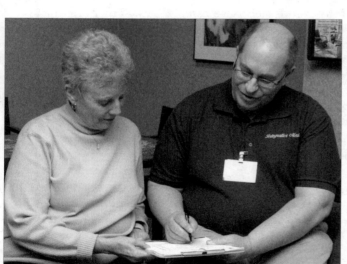

Figure 10.1 Sit at the client's level when doing intake.
Photograph by David J. Lawton

- Curb the desire to ask questions out of idle curiosity. Think through the questions to be asked beforehand. Quizzing patients about the stage of their cancer, the prognosis, or how their children are coping, could be startling or hurtful to them.

- Leave your "pity" face at home. Receive the information with an open, friendly expression. When patients reveal something that is distressing, keep your face relaxed rather than looking horrified.

- Being overly positive and upbeat can be annoying to patients. A kind listener is what many people prefer.

- Create a script to help remind you of the questions to be asked. Note the sample form in the adjacent Info Box. This intake form serves as a script for the hospital massage therapists who give seated massage in the radiation oncology department. They sometimes also give it to the patient to fill out while waiting.

SAMPLE INTAKE DIALOGUE

In previous chapters, a framework revolving around pressure, site, and positioning adjustments was used to help bodyworkers categorize in their minds the various side effects of cancer treatments. The same structure can also be applied to the interview process. Notice how the following interview between the massage therapist and her client, June, revolves around the pressure, site, and position categories. (See the sample intake form on pages 214–215 for an example of a form that revolves around the three categories.)

Th: June, I know you are eager to get on the table, but the first session with new clients, I spend extra time to do a complete health history. In the future then, we will just spend a moment before you get on the table to see how you are feeling.

Let me review the general health history form that you filled out and then I'll ask you some other questions specific to your cancer treatment. [Therapist reviews health history form that the client did in writing, asking client for any clarifications.]

Tell me about the kind of treatments you've received and the type of cancer they are for.

Cl: Last summer I had been really tired, but didn't think too much about it. I had to take a physical as part of applying for life insurance. The blood work showed that my white blood count was really elevated. I went to a hematologist who diagnosed me with chronic myelogenous leukemia. So now, I am being given chemotherapy every three weeks. I have two rounds to go. I missed last week because my white count was low. It's kind of funny, my white count went from too high to too low.

Th: It must've been surprising to be told all of this.

Cl: It was, because I am very active, I don't smoke, and I eat fairly well. I was doing all of the right things. I used to be a white-water rafter.

Th: I can't even imagine. I think you're going to find the massage sessions to be really supportive as you go through the treatment and recovery process. I want to ask you some specific questions that will help us plan the massage session. You indicated on the general intake form that you bruise easily. Is that due to low platelets?

INFO BOX

SEATED MASSAGE INTAKE FORM

Name: _____

Phone: _____ Date: _____

Are you currently receiving chemotherapy?   Yes __ No __

Are you currently receiving radiation treatments?   Yes __ No __

Have you had surgery in the last 8 weeks?   Yes __ No __

Do you have any neck or spine problems?   Yes __ No __

Do you bruise easily? Yes __ No __

Are you taking any medication for pain?   Yes __ No __

Do you have fatigue? Yes __ No __

Have you had lymph nodes removed?   Yes __ No __

Have you recently had blood clots?   Yes __ No __

Do you have chronic pain?   Yes __ No __

Do you have fragile bones?   Yes __ No __

Do you have neuropathy?   Yes __ No __

Do you have any medical devices?   Yes __ No __

Do you have any heart conditions?   Yes __ No __

© Tony Borcich,
Providence St. Vincent Medical Center

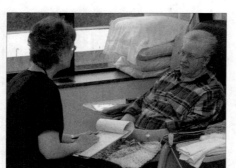

Figure 10.2 Massage therapist gathers information before massaging patient in the chemotherapy clinic.

Photograph by David J. Lawton

Cl: Yes, they have been running between 75 and 90.

Th: That will be one of the reasons we will use just a moderate pressure. What about your energy level? Is the chemotherapy causing fatigue?

Cl: I am fairly tired most of the time. People don't realize it because I look so normal.

Th: Are you able to exercise at all?

Cl: Not often. Sometimes my husband and I walk after dinner.

Th: You said your white blood count is low.

Cl: Yes. I was supposed to get chemo this week, but my count was too low. They've given me Neupogen to bring it back up. Hopefully next week I can get it.

Th: Do you receive your chemo through a catheter in your chest?

Cl: I have a port right here. [Client points to right side of chest.]

Th: I'll be sure to stay well away from that spot. Is your skin fragile or sensitive in any places?

Cl: No. Just my feet, they've always been sensitive.

Th: Speaking of your feet, did the chemo cause numbness or tingling? The doctors call it neuropathy.

Cl: The tips of some of my fingers are starting to tingle.

Th: Have you noticed any unusual swelling in the body, particularly in the arms or legs? [This is being asked in order to assess whether there could be a blood clot related to the port, infection, or edema due to chemotherapy.]

Cl: No.

Th: How about your bone density? Do you have any areas that you know of that are fragile?

Cl: The last time I had a bone scan, which was about two years ago, the doctor said that I have osteopenia in my lower spine and hips. It's not related to the leukemia, just age.

Th: I'm not going to give you a heavy massage today, but I'll stay mindful of those areas. Are there any areas of your body that are painful or have discomfort?

Cl: No, just my neck is really stiff.

Th: I can give that a bit more attention, if you would like?

Cl: That sounds good, along with my back.

Th: Besides the port, do you have any other medical devices?

Cl: No.

Th: How about any recent history of a blood clot?

Cl: No, nothing.

Th: Just a few more questions to cover. Do you think you'll be comfortable on the massage table face down on the port or would it be better to position you on your side?

Cl: I'm not sure, I haven't had a massage since the port was put in. I want to try to lay face down because I really want my back massaged.

Th: What I'll do is put a wash-cloth above the port, like so [demonstrates to client]. That will take the pressure off of the port.

Cl: That sounds good.

Th: Besides your back, what other parts of your body should I spend time on?

Cl: My feet and hands.

Th: How about your head and face?

Cl: That sounds wonderful!

Th: The pressure I am going to use will be much lighter than the massages you've had before your diagnosis. The goal today is just to get used to each other, to help you relax and rest, and to help you have more energy. If I used too much pressure, you would probably feel like you'd been hit by a truck. Massage can be very beneficial as you are going through treatment. Many people find they have less anxiety and pain and that they feel more whole and connected. But, in order to accomplish this, less pressure, less demand is better. Your liver, kidney, intestines, lymphatic system, all of them are working overtime just to keep up with the side effects of the chemo. This first session, we are trying to find your "new normal."

Cl: That makes total sense.

LONG-TERM SURVIVORS

The success rate for many cancer treatments is on the rise, which means more and more long-term survivors. It is inevitable that massage therapists will encounter a number of these people in the span of their career. All of them, with the right adjustments, are eligible to receive massage. The intake process with a long-term survivor will be less detailed than with the person in treatment. Because a number of side effects from treatment linger or last a lifetime, therapists still need to inquire about the following information:

- What type of cancer was the client treated for?
- What treatments were received?
- How long ago did treatment end?
- When was the client last seen by the oncologist? and how often does he have a check-up with the doctor?

Offering Advice

Therapists in private practice think nothing of advising clients to drink more water, eat fruits and vegetables, or apply a certain preparation onto a sore muscle. It is not advisable to be so free with casual suggestions to people with cancer. Some of a practitioner's suggestions may go against the doctor's instructions. For example, suggesting a skin care product to a radiation patient might go against doctor's orders to apply nothing but the clinic's recommended lotion. Advising a certain herbal supplement for the immunosuppressed patient may not be compatible with their other treatments. Advising a chemo patient who is on diuretics to drink quantities of cranberry juice to flush out the toxins may leave the person dehydrated with electrolyte imbalances.

The story of Susan really illustrates the need to avoid offering advice. Her nutritionist suggested a colonic to help Susan detoxify following chemotherapy and radiation. The procedure was so demanding on her that Susan ended up in the ER the night after the colonic.

- Are there any long-term side effects from treatment such as:
  - ○ easy bruising
  - ○ fatigue
  - ○ peripheral neuropathy
  - ○ swelling
  - ○ pain
  - ○ decreased ROM or function
  - ○ loss of bone density
  - ○ low blood counts

> ### Katherine
>
> Katherine had ovarian cancer eight years ago and had been cancer-free during that time. She thought nothing of it when making an appointment with a new massage therapist. The session, however, never happened. The practitioner refused to work with Katherine without a doctor's permission. While the therapist is to be praised for a cautious approach, there is such a thing as going overboard. When the incidence of cancer is years in the past and a clean bill of health has been given, the client should be approached in the same manner as all clients. Rather than refusing to massage a first-time client, administer a comfort-oriented, relaxation massage.
>
> — AUTHOR

NO TIME TO DO INTAKE!

Often, bodyworkers aren't given enough time by employers or are discouraged by them from performing a health history. Or, the venue doesn't easily lend itself to the interview process. Despite time issues or employer practices, it is still possible to gather enough information through an abbreviated verbal interview to give a safe session. The Info Box on page 207 lists a few questions that can be used in situations in which the time for intake is limited, such as for a seated massage event or in a spa setting.

The interview process could begin as the therapist and client are walking toward the massage room. Begin with casual inquiries that can be discussed in the hearing of others, such as the client's massage history. Move next to the unobtrusive health questions, such as easy bruising, condition of spine and neck, and medication use for inflammation or pain. More private questions should be asked once the client has entered the massage room. An example is, "Are you being treated for any medical conditions?" Or, "Have you ever had lymph nodes removed?"

Another option is for the receptionist to ask the client to fill out a very brief health history checklist while the therapist is setting up the room. This list could be printed on a laminated sheet of paper and then wiped clean after the massage, ready to be used by another client. The therapist can then quickly peruse the form, asking for clarification or amplification where needed. This process can be done in minutes and is surely well worth that time.

FOLLOW UP

Typically, bodyworkers follow up with clients the next time they see them. The time gap between appointments might be a week but more often is two or more weeks or even a month. When the time gap is too great, clients don't recall how the touch session affected them. In order to get specific feedback, follow-up is best done within 24–48 hours. A quick follow-up also helps the client to tune into how the massage affected them, such as better sleep that night or increased energy for the remainder of the day.

Following up by phone is the ideal, but e-mail or voice mail are also options. It should be done after each session. At the very least, therapists should phone the clients after the first three to four sessions, and thereafter check in with clients after major changes are made in the massage treatment plan. For example, when the focus shifts from comfort-oriented to treatment-oriented, the practitioner should resume follow-ups until the sessions reach a plateau again.

Patients are usually surprised and appreciative to have a practitioner who follows up. The advantage to the practitioner is that he begins to gauge the effects of his work, both positive and negative. If the sessions are too demanding on clients, the quick follow-up will help the practitioner make speedy course corrections on other clients. Most often what therapists hear is how wonderful the massage felt. Perhaps the client slept well the next two nights, had the energy to run errands, or had a two-day reprieve from the neuropathy in their feet. Much of that specific feedback is lost when follow-up isn't done soon after the massage.

Some working situations, such as a spa, make follow-up phone calls difficult or impossible. While it would be overwhelming for therapists to check on each of the massage recipients they saw that day, a special effort could be made to follow up with the more fragile clients so that the therapists can learn from their work. In the spa setting, perhaps the guest could be given a comment card that is returned to the front desk at their convenience or when checking out.

When I called to follow up with my client, her feedback blew me away. She shared how she had never experienced a massage where she could feel the love pouring through the hands.

— CAROLYN CRUZ, LMT
FLORENCE, OREGON

SUBSEQUENT MASSAGES

A comprehensive intake is the best practice prior to the first bodywork session. As part of subsequent visits, the therapist should have a short check-in period each time. This is especially true when clients are in treatment. Energy levels, blood counts, or emotional status can all change from day to day, let alone week to week. Each time, the therapist should inquire about the following: energy level, new symptoms, status of previous symptoms, and recent lab work or diagnostic scans.

There is no predictability for those in treatment. Bodywork sessions can change drastically from week to week. One week the client may thrive on the use of gentle effleurage with superficial muscle contact. The following week, they may have a neutropenic fever and want a low-impact modality such as Healing Touch or Reiki.

As people get further from the end of treatment, they become more stable. The preliminary check-in period becomes shorter and bodywork sessions will become more predictable.

MASSAGE AT SPECIAL EVENTS

Marsha, a massage therapist who is also cancer survivor, attended a special cancer survivors' event. Seated massage was one of the activities attendees could participate in. When the therapist/survivor sat down to receive a 15-minute neck and shoulder massage, the only question that the therapist asked was, "Have you ever received a massage?" Unfortunately, this type of question is common at special events, such as wellness fairs and even cancer-related special events. While it is a fine introductory question, it does not suffice as an adequate intake.

Because the sessions are shorter and the atmosphere is more hurried, touch practitioners often bypass the interview process or forget about it in their hurry to get to the massage. But it is necessary, even in these situations, to gather data about clients' health profiles. Massage sessions at special events are often given in a massage chair, which makes the sessions inherently more vigorous. All the more reason for inquiring about a person's health. Even if the session is a 15-minute neck and shoulder massage, therapists must adjust for the side effects of treatment, such as easy bruising, elevated toxicity, or the risk for lymphedema. Adrienne, the nursing assistant introduced at the beginning of this chapter, is a good example of this need.

A lengthy interview isn't required to gather the information needed to perform a safe massage. Notice the questions used in the adjacent Info Box. They can be accomplished in one to two minutes.

Some therapists prefer to do a verbal intake at special events. This allows them to quickly develop rapport with the massage recipient as well as to observe them face-to-face. This position gives the therapist

---

General Seated Massage Intake

Performance of a health intake before the massage is vital for all recipients. It is not uncommon to encounter such conditions among the general population as diabetes, prior cancer treatment, breathing disorders, fibromyalgia, or even mild congestive heart failure. People in treatment for cancer, as the reader now knows, can have a whole host of problems. For a sample of a seated massage intake tailored to cancer patients, see page 207.

Inquire about the following:

- General energy level at the moment
- Present medical treatment
- Pregnancy
- Skin health in the area to be massaged

- Health of the neck and spine
- Easy bruising
- Use of pain or anti-inflammatory medications
- Lymph node removal and/or radiation*

*All clients should be asked about lymph node removal. Asking is the only way to find out. This can be done in a gentle but direct way. Because so many women have a prior history of breast cancer treatment, it is imperative to ask this question. Breast cancer treatment nearly always involves the removal of lymph nodes and/or radiation to them. Both interventions put them at risk for lymphedema, which can be triggered by a short shoulder massage. The consequences of lymphedema are so significant, that it pays to be diligent about asking this question. Lymph nodes also may be removed for other reasons, as therapists will learn when they start asking this question.[4]

a lot of immediate information. The color of the skin and brightness of the eyes give clues about the client's immediate sense of well-being.

Other therapists prepare a question card for clients to complete while waiting in line. This has the advantage of greater speed. One bodyworker has the intake questions printed on a postcard. On one side is information about the practitioner's massage business; on the opposite side are the health profile questions. The client is then given the card after the massage as a promotional device. Another bodyworker has a laminated page of the intake questions on a clipboard. While clients wait in line, they fill out the questionnaire with an erasable pen. After the massage, the bodyworker wipes the page clean, leaving the laminated board ready for use by another waiting client. These innovative strategies are proof that the health intake process need never be abandoned.

FINAL THOUGHTS

The span of people now receiving massage is extremely broad, which means that the spectrum of health conditions is as well. Therefore, all clients need to be interviewed about their health prior to a massage, no matter the length of the session, the type of touch technique or the venue used. No matter whether the massage is given in a physician's office, a wellness fair, or a private practitioner's office, massage precautions must be observed. Even a 15-minute neck and shoulder massage can have profound outcomes.

REFERENCES

1. Cancer Patients Hide Their Use of Complementary and Alternative Treatments from Their Doctors. American Society for Therapeutic Radiology and Oncology.
    http://www.astro.org/annual_meeting/media_corner/
    annual_meeting_press_releases/101605hide.htm
    Accessed Dec. 1, 2005.

2. Sparber A, Bauer L, Curt G, et al. Use of Complementary Medicine by Adult Patients Participating in Cancer Clinical Trials. *Oncology Nursing Forum.* 2000;27(4):623-630.

3. Yates JS, Mustian KM, Morrow GR, et al. Prevalance of Complementary and Alternative Medicine Use in Cancer Patients During Treatment. *Supportive Care in Cancer.* 2005;13(10):806-811.

4. MacDonald G. *Massage for the Hospital Patient and Medically Frail Client.* Philadelphia, PA: Lippincott Williams and Wilkins, 2005.

SAMPLE

Your name   Date

Address

Telephone # (day)   (eve)   Date of Birth

1. Have you had Massage Therapy before?   **Yes / No**   If yes, was there anything that you liked or didn't like?

2. When were you first diagnosed with cancer?   What type of cancer?

3. Where was/is it located?

4. Are you being treated now?   **Yes / No**   If no, what was the date of your last treatment?

    NOTE: if you are currently in treatment, between treatments, or if your last treatment session was within one year of the date of the massage session, please have your physician complete the MD permission form.

5. What treatments have you undergone, when? **Please supply dates and types of surgery and other treatments.**

6. Current medications, not described above:

7. Did your treatment include any removal or radiation of lymph nodes? *(If yes, please describe where)*

8. Did your treatment include radiation therapy? *(If yes, please describe where)*

9. Do you have any site restrictions due to:

    incisions, open wounds, drains or dressings,

    skin sensitivity, rash or skin condition,

    IV, port, ostomy, catheter, or other device (circle)

    a tumor site   radiation site

    bone or spine metastasis   neuropathy

    fracture history   area of infection

    history or risk of blood clots or phlebitis

    other (please describe below)

10. Do you have any pressure restrictions due to:

    history or risk of lymphedema **(circle which)**

    anticoagulants   low platelet count

    bone or spine metastasis   steroid medication

    fragile/sensitive skin   fragile veins

    area of pain or burning   fatigue

    recent surgery   infection or fever

    other (please describe below)

INTAKE FORM

Your name again: _____   Client Health Form, Page 2 of 2

11. Do you have any **position restrictions** due to:

incision   medication   ostomy   tumor site   difficulty breathing   tender skin

swelling or risk of swelling (any body area need elevating?) *please describe*

medical devices *please describe*

discomfort *please describe*

12. Has cancer or cancer treatment affected any of the following functions in your body?

Lungs   Liver   Nervous system   Heart   Kidney   Blood counts   Energy Level

Circle any that you are currently experiencing and describe.

General Signs and Symptoms Check "yes" and add comments if you have or have had any of the following:

	Yes	No	Comments
13. Any **swelling** or **tendency** to swell anywhere in your body?			
14. Any sites of **pain** or **tenderness** anywhere in your body?			
15. Any sites of **numbness** or **reduced sensation** anywhere in your body?			
16. Any areas of **inflammation?**			

Other Medical Conditions	Yes	No	Comments
17. **Skin conditions** (rashes, infections, itching)			
18. Known **allergies** or **sensitivities** (if you use any physician-approved lotion on your skin, please bring it for the massage therapist to use)			
19. **Cardiovascular conditions** (history of heart condition, high blood pressure, angina, hardening of the arteries, stroke, varicose veins, blood clots)			
20. **Liver or kidney conditions** (for example: kidney failure, hepatitis, portal hypertension, etc.)			
21. **Respiratory or lung** conditions			
22. **Diabetes** (describe type, any medication, whether blood sugar is well-controlled, any complications.)			
23. **Injuries** (any back problems, knee problems, tendonitis, disc injuries, neck problems, recent fractures)			
24. **Arthritis or Joint problems**			
25. **Digestive problems**			
26. **Surgery**			

Created by Tracy Walton and Gayle MacDonald

Chapter 11

Companions
on the Journey

Who Gives? Who Receives?

When it comes to healing, how we feel is at least as important as what we know. This is true for both patient and healer because both must connect with feeling if they are to maximize their shared healing journey.

— CARL A. HAMMERSCHLAG, MD, AND HOWARD D. SILVERMAN, MD, *HEALING CEREMONIES: CREATING PERSONAL RITUALS FOR SPIRITUAL, EMOTIONAL, PHYSICAL AND MENTAL HEALTH*

The clinical knowledge practitioners bring to their work is, without a doubt, a vital ingredient. Understanding how cancer arises and spreads, cognizance of the research, and familiarity with indications and contraindications are essential. But another important resource practitioners bring to the experience is themselves. Just as important as massage skills or familiarity with medical terminology, is a therapist's way of being, who they are in relationship to themselves and how they relate to those who are ill.

Bodyworkers are drawn toward working with different groups. Some have an affinity for athletes, others for the elderly, and those reading this book possibly feel an inclination toward cancer patients or the seriously ill. Practitioners are attracted to certain groups by a complex set of motivations, many conscious and others well below the surface. Some people are drawn to be with the seriously ill as a means of healing their own grief about the death of a loved one. For others it is part of a spiritual passage or the quest for a deeper and more meaningful life.

The most conscious motivation is the desire to help. Nearly always when students share their reasons for wanting to work with cancer patients in the hospital, common answers include: to ease the physical pain, to transform hospitals into caring places, or to be a soothing, nurturing presence. The students' focus is on what they have to give. But as soon as the work with patients begins, they realize how much there is to receive. Time on a cancer unit changes their lives forever. They, too, are transformed and healed.

CHAPTER 11
COMPANIONS ON THE JOURNEY:
WHO GIVES? WHO RECEIVES?

217

> ### Only Love
>
> My dreams seem to be coming into play with whatever it is that is trying to break through in my life right now. I dreamed about being in a hospital, walking through long halls, seeing patients, while feeling and being told that there was no way I could help them. I felt the frustration for days after the dream. My whole life I've wanted to serve, to help, and in the past I haven't always felt that I could make any difference. It's all connected, my feelings about myself, helping myself, and being able to help others. I've been questioning everything in my life – my beliefs, who I am, what my life is all about. The night before going to the hospital, I felt anxious. Would I be able to make a difference? Is this my path? My head was spinning with questions. I went to sleep and had the sweetest, simplest dream. I was a child on a big swing, going back and forth, free, my legs kicking, hair flying. Over and over I heard the same words – *only love, only love, only love.* Sounds kind of corny, but it make me feel wonderful! It reminded me that it is that simple. My intent now is to give love and to serve, helping myself as well as others. I feel like this whole experience is some kind of resolution to a learning that has been ongoing for years. It's not done, but something major has happened. My perspective has changed. I have changed. This life is as much about my healing as it is about others'. Finally I feel the importance of my own healing being the key to helping others.
>
> — Diane Hutson, LMT, Scappoose, Oregon

Equal Partners

Why take the time and effort to dive below the surface and examine the less conscious motivations that pull us toward working with cancer patients? Isn't it enough to just want to help others, to ease their discomfort? To be sure, this is a noble stance from which to work, but it is a one-way dynamic: the therapist is the helper, the patient is the one being helped. This is a hierarchical, linear relationship rather than a holistic one. The practitioner is on top in the power position and the patient is on the bottom in the powerless role. The person who is sick is the receiver, the taker; they are needy or broken. These are qualities that have lesser value. The therapist, meanwhile, is the helper, the useful one, the giver, the strong, healthy, and energetic one – characteristics that are considered to be superior.

Wanting to help or comfort is a good starting point, but bodyworkers must go deeper into their motivations. This is the only way to have a complete and whole relationship with themselves and their patients. Through this exploration, fuller access is gained to deeper capacities and special innate gifts. Therapists see not only what they give, but what they receive. In this paradigm, massage therapist and client become equal partners, their journeys inextricably woven together.

The novelist Isabelle Allende commented that she uses writing to explore her soul. Are bodyworkers exploring something in their souls by working with cancer patients? Why would it be healing or soulful

The more you think of yourself as a "therapist," the more pressure there is on someone to be a "patient." The more you identify as a "philanthropist," the more compelled someone feels to be a "supplicant." The more you see yourself as a "helper," the more need for people to play the passive "helped."

— Ram Dass and Paul Gorman, *How Can I Help: Stories and Reflections on Service* to give massage to cancer patients? Are there qualities within their experience that practitioners yearn for in their own lives? When they are with the ill, are practitioners able to to let certain qualities within themselves come to the surface that aren't normally experienced? Try the following exercise in order to answer this question. (It will be most helpful if another person reads the exercise out loud.)

Exercise 1:
Who are you in the presence of the ill?

Imagine a setting where you are with someone who is sick. Notice how you greet them. As you are with them, what is your demeanor? Happy? Fearful? Calm? Grateful? Pitying? Now move your attention to the body. What sensations are discernable? Are you relaxed? Tense? Open? Closed? Does your physical energy concentrate in any certain place?

Does this setting bring out parts of your being not normally in evidence? Does it allow you to experience yourself in a different way? Are there any of these qualities that you would like to take with you from this world and integrate into other worlds, such as work, family, or friends?

When Valeri imagined being in the presence of someone who is ill, she no longer felt a need to have all of the answers. Her stomach was calm and she could just "be." Cliff felt less judged. Michelle was calmer and moved more slowly. Carol was more gracious and full of humor. Being with someone who is ill moved Gayle to greater tenderness. Her heart radiated with a golden light that enveloped her chest, shoulders, and head. What would it be like to bring that tenderness and radiant light into the relationships with family, friends, and colleagues?

A life-threatening illness that happens to someone close to us, takes us into the underworld as a companion on the journey, and in as much as it will take us into our own depths of feeling and meaning, there are consequences for us as well.

JEAN SHINODA BOLEN, MD,
CLOSE TO THE BONE

Serious illness brings with it a new way of being in the world, a new identity, qualities often not cultivated during times of health, such as quietude, stillness, dependency, or "being" rather than "doing." The focus turns inward, masks are stripped away, self-worth can no longer be measured by what is produced in the world. Patients are forced to find new answers to the question, "Who am I?" Perhaps it is this same question that bodyworkers are examining through their work with cancer patients. Explore this question for yourself by doing Exercise 2.

Exercise 2:
Exploring the Qualities of Illness

CHAPTER 11
COMPANIONS ON THE JOURNEY:
WHO GIVES? WHO RECEIVES?

219

Take a moment to explore the experience of illness. Put down the book. Close your eyes. Imagine you are deeply ill. Sink into the physical sensations of being sick. Notice your energy, strength or weakness, whether you are heavy or light, still or agitated. Which feelings surface in this state of being? Are there moments of fear? joy? frustration? satisfaction? How do you view the world from this position? Let these sensations unfold for several moments, allowing in everything, pushing away nothing.

Return now to your present health status. Were there any of these qualities that you would like to integrate into your life? Perhaps you would bring back the quality of softness, increased vulnerability, slowness, or less ambition? When we open to the experience of illness, we see the opportunities within it and no longer see the ill as victims to be pitied.

Christy felt empty as she imagined being ill. In this state, she was happy and uncluttered. Now she could decide consciously which people, places, and things to keep in her life and which to let go of. Vaughn wanted to slow down. Illness was the only way to accomplish this and the only way to create the time to ruminate about his life. For Gill, sickness gave him permission to rest and have the occasional quiet that he yearned for.

Although bodywork is potentially one of the ultimate holistic modalities, without a conscious effort, its training and method of practice can be done in a dualistic and hierarchical manner. The bodyworker can easily take on the attitude of being in a one-up position of helper, provider, or giver, forgetting that they too are being healed, that they too are receiving. In a holistic relationship, therapist and patient are collaborators.

Not only does wholeness need to be created between the therapist and patient, but it must happen within the therapist as well. If bodyworkers are to provide a holistic experience, they must be a microcosm of it. All of the self must be brought to the encounter, not just the parts that are energetic, cheerful, serene, or healthy, but also those that are tired, depressed, confused, or wounded.

Often therapists erroneously believe that if they are tired or lacking in enthusiasm, they should not touch clients, fearing that these qualities will leach into the patient. And yet, when the therapist acknowledges all of himself, he gives patients permission to do the same. Space is created for the whole, for the truth. Interestingly, when a therapist who is tired or depressed allows those sensations into her state of being as she is massaging a client, the feelings transmute quickly into high energy and appreciation.

Service is a relationship between two equals…. Our service serves us as well as others. That which uses us strengthens us. Over time, fixing and helping are draining, depleting. Over time, we burn out. Service is renewing. When we serve, our work itself will sustain us.[1]

— RACHEL NAOMI REMEN, MD

It is not being suggested that practitioners share their sorrows or fatigue with patients. What is being proposed is that therapists be open to what they are feeling within themselves. To be sure, the focus of the massage session must remain on the patient and her needs. Otherwise the risk is too great that the patient will try to take care of the therapist. Practitioners must find other outlets for what they are experiencing – a mentor, a supervisor, or journal.

TELLING OUR STORIES

During a lecture, Thomas Moore said, "We can't heal anybody, we're just here to share our stories with each other, to have a conversation." Just as patients need to tell their stories, so, too, do those who work with them. Touch practitioners often live a solitary professional life and can suffer from the absence of colleagues with whom to interact on a regular basis. Forming alliances or mentoring relationships is important in order to have people to whom they can tell their stories. Through the telling, the experience becomes complete and whole and practitioners come to better understand the events of their lives. Without someone to hear and understand, they are isolated in the experience.

The power of having someone to share with is evident in the unexpected results of Dr. David Spiegel's study of women with metastatic breast cancer. The group who attended a weekly support group, in addition to receiving their medical regimen, survived twice as long as the group who did not attend a support group. Therapists, too, need a place to share their experiences, or they shall not survive.

Whether the stories are told through poetry, journaling, drawing, sculpting, or dance, the attempt takes the practitioner inside, to the deeper layers of the event. In trying to write it, draw it, or dance it, they must look closer and more keenly. The senses become more alert to the experience for both the therapist and the patient.

Wrapped in White Deer Hide

I am finding that when I write about my hospice experiences in story format or in a poem, it gives me clarity and peace. It's like putting the gift of the experience to be safely stored away. I imagine in my mind's eye that the story is being wrapped with white deer hide in Navajo way like my people do with a precious piece of silver and turquoise jewelry to be treasured or worn at a later time.

—YOLANDA TALBERT, RN, LMT, CHUGIAK, ALASKA

Alone

An episode happened today while I was on my way out of the clinic and I need to share. In fact I was needing to share right after it happened but to no avail; I was on my own. I saw "Janet" in the waiting room and greeted her and asked her if she was coming in the afternoons now (I went to the chemo clinic in the afternoon today) and she told me, no, she's not coming any longer because the chemo "didn't take." Then she went on about my fabulous foot massages. I wished her well and gave her the most heartfelt hug I could muster. Then I turned around and saw her friend who accompanied her to the clinic; she had tears in her eyes. I hugged her and told her to keep giving her friend foot massages.

I can't tell you how alone I felt after walking out of that clinic. Alone in my experience. Alone in the grief. Who could I talk to at that time to unload? So there you have it. I'm crying now, finally, but I must say that this path can be tougher than I imagined. I know this for the mere reason that I'm a sensitive person. I also know that I gave the rest of my energy away at that moment in the waiting room. I had nothing left to give for the remainder of the day.

— EILEEN HICKEY, LMT, PORTLAND, OREGON

Not only do bodyworkers need a chance to tell their stories, but they also need the opportunity to hear the experiences of others. Through stories, practitioners are taught, inspired, guided, and affirmed. Personal stories, like myths, provide guideposts for the journey that lies ahead. Their own process is quickened by listening to the experiences of others. Through others' experiences, practitioners learn what works and what to avoid. New possibilities surface, as do affirmations that they are on the right track.

CHAPTER 11
COMPANIONS ON THE JOURNEY:
WHO GIVES? WHO RECEIVES?

221

IDEAS FOR CREATING HOLISM AND EXPLORING OUR EXPERIENCES

Carl Jung believed that the unconscious pulls people toward that which will be healing. It is only by delving into this area that individuals become whole. In order to access the deeper, unconscious parts of the self, its language must be deciphered. The unconscious can speak through dreams, yearnings, movement, stories, symbols, places, colors, or poems. The following ten exercises will help reveal parts of the self that unknowingly reside in uncharted waters.

- Keep a bodywork story journal.

- Cultivate a relationship with a bodyworker who is doing similar work. Have a regular meeting time over tea or a meal to swap stories.

- Start a monthly support group for bodyworkers with the focus on telling the stories from your work, sharing poems, or deepening awareness of the yearnings of your soul.

- Write a short story or case history about a patient for submission to a professional periodical or hospital newsletter.

- Set aside one day or one bodywork session where you let go of your identity as a healer or therapist. Instead, give massage as if you were the receiver, or the student, or the one in need of healing.

- Pretend you are a poet. Give touch from this poet-self.

- Assume an outlook of gratitude. Massage a patient from this place.

- Meditate on cancer. Notice the physical sensations the word evokes. Say the word "cancer" several times inside your head. Notice the tone and feelings with which you say it. If cancer were a symbol, what would it look like? Feel the energy of it in your body. Draw the symbol. Is this symbol relevant in your own life?

- Write or imagine a fairy tale about someone who has a gift for using touch to comfort the ill. What is the setting of the story? When does it take place? What does the central figure look like? What qualities does it possess? Imagine in detail this character giving healing touch to someone who is ill. Are there parts of this fairy tale that you wish were true for you?

Additional Resources

- Barsch M. *The Healing Path: A Soul Approach to Illness.* Arkana, 1993
- Cancer as a Turning Point Conferences www.healingjourneys.org
- Commonweal Cancer Help Program www.commonweal.org
- *Her Soul Beneath the Bone: Women's Poetry on Breast Cancer.* Edited by Leatrice H. Lifshitz. University of Illinois Press, 1988
- LeShan L. *Cancer as a Turning Point.* Plume/Penguin Books, 1989
- Steingraber S. *Post-Diagnosis.* Firebrand Books, 1995
- Woodman M. *Bone: Dying Into Life.* Viking/Penguin, 2000
- WIT (2001) an HBO film by Mike Nichols, starring Emma Thompson. Available on DVD

- Pretend a friend or loved one has cancer. Imagine spending a few hours, or even the day, together. Hear the conversations you might have. Envision your actions. Sense your feelings. Are there ways in which you are different? What parts of this scenario would you like to integrate into your real-life relationship with this person?

FINAL THOUGHTS

What does it mean to be a "companion on the journey" to someone with cancer? It means being open to their diagnosis just as it is, not wishing it were different; it means being with the person just as they are – nauseated, confused, luminous, or hopeful. We are walking the path together when we don't pity the client or suggest that they do things differently. We approach patients as equal partners, seeing the medicine they have to offer us. We allow them to be the teacher, the giver, the expert, and the useful one. There is no separation between student and teacher, giver and taker, useful and useless, expert and novice. This is wholeness, which is the root of healing.

REFERENCES

1. Remen R. In the Service of Life. *Noetic Sciences Review*. Spring 1996, p.24-25.

INDEX

Introducing the 2nd revised and updated edition of

FROM THE HEART
THROUGH THE HANDS:
THE POWER OF TOUCH IN CAREGIVING

BY DAWN NELSON

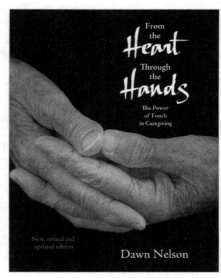

"This book is a treasure that every caregiver and health professional should read."
—Dr. Bernie Siegel, author of *Love, Medicine and Miracles*

"In this book you will find food for the head, hands, and heart. It is comprehensive, practical and inspiring."
—Gayle MacDonald, author of *Medicine Hands: Massage Therapy for People with Cancer*

"Here are the tools for revolutionizing geriatric care and utterly transforming the experience of aging."
—Deane Juhan, author of *Job's Body*

This book is for people who feel comfortable communicating through their hands and for those who wish to feel more ease in transmitting care through touch. It is for people whose responsibility or job or gift is to oversee or to help care for the elderly and ill members of our society. It is for sons and daughters caring for aging parents with physical impairments that effect a role reversal in a lifetime of relating. It is for the courageous men and women who continue caring for spouses or mothers or fathers with dementia-related diseases such as Alzheimer's after such a disease has robbed that loved one of the ability to remember the relationship he or she once shared with the caregiver. It is for companions and family members struggling and sometimes sacrificing to provide care for their loved ones at home.

This book is for doctors who have forgotten or never learned that touch is medicine and for those who are wise enough to know that a five-second hug, offered as a gesture of shared humanity, can often do more to assuage fear and anxiety than a five-minute lecture. It is for nurses and nursing assistants who, once trained in giving back rubs to hospitalized patients to reduce discomfort and induce sleep, in current care systems may be more often in contact with equipment than with people, or spend most of their time dispensing medicines and completing paperwork. It is for the restorative aides, the occupational and physical and recreational therapists in extended care facilities who are searching for more effective and affirming ways of relating to those whom they serve. It is for hospice professionals and volunteers, hired companions, geriatric consultants, guardians, home health aides and others who want to help improve quality of life for their charges and clients. It is for chaplains and social workers and grief counselors who wish to reclaim the power of intentional touch in ministering to the frail, the distraught and the bereaved. It is for massage therapy students desiring to build careers in arenas that combine service with professional and personal growth and for practitioners whose hearts and hands lead them to forge new paths in venues where their skills are sorely needed. It is for anyone who wishes to use touch more consciously and compassionately in relating to the elderly, the ill and the dying

Dawn Nelson is an internationally recognized speaker, workshop leader and touch educator. Founder of COMPASSIONATE TOUCH® for those in Later Life Stages, author of four books and co-producer of several award-winning videos, Dawn is also a meditation teacher and couples communications counselor. An ovarian cancer survivor, Dawn has three children and three grandchildren. She lives with her husband in northern California and continues to be interested in helping to enhance the quality of life for the elderly, the ill and the dying.

ISBN 978-1-84409-083-9